MEASURING AGREEMENT

MEASURING AGREEMENT
Models, Methods, and Applications

Pankaj K. Choudhary
The University of Texas at Dallas

Haikady N. Nagaraja
The Ohio State University

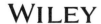

The rights of Pankaj K. Choudhary and Haikady N. Nagaraja to be identified as the authors of this work has been asserted in accordance with law.

Registered Office
John Wiley & Sons, Inc., 111 River Street, Hoboken, NJ 07030, USA

Editorial Office
111 River Street, Hoboken, NJ 07030, USA

For details of our global editorial offices, customer services, and more information about Wiley products visit us at www.wiley.com.

Wiley also publishes its books in a variety of electronic formats and by print-on-demand. Some content that appears in standard print versions of this book may not be available in other formats.

Library of Congress Cataloging-in-Publication Data
Names: Choudhary, Pankaj K. (Pankaj Kumar), 1975- author. | Nagaraja, H. N.
    (Haikady Navada), 1954- author.
Title: Measuring agreement : models, methods, and applications / by Pankaj K.
    Choudhary, Haikady N. Nagaraja.
Description: Hoboken, NJ : John Wiley & Sons, 2017. | Series: Wiley series in
    probability and statistics | Includes bibliographical references and
    index. | Description based on print version record and CIP data provided
    by publisher; resource not viewed.
Identifiers: LCCN 2017022085 (print) | LCCN 2017037255 (ebook) | ISBN
    9781118553145 (pdf) | ISBN 9781118553244 (epub) | ISBN 9781118078587
    (cloth)
Subjects: LCSH: Statistics--Methodology.
Classification: LCC QA276.A2 (ebook) | LCC QA276.A2 C46 2017 (print) | DDC
    001.4/22--dc23
LC record available at https://lccn.loc.gov/2017022085

Cover images: (Background) © BlackJack3D/Gettyimages; (Graph) Courtesy of Pankaj K. Choudhary and
    Haikady N. Nagaraja
Cover design by Wiley

10 9 8 7 6 5 4 3 2 1

To:
My parents, and Swati,
Aalo, and Arushi—PKC
Jyothi—HNN

CONTENTS

Preface   xv

1   Introduction   1

   1.1   Preview   1

   1.2   Notational Conventions   1

   1.3   Basic Characteristics of a Measurement Method   2

      1.3.1   A Statistical Model for Measurements   3

      1.3.2   Quality Characteristics   3

   1.4   Method Comparison Studies   5

   1.5   Meaning of Agreement   6

   1.6   A Measurement Error Model   8

      1.6.1   Identifiability Issues   9

      1.6.2   Model-Based Moments   10

      1.6.3   Conditions for Perfect Agreement   10

      1.6.4   Link to Test Theory   11

   1.7   Similarity versus Agreement   11

      1.7.1   Evaluation of Similarity   11

      1.7.2   Evaluation of Agreement   12

   1.8   A Toy Example   13

   1.9   Controversies and Our View   14

   1.10   Concepts Related to Agreement   15

1.11	Role of Confidence Intervals and Hypotheses Testing	16
	1.11.1 Formulating the Agreement Hypotheses	16
	1.11.2 Testing Hypotheses Using Confidence Bounds	17
	1.11.3 Evaluation of Agreement Using Confidence Bounds	17
	1.11.4 Evaluation of Similarity Using Confidence Intervals	18
1.12	Common Models for Paired Measurements Data	18
	1.12.1 A Measurement Error Model	19
	1.12.2 A Mixed-Effects Model	20
	1.12.3 A Bivariate Normal Model	21
	1.12.4 Limitations of the Paired Measurements Design	22
1.13	The Bland-Altman Plot	23
	1.13.1 The Ideal Plot	23
	1.13.2 A Linear Trend in the Bland-Altman Plot	25
	1.13.3 Heteroscedasticity in the Bland-Altman Plot	26
	1.13.4 Variations of the Bland-Altman Plot	27
1.14	Common Regression Approaches	29
	1.14.1 Ordinary Linear Regression	29
	1.14.2 Deming Regression	31
1.15	Inappropriate Use of Common Tests in Method Comparison Studies	34
	1.15.1 Test of Zero Correlation	34
	1.15.2 Paired t-test	36
	1.15.3 Pitman-Morgan and Bradley-Blackwood Tests	36
	1.15.4 Test of Zero Intercept and Unit Slope	38
1.16	Key Steps in the Analysis of Method Comparison Data	39
1.17	Chapter Summary	40
1.18	Bibliographic Note	41
	Exercises	47
2	**Common Approaches for Measuring Agreement**	**53**
2.1	Preview	53
2.2	Introduction	53
2.3	Mean Squared Deviation	54
2.4	Concordance Correlation Coefficient	54
2.5	A Digression: Tolerance and Prediction intervals	57
	2.5.1 Definitions	57
	2.5.2 Normally Distributed Data	58
2.6	Lin's Probability Criterion and Bland-Altman Criterion	59
2.7	Limits of Agreement	60
	2.7.1 The Approach	60
	2.7.2 Why Ignore the Variability?	61
	2.7.3 Limits of Agreement versus Prediction and Tolerance Intervals	62

2.8		Total Deviation Index and Coverage Probability	62
	2.8.1	The Approaches	62
	2.8.2	Normally Distributed Differences	63
2.9		Inference on Agreement Measures	64
2.10		Chapter Summary	64
2.11		Bibliographic Note	65
		Exercises	66

3 A General Approach for Modeling and Inference — **71**

3.1		Preview	71
3.2		Mixed-Effects Models	71
	3.2.1	The Model	72
	3.2.2	Prediction	73
	3.2.3	Model Fitting	74
	3.2.4	Model Diagnostics	75
3.3		A Large-Sample Approach to Inference	76
	3.3.1	Approximate Distributions	77
	3.3.2	Confidence Intervals	78
	3.3.3	Parameter Transformation	80
	3.3.4	Bootstrap Confidence Intervals	81
	3.3.5	Confidence Bands	83
	3.3.6	Test of Homogeneity	83
	3.3.7	Model Comparison	84
3.4		Modeling and Analysis of Method Comparison Data	85
3.5		Chapter Summary	88
3.6		Bibliographic Note	89
		Exercises	89

4 Paired Measurements Data — **95**

4.1		Preview	95
4.2		Modeling of Data	95
	4.2.1	Mixed-Effects Model	95
	4.2.2	Bivariate Normal Model	97
4.3		Evaluation of Similarity and Agreement	98
4.4		Case Studies	99
	4.4.1	Oxygen Saturation Data	99
	4.4.2	Plasma Volume Data	101
	4.4.3	Vitamin D Data	103
4.5		Chapter Summary	106
4.6		Technical Details	106
	4.6.1	Mixed-Effects Model	106

		4.6.2	Bivariate Normal Model	107
	4.7		Bibliographic Note	108
			Exercises	108

5   Repeated Measurements Data   111

	5.1		Preview	111
	5.2		Introduction	111
		5.2.1	Types of Data	112
		5.2.2	Individual versus Average Measurement	113
		5.2.3	Example Datasets	113
	5.3		Displaying Data	114
		5.3.1	Basic Plots	114
		5.3.2	Interaction Plots	116
	5.4		Modeling of Data	117
		5.4.1	Unlinked Data	118
		5.4.2	Linked Data	121
		5.4.3	Model Fitting and Evaluation	123
	5.5		Evaluation of Similarity and Agreement	123
	5.6		Evaluation of Repeatability	124
		5.6.1	Unlinked Data	125
		5.6.2	Linked Data	125
	5.7		Case Studies	126
		5.7.1	Kiwi Data	126
		5.7.2	Oximetry Data	129
	5.8		Chapter Summary	133
	5.9		Technical Details	134
		5.9.1	Unlinked Data	134
		5.9.2	Linked Data	134
	5.10		Bibliographic Note	135
			Exercises	137

6   Heteroscedastic Data   141

	6.1		Preview	141
	6.2		Introduction	141
		6.2.1	Diagnosing Heteroscedasticity	142
		6.2.2	Example Datasets	143
	6.3		Variance Function Models	144
	6.4		Repeated Measurements Data	146
		6.4.1	A Heteroscedastic Mixed-Effects Model	147
		6.4.2	Specifying the Variance Function	149
		6.4.3	Model Fitting and Evaluation	150

	6.4.4	Testing for Homoscedasticity	151
	6.4.5	Evaluation of Similarity, Agreement, and Repeatability	151
	6.4.6	Case Study: Cholesterol Data	152
6.5	Paired Measurements Data		162
	6.5.1	A Heteroscedastic Bivariate Normal Model	162
	6.5.2	Specifying the Variance Function	163
	6.5.3	Model Fitting and Evaluation	164
	6.5.4	Testing for Homoscedasticity	164
	6.5.5	Evaluation of Similarity and Agreement	164
	6.5.6	Case Study: Cyclosporin Data	165
6.6	Chapter Summary		171
6.7	Technical Details		171
	6.7.1	Repeated Measurements Data	171
	6.7.2	Paired Measurements Data	173
6.8	Bibliographic Note		174
	Exercises		174

7 Data from Multiple Methods — **177**

7.1	Preview		177
7.2	Introduction		177
7.3	Displaying Data		179
7.4	Example Datasets		179
	7.4.1	Systolic Blood Pressure Data	180
	7.4.2	Tumor Size Data	180
7.5	Modeling Unreplicated Data		184
7.6	Modeling Repeated Measurements Data		186
	7.6.1	Unlinked Data	186
	7.6.2	Linked Data	187
7.7	Model Fitting and Evaluation		189
7.8	Evaluation of Similarity and Agreement		190
7.9	Evaluation of Repeatability		191
7.10	Case Studies		192
	7.10.1	Systolic Blood Pressure Data	192
	7.10.2	Tumor Size Data	195
7.11	Chapter Summary		198
7.12	Technical Details		198
7.13	Bibliographic Note		200
	Exercises		200

8 Data with Covariates — **205**

| 8.1 | Preview | | 205 |

8.2	Introduction		205
8.3	Modeling of Data		206
	8.3.1	Modeling Means of Methods	206
	8.3.2	Modeling Variances of Methods	207
	8.3.3	Data Models	208
	8.3.4	Model Fitting and Evaluation	211
8.4	Evaluation of Similarity, Agreement, and Repeatability		211
	8.4.1	Measures of Agreement for Two methods	212
	8.4.2	Measures of Agreement for More Than Two Methods	213
	8.4.3	Measures of Repeatability	213
	8.4.4	Inference on Measures	214
8.5	Case Study		214
8.6	Chapter Summary		224
8.7	Technical Details		225
8.8	Bibliographic Note		226
	Exercises		226

9 Longitudinal Data — **229**

9.1	Preview		229
9.2	Introduction		229
	9.2.1	Displaying Data	231
	9.2.2	Percentage Body Fat Data	231
9.3	Modeling of Data		234
	9.3.1	The Longitudinal Data Model	236
	9.3.2	Specifying the Mean Functions	237
	9.3.3	Specifying the Correlation Function	237
	9.3.4	Model Fitting and Evaluation	240
9.4	Evaluation of Similarity and Agreement		241
9.5	Case Study		242
9.6	Chapter Summary		247
9.7	Technical Details		247
9.8	Bibliographic Note		249
	Exercises		250

10 A Nonparametric Approach — **253**

10.1	Preview		253
10.2	Introduction		253
10.3	The Statistical Functional Approach		255
	10.3.1	A Weighted Empirical CDF	256
	10.3.2	Distributions Induced by Empirical CDF	256
10.4	Evaluation of Similarity and Agreement		258

	10.5	Case Studies	259
		10.5.1 Unreplicated Blood Pressure Data	259
		10.5.2 Replicated Blood Pressure Data	263
	10.6	Chapter Summary	267
	10.7	Technical Details	267
		10.7.1 The Ω Matrix	268
		10.7.2 Estimation of Ω	269
		10.7.3 Influence Functions for the Measures	270
		10.7.4 TDI Confidence Bounds	270
		10.7.5 Summary of Steps	271
	10.8	Bibliographic Note	271
		Exercises	272
11	**Sample Size Determination**		**279**
	11.1	Preview	279
	11.2	Introduction	279
	11.3	The Sample Size Methodology	281
		11.3.1 Paired Measurements Design	281
		11.3.2 Repeated Measurements Design	281
	11.4	Case Study	282
	11.5	Chapter Summary	286
	11.6	Bibliographic Note	286
		Exercises	287
12	**Categorical Data**		**289**
	12.1	Preview	289
	12.2	Introduction	289
	12.3	Experimental Setups and Examples	290
		12.3.1 Types of Data	290
		12.3.2 Illustrative Examples	290
		12.3.3 A Graphical Approach	292
	12.4	Cohen's Kappa Coefficient for Dichotomous Data	293
		12.4.1 Definition and Basic Properties: Two Raters	293
		12.4.2 Sample Kappa Coefficient	297
		12.4.3 Agreement with a Gold Standard	298
		12.4.4 Unbiased Raters: Intraclass Kappa	299
		12.4.5 Multiple Raters	300
		12.4.6 Combining and Comparing Kappa Coefficients	301
		12.4.7 Sample Size Calculations	302
	12.5	Kappa Type Measures for More Than Two Categories	303
		12.5.1 Two Fixed Raters with Nominal Categories	303

	12.5.2	Two Raters with Ordinal Categories: Weighted Kappa	303
	12.5.3	Multiple Raters	304
12.6	Case Studies		305
	12.6.1	Two Raters with Two Categories	305
	12.6.2	Weighted Kappa: Multiple Categories	306
12.7	Models for Exploring Agreement		306
	12.7.1	Conditional Logistic Regression Models	306
	12.7.2	Log-Linear Models	307
	12.7.3	A Generalized Linear Mixed-Effects Model	308
12.8	Discussion		309
12.9	Chapter Summary		310
12.10	Bibliographic Note		311
	Exercises		312
References			319
Dataset List			331
Index			333

PREFACE

This book presents statistical models and methods for analyzing common types of data collected in method comparison experiments and illustrates their application through detailed case studies. The main aim of these trials is to evaluate agreement between two or more methods of measurement. Although such studies are particularly abundant in health-related fields, they are also conducted in other disciplines, including metrology, ecology, and social and behavioral sciences.

Currently, at least six books cover the topic of agreement evaluation, including von Eye and Mun (2004), Carstensen (2010), Dunn (2004), Shoukri (2010), Broemeling (2009), and Lin et al. (2011). Of these, the first focuses exclusively on categorical data, and the second on continuous data. Others consider both types of data with varying levels of depth and choice of topics. Our book also considers both but with a primary focus on continuous data and one chapter devoted to categorical data. By providing chapter-length treatments of the common types of continuous data, it offers a comprehensive coverage of the topic, and its scope is broader than any other book currently available. It, however, by no means offers a complete survey of the literature. For example, measurement error models, Bayesian methods, and approaches based on generalized estimating equations are not included.

Essentially two principles guided us while writing this book. The first was to view the analysis of method comparison data as a two-step procedure where, in step 1, an adequate model for the data is found, and in step 2, inferential techniques are applied for appropriate functions of the parameters of the model found in step 1. For modeling of data, we primarily rely on mixed-effects models because they capture dependence in a subject's measurements in an intuitively appealing manner by means of random subject effects; and they also offer a unified framework for dealing with a variety of data types. Besides, they can be fit by the maximum likelihood method using any commonly available statistical software package. For inference, we use the standard large-sample theory and invoke a bootstrap approach whenever the sample size seems too small for the asymptotic methods to be accurate. The second principle was to strive to make the presentation accessible to a wide audience while at the same time making the book theoretically rigorous and self-contained with necessary technical details and references. We have attempted to strike this balance by separating the technical details from the methodological descriptions, forgoing the references in favor of a bibliographic note at the end of each chapter, and by presenting detailed analyses of several real datasets.

The book is organized into twelve chapters. The first eleven are concerned with continuous data while the last covers categorical data. Chapter 1 provides a general introduction to studies comparing two measurement methods and discusses key concepts and statistical issues and tools involved in their analysis. Chapter 2 introduces various measures of agreement for continuous data. Chapter 3 describes mixed-effects models in general and presents the large-sample approach for inference. It provides the technical foundation for the rest of the book and can be skipped by a reader interested in applications. Chapters 4 through 9 consider continuous data collected from various types of experiments, with study designs becoming increasingly more complex. In order, these chapters are devoted to designs with paired measurements, repeated measurements, heteroscedastic measurements, more than two methods, covariates, and longitudinal data. Chapter 10 presents a nonparametric approach for data that do not satisfy assumptions of a mixed-effects model. Chapter 11 considers sample size determination for designing a method comparison study with continuous data. Chapter 12 takes up the question of agreement with categorical data.

Even though the presentation is self-contained, some statistical background is expected from the readers. Familiarity with basic statistical concepts such as maximum likelihood estimation, hypothesis testing, confidence intervals, correlation, and linear regression is necessary. A prior introduction to mixed-effects models and linear algebra will enhance the understanding of the technical details.

The free statistical software R (R Core Team, 2015) has been used to perform all the computations and to generate all the graphics presented in this book. However, the R code is not presented. Much of the code and many of the datasets used here are publicly available at the companion website:

http://www.utdallas.edu/~pankaj/agreement_book/

Some familiarity with R programming is assumed for following the code and understanding the output produced. In addition to the base and graphics packages of R, the the following packages and their dependencies have been used in preparing this book: lattice (Sarkar, 2008), latticeExtra (Sarkar and Andrews, 2013), Matrix (Bates and Maechler, 2015), mvtnorm (Genz et al., 2015), multcomp (Hothorn et al., 2008), nlme (Pinheiro et al., 2015), numDeriv (Gilbert and Varadhan, 2015), tikzDevice (Sharpsteen and Bracken, 2015), and xtable (Dahl, 2016).

The book is targeted primarily towards two groups of researchers. The first consists of biomedical and social and behavioral scientists interested in the development and validation of measurement methods. The second includes statisticians engaged in the design and analysis of method comparison studies and in the development of associated statistical methodologies. It can also serve as a textbook for a semester-long special topics course at the graduate level. With that purpose, we have incorporated numerous theoretical and data-centric exercises at the end of the chapters that expand on the material covered in the main body. These exercises provide practice for mastering methodological details and applying the results.

We appreciate the support from our institutions as we marched through this project and for their outstanding library and computing facilities. We thank all those scientists whose dedicated research we were able to highlight in this work. We thank our long-time friends and colleagues for their advice and encouragement, including Professors Babis Papachristou (Rowan University), Michael Baron (American University), Vladimir Dragovic and Vish Ramakrishna (UT Dallas), and Tom Santner and Doug Wolfe (Ohio State University). We thank Professor Phill Cassey (University of Adelaide) for introducing us to applications in ecology and providing datasets, and Professor Chaitra Nagaraja (Fordham University) for producing the plots in Chapter 12. We also thank Professors Huiman Barnhart (Duke University), Douglas Hawkins (University of Minnesota), Vernon Chinchilli (Pennsylvania State University), and Michael Haber (Emory University) for sharing their datasets.

We are grateful to Professors Mohamed Shoukri (King Faisal Specialist Hospital and Research Centre) and Tony Ng (Southern Methodist University) for reading an earlier draft of the manuscript and providing valuable comments. We thank Susanne Steitz-Filler, Allison McGinniss, and Melissa Yanuzzi from John Wiley for guiding the project from start to finish and for their patience and perseverance. We invite the input of our readers on the coverage and presentation here as well as on the companion website as there is always room for improvement.

This book would not have been possible without the support of our family members. They gracefully sacrificed their time with us to allow us to work on a project that seemed to take forever. We take this opportunity to thank them all from the bottom of our hearts.

P. K. CHOUDHARY & H. N. NAGARAJA

Richardson, Texas
Columbus, Ohio
July, 2017

CHAPTER 1

INTRODUCTION

1.1 PREVIEW

This chapter focuses on method comparison studies involving two methods of measurement of a quantitative variable. It introduces the companion problems of evaluation of similarity and evaluation of agreement between the methods, reviews the related concepts, critically examines the currently popular statistical tools, and describes a model-based approach for data analysis. It also points out the inadequacy of the widely used paired measurements design for data collection for the purpose of measuring agreement. To keep the flow of the text smooth, specific references are provided in the bibliographic note section at the end of the chapter. This practice is followed throughout the book.

1.2 NOTATIONAL CONVENTIONS

We generally use uppercase roman letters for random quantities whose values can be observed, for example, measurements made by medical devices. Lowercase roman letters are generally used for random quantities whose values cannot be observed (e.g., measurement errors) and for observed values of observable random quantities. Vectors and matrices are denoted by boldface letters. Their dimensions are clear from the context. By default, a vector is a column vector, and its transpose is denoted by attaching the superscript T to its symbol. For example, $\mathbf{x}$ is a column vector, $\mathbf{x}^T$ is the transpose of $\mathbf{x}$, and $\mathbf{X}$ is a matrix. We also use $\mathbf{I}$ for an identity matrix, $\mathbf{1}$ for vectors and matrices of ones, and $\mathbf{0}$ for vectors and

Measuring Agreement: Models, Methods, and Applications. By P. K. Choudhary and H. N. Nagaraja
Copyright © 2017 John Wiley & Sons, Inc.

matrices of zeros. We often attach a subscript to these symbols for clarity. For example, $\mathbf{I}_n$ denotes an $n \times n$ identity matrix and $\mathbf{1}_n$ denotes an $n \times 1$ vector of ones. A diagonal matrix is denoted as diag$\{x_1, \dots, x_n\}$. If $\mathbf{A}_1, \dots, \mathbf{A}_n$ are matrices, diag$\{\mathbf{A}_1, \dots, \mathbf{A}_n\}$ denotes a block-diagonal matrix. Further, tr$(\mathbf{A})$, $|\mathbf{A}|$, and $\mathbf{A}^{-1}$, respectively, denote the trace, determinant, and inverse of a (square) matrix $\mathbf{A}$.

Generally, the unknown scalar and vector parameters are denoted by lowercase Greek letters. An exception to this rule is the letter α, which is used as a known level of significance of a test of hypothesis and $100(1 - \alpha)\%$ represents level of confidence of a confidence interval or bound. Matrices of unknown parameters as well as known quantities (e.g., the design or the regression matrix) are denoted by uppercase roman letters in boldface. A "hat" over an unknown parameter denotes its estimate, whereas a "hat" over a random quantity denotes its predicted or fitted value. The (estimated) standard error of the estimator $\hat{\theta}$ of an unknown parameter θ is denoted by SE$(\hat{\theta})$.

We also use the convention that if, say, Y is a random quantity, then $Y_1, Y_2, \dots$ denote observations from the distribution of Y. Similarly, if Y_j is a random quantity, then Y_{ij}, $i \geq 1$, denote observations from the distribution of Y_j.

We use $\mathcal{N}_1(\mu, \sigma^2)$ for a univariate normal distribution with mean μ and variance σ^2. A multivariate normal distribution having p components with mean vector $\boldsymbol{\mu}$ and covariance matrix $\mathbf{V}$ is denoted as $\mathcal{N}_p(\boldsymbol{\mu}, \mathbf{V})$. We also use z_α, $t_{k,\alpha}$, $\chi^2_{k,\alpha}$, and $f_{k_1, k_2, \alpha}$ to, respectively, denote the (100α)th percentiles of a $\mathcal{N}_1(0, 1)$ distribution, a t distribution with k degrees of freedom, a χ^2 distribution with k degrees of freedom, and an F distribution with k_1 and k_2 as numerator and denominator degrees of freedom, respectively. We further use $\chi^2_{k,\alpha}(\delta)$ and $t_{k,\alpha}(\delta)$, respectively, to denote the (100α)th percentiles of noncentral χ^2 and t distributions with k degrees of freedom and noncentrality parameter δ. Finally, log refers to natural logarithm throughout the book.

1.3   BASIC CHARACTERISTICS OF A MEASUREMENT METHOD

Measurements are fundamental to any scientific endeavor. In particular, in health-related fields, measurements of clinically important quantities form the basis of diagnostic, therapeutic, and prognostic evaluation of patients. The quantity being measured may be *continuous* (or quantitative), for example, level of cholesterol, blood pressure, and concentration of a chemical. The quantity may also be *categorical* (or qualitative), for example, presence or absence of a medical condition and severity of a disease as identified by stage. Although this chapter is concerned with continuous measurements, it is obvious that any measurement process is prone to errors, regardless of whether its outcome is continuous or categorical. The errors in measurement cause the observed values to differ from the true underlying values. The relationship between the observed and the true values can be studied using statistical models.

Before describing such a model, let us set up some notation. Let the random variable Y represent the observed measurement from a method of measurement on a randomly selected subject from a population. We use the term "measurement method" in a generic sense. It may refer, for example, to an instrument, an assay, a medical device, a technician, or a clinical observer. The term "subject" is used here to refer to the entity on which the measurements are taken. For example, it may be a patient, a specimen, or a blood sample. Next, let the random variable b denote the true measurement of the subject associated with

Y. The true value is well defined, albeit it may be hard to measure directly (e.g., blood pressure); or it may be unobservable. In either case, the true value is not observed; and it is treated like a *latent variable* or a *random effect*.

1.3.1 A Statistical Model for Measurements

A commonly used model relating the observed Y to the true b is the classical linear model. It assumes

$$Y = \beta_0 + \beta_1 b + e, \qquad (1.1)$$

where β_0 and β_1 are fixed constants specific to the measurement method; and e is the random error of the method. The following assumptions are also made:

(*i*) The true value b has a probability distribution over the population of subjects. This distribution has mean (or expected value) μ_b and variance σ_b^2. The variance σ_b^2 is called the *between-subject variance* as it represents subject to subject variability in the true values—that is, the heterogeneity in the population.

(*ii*) The error e has a probability distribution with mean zero and variance σ_e^2. This distribution is over replications of the same underlying measurement by the same method on the same subject under identical conditions. For this reason, the error variance σ_e^2 is also called the *within-subject variance*. The square root of this variance is often known as the *repeatability standard deviation* or the *analytical standard deviation* of the measurement method.

(*iii*) The distributions of errors and true values are independent.

This model assumes that the error variance remains constant throughout the range of the value being measured. Often, this is not the case as the error variance may depend on the magnitude of measurement. An extension of the above model that accommodates such heteroscedastic errors is presented in Chapter 6.

A distinction is made between the true value of the *subject* and the true (i.e., error-free) value of the *measurement method*. The true value of the subject is b, whereas the true value produced by the measurement method is $\beta_0 + \beta_1 b$. These true values are linearly related in our model.

1.3.2 Quality Characteristics

The intercept β_0 in the model (1.1) is called *fixed bias* of the measurement method. It is a constant that the method adds to its measurements regardless of the true value being measured. The slope β_1 is called *proportional bias* or *level-dependent bias*. Instead of correctly measuring the true b, the method measures it as $\beta_1 b$. In other words, β_1 is the amount of change observed by the method if the true b changes by 1 unit. Both the fixed bias β_0 and the proportional bias β_1 cause systematic errors in measurement.

Under the model (1.1), the conditional mean and variance of Y given b are

$$E(Y|b) = \beta_0 + \beta_1 b, \ \operatorname{var}(Y|b) = \sigma_e^2, \qquad (1.2)$$

respectively. These quantities essentially represent the average and the variance of an infinitely large number of replications produced by the method while evaluating the same subject under identical conditions. The conditional mean is also what we have called the error-free value of the method.

A measurement method is said to be *accurate* if it has no bias in estimating the true value b. The biases β_0 and β_1 measure the magnitude of the lack of accuracy of the method. Consequently, a method is accurate if $(\beta_0, \beta_1) = (0, 1)$. In this case, the method has neither fixed nor proportional bias and its error-free value always matches the true value. Turning this interpretation around, we can say that the true value of a subject is the average of a large number of replications made on the subject under identical conditions by a method that has no bias.

The *precision* of a measurement method is related to the size of the random errors in measurement. The variance σ_e^2 of these errors measures variability in the observed Y around the error-free value of the method. Thus, σ_e^2 is a measure of the precision of the method and sometimes is formally defined as the reciprocal of the error variance. The method is *fully precise* if $\sigma_e^2 = 0$. In this case, the method has no measurement error—its observed value equals its error-free value.

A measurement method may appear highly precise merely because it is too crude to discern small changes in the true value. The ability of a method to discern small changes is measured by a relative measure of precision known as *sensitivity*. The notion of sensitivity combines the rate of change and the precision of a measurement method in a single index. For the model (1.1), it is given by $|\beta_1|/\sigma_e$. To understand the motivation behind this index, recall that the slope β_1 represents the rate of change in the error-free measurement of the method with respect to the true b. Thus, if $|\beta_1|$ is large, a small change in b will cause a comparatively large change in its measured value, resulting in increased sensitivity. Also, if the error variance is small, the observed measurement Y will be precise and the sensitivity will be large. In either case, it will be relatively easy to distinguish b from its nearby values on the basis of the observation Y. The larger the sensitivity, the more effective is the measurement method. Often when the interest is in comparing two methods, the square of the sensitivity is considered the precision of a method (Section 1.7.1).

It can be seen that the marginal mean and variance of Y are (Exercise 1.1)

$$E(Y) = \beta_0 + \beta_1 \mu_b, \ \text{var}(Y) = \beta_1^2 \sigma_b^2 + \sigma_e^2, \tag{1.3}$$

respectively. These quantities represent the average and variance of the measurements in the population from which the subject is being sampled. The expression for the variance also shows that there are two sources of variation—the true values in the population and the random errors. The variance is also affected by the proportional bias (β_1) of the method.

The *reliability* of a measurement method is defined as the proportion of variation in observed measurements that is not explained by the error variation inherent in the method. The reliability of a method following the model (1.1) is

$$1 - \frac{\text{var}(e)}{\text{var}(Y)} = 1 - \frac{\sigma_e^2}{\beta_1^2 \sigma_b^2 + \sigma_e^2} = \frac{\beta_1^2 \sigma_b^2}{\beta_1^2 \sigma_b^2 + \sigma_e^2} = \frac{1}{1 + \sigma_e^2/(\beta_1^2 \sigma_b^2)}, \tag{1.4}$$

where the variance of Y is substituted from (1.3). It can also be interpreted as the correlation between two independent replications of the same underlying measurement (Exercise 1.1). Thus, the reliability is actually an *intraclass correlation*. It ranges between zero and one. It increases as the error variance σ_e^2 decreases in relation to the variance $\beta_1^2 \sigma_b^2$ in the error-free measurements. This way the reliability of a method is a measure of its relative precision. A high value of reliability indicates that the error variation is small compared to the variation in the error-free values.

The expression for reliability shows that it depends on the error variation of the method as well as the heterogeneity (or the between-subject variation) in the population. In particular, the reliability increases as the population heterogeneity increases even if the precision of the method does not change. Thus, care must be taken in interpreting reliability.

1.4 METHOD COMPARISON STUDIES

Method comparison studies are designed to compare two competing methods of measurement of the same quantity, having a common unit of measurement. The measurements are taken by each method on every subject in the study, and there may or may not be replications. In this book, we are primarily concerned with the case when the methods under consideration are assumed to be fixed rather than a random sample from a population of methods. The case of randomly selected methods providing categorical measurements is discussed in Chapter 12.

A distinguishing feature of method comparison studies is that none of the methods in the study is assumed to be producing the true values. The true values remain unknown and the methods involved measure them with error. Usually, one of the methods is a new test method and other is an established standard method, which is often called the *gold standard* or the *reference* method. However, the gold standard designation does not mean that the method is free of systematic and random errors. It is also understood that future improvements in the measurement technique may render a current gold standard obsolete.

Generally, there are two goals for a method comparison study. The primary one is to quantify the extent of agreement between the measurement methods and determine whether they have sufficient agreement so that we can use them "interchangeably" for a particular purpose. By interchangeable use we mean that a measurement from one method on a subject can be replaced by a measurement from another method without causing any difference in the *practical* use of the measurement. In other words, it does not matter which method is being used to take the measurement as both give practically the same value. If two methods agree well enough to be used interchangeably, we may prefer the one that is cheaper, faster, less invasive, or is simply easier to use. This is also the motivation behind method comparison studies.

A secondary goal of a method comparison study is to compare characteristics of the measurement methods—such as their biases, precisions, and sensitivities—to find the differences in the methods that cause them to disagree. We refer to this comparison as *evaluation of similarity*. Understanding why the methods disagree is important. For example, we may discover that a new method does not agree well with a standard method because it is much more precise than the standard method.

The two putative goals of a method comparison study—evaluation of agreement and evaluation of similarity—are closely related. For example, when the methods agree well, it generally implies that their characteristics are similar as well. Likewise, when one method is substantially more precise than the other or when the methods have quite different characteristics, the issue of agreement evaluation may be moot. However, the methods may not agree well despite having similar characteristics. Furthermore, when the methods do not agree well, a comparison of their characteristics reveals why the methods disagree.

This information is helpful in determining whether one method is clearly superior to the other. It may also suggest corrective actions that may improve the extent of agreement between the methods. Often, a simple addition of a constant to one method or its rescaling may be all that is needed.

A method comparison study may seem similar to a calibration study, but their goals are different. In a typical calibration study, subjects with known measurements of a variable obtained from a highly accurate method that has negligible measurement error are also measured by a test method to develop an equation that converts a measurement from the test method into a predicted true measurement. In contrast, in a method comparison study, the methods being compared are already calibrated. Although there may be a standard method in the comparison, it is not assumed to be error free. If, however, the methods do not agree well, then an equation may be developed to transform measurements from one method for better agreement with the other.

1.5 MEANING OF AGREEMENT

To fix ideas, assume that the two methods are labeled as "1" and "2." Let Y_1 and Y_2, respectively, denote the paired measurements from methods 1 and 2 on a randomly selected subject from the population. It may be helpful to think of (Y_1, Y_2) as paired measurements on a typical subject. We assume that (Y_1, Y_2) has a continuous bivariate distribution with mean (μ_1, μ_2), variance (σ_1^2, σ_2^2), covariance σ_{12}, and (Pearson or product-moment) correlation ρ. The correlation is typically positive in practice. Let $D = Y_2 - Y_1$ denote the difference in the measurements. It follows a continuous distribution with mean $\xi = \mu_2 - \mu_1$ and variance $\tau^2 = \sigma_1^2 + \sigma_2^2 - 2\rho\sigma_1\sigma_2$.

Agreement between two methods refers to closeness between their measurements. The methods have *perfect agreement* in the ideal case when $P(Y_1 = Y_2) = 1$. In this case, the bivariate distribution of (Y_1, Y_2) is concentrated on the line of equality—the $45°$ line, causing the distribution of the difference to be degenerate at zero. This will be reflected in the scatterplot of Y_2 versus Y_1 if all (Y_1, Y_2) values fall on the line of equality. See panel (a) of Figure 1.1 for such a scatterplot of simulated data. In this case, all the differences are zero. Thus, perfect agreement corresponds to any of the following two equivalent conditions (Exercise 1.2):

(*i*) $\{\mu_1 = \mu_2, \sigma_1^2 = \sigma_2^2, \rho = 1\}$, that is, the methods have equal means, equal variances, and correlation one, or

(*ii*) $\{\xi = 0, \tau^2 = 0\}$, that is, the difference has zero mean and zero variance.

However, it is unrealistic to expect this ideal condition to hold in practice and some deviation from perfect agreement is inevitable. In fact, some degree of lack of agreement is acceptable as this is the very premise of a method comparison study.

The notion of perfect agreement is quite restrictive. For example, the methods may have equal means ($\xi = 0$). But this may not be enough for good agreement because the two variances may differ considerably, causing unacceptably large variability in the differences around zero (i.e., large τ^2) even when the correlation between the measurements is high. Having equal variances in addition to equal means may also not be enough for good agreement because if the correlation is small, one would again obtain a large τ^2. (Recall from Exercise 1.2 that $\tau^2 = 0$ if and only if $\sigma_1^2 = \sigma_2^2$ and $\rho = 1$.) Moreover, the methods

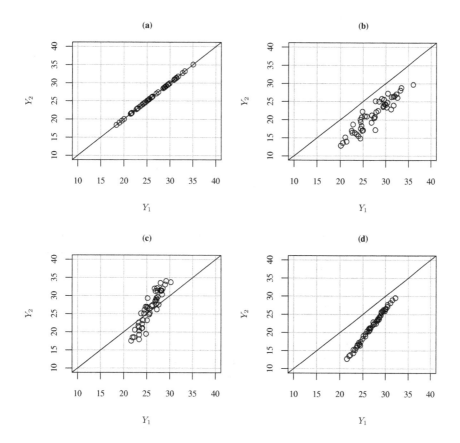

Figure 1.1   Scatterplots of simulated paired measurements data with high correlations superimposed with the line of equality. (a) The methods have perfect agreement. (b) The methods have unequal means but equal variances. (c) The methods have unequal variances but equal means. (d) The methods have unequal means and variances.

may have poor agreement despite having a perfect correlation ($\rho = \pm 1$) as it is a necessary but not sufficient condition for perfect agreement. This happens because the correlation is a measure of linear relationship, not of agreement. A perfect linear relationship simply means $Y_2 = \tilde{\beta}_0 + \tilde{\beta}_1 Y_1$, where $\tilde{\beta}_0$ and $\tilde{\beta}_1$ are constants. In this case, $\mu_2 = \tilde{\beta}_0 + \tilde{\beta}_1 \mu_1$ and $\sigma_2^2 = \tilde{\beta}_1^2 \sigma_1^2$. Thus, depending upon how far away $\tilde{\beta}_0$ is from zero and $\tilde{\beta}_1$ is from one, the methods may have substantially different means and variances, implying large ξ and τ^2, and hence poor agreement. See panels (b)–(d) of Figure 1.1 for scatterplots of simulated data for the following scenarios: unequal means but equal variances, equal means but unequal variances, and nearly perfect correlation but unequal means and unequal variances.

For a familiar example of perfect correlation but poor agreement, consider measuring temperature using a thermometer calibrated in Celsius (method 1). Take method 2 as the method that simply transforms the method 1 measurements into Fahrenheit, that is, $Y_2 = 32 + (9/5)Y_1$. These two methods are perfectly correlated, but they obviously have poor agreement. Nevertheless, in this case a simple recalibration of method 2 as $5(Y_2 - 32)/9$ will make the methods agree perfectly.

If the notion of agreement appears unduly restrictive, recall that some deviation from perfect agreement is acceptable provided the deviation is not too large to prohibit interchangeable use of the methods. Essentially, this means that some difference in means and variances and a non-perfect correlation is acceptable as long as the methods can be considered to have sufficient agreement for the intended purpose.

To evaluate agreement, we do two things. First, we quantify the extent of agreement by measuring how far the paired measurements are from the line of equality. The *measures of agreement* are used for this purpose. They are specific functions of parameters of the bivariate distribution of (Y_1, Y_2) and perfect agreement corresponds to appropriate ideal boundary values for these measures. Some common agreement measures are described in Chapter 2. Second, we determine whether the agreement is sufficiently strong to justify interchangeable use of the methods for the purpose at hand. This can be done by comparing the observed value of the agreement measure to a threshold value that represents acceptable agreement. The threshold, however, depends upon the intended use of the measurement and has to be clarified on a case-by-case basis. It is entirely possible for the methods to agree while both being wrong.

1.6   A MEASUREMENT ERROR MODEL

To explain how the notion of agreement is related to the characteristics of the two methods, we first need a model that links the observed (Y_1, Y_2) to the true value being measured and the measurement errors associated with the methods. It is common to assume the classical model (1.1) that leads to the following setup for the bivariate data:

$$Y_j = \beta_{0j} + \beta_{1j}b + e_j, \quad j = 1, 2, \tag{1.5}$$

where the intercept β_{0j} is the fixed bias of the jth method; the slope β_{1j} is its proportional bias; and e_j is its measurement error. As before, b is the true measurement of the subject. The assumptions regarding b are the same as those for model (1.1). The error e_j is assumed to have a mean of zero and variance σ_{ej}^2 that depends on the method. The errors are mutually independent of each other and of the true value. Later, the errors and the true values will be assumed to follow normal distributions (see Section 1.12); but these distributional assumptions are not needed at this time.

In this model, the error-free values of the methods, namely, $\beta_{01} + \beta_{11}b$ and $\beta_{02} + \beta_{12}b$, are linearly related to the true underlying value, and hence are linearly related to each other. This relationship between the error-free values induces dependence in the observed Y_1 and Y_2 since they share the common b, which itself is a random variable. However, conditional on b, Y_1 and Y_2 are independent.

When the two methods have different proportional biases, that is, $\beta_{11} \neq \beta_{12}$, we can interpret the situation as the methods having different *measurement scales*. This means that a unit change in the true value of the subject does not cause equal change in error-free values of both methods. As a result, the difference in the error-free values, $\beta_{02} - \beta_{01} + (\beta_{12} - \beta_{11})b$, is not a constant. Methods with different scales also have unequal variabilities in their error-free values ($\beta_{11}^2 \sigma_b^2$ versus $\beta_{12}^2 \sigma_b^2$). The terms "difference in proportional biases" and "difference in scales" are used interchangeably in this book.

Familiar examples of methods with obviously different scales include thermometers calibrated in Fahrenheit and Celsius, and weighing scales calibrated in ounces and grams.

Although in both these examples, the units of measurement are also different, it may happen that methods have different scales despite having a common nominal unit (Section 1.8).

1.6.1 Identifiability Issues

Although so far we have called b as *the* true measurement, the absolute truth is not available in *most* method comparison studies. Under our model assumptions, the true value is identifiable only up to a linear transformation. This is because the same linear model (1.5) results if b in (1.5) is replaced by its linear transformation $\beta_0^* + \beta_1^* b$, and (β_{0j}, β_{1j}) are redefined as $(\beta_{0j} + \beta_0^* \beta_{1j}, \beta_1^* \beta_{1j})$. The practical implication of this lack of identifiability is that the method-specific fixed and proportional biases cannot be determined. As a result, we cannot evaluate how close β_{0j} is to zero or β_{1j} is to one, meaning that we cannot ascertain how accurate the jth method is. With appropriate data, however, we can determine how close the bias differences $\beta_{02} - \beta_{01}$ and $\beta_{12} - \beta_{11}$ are to zero. This serves the purpose of method comparison because we are generally not interested in determining how accurate the individual methods are, but rather in comparing the methods and evaluating their agreement.

We can resolve the identifiability problem by assuming, without any loss of generality, that one of the methods (say, method 1) is the *reference method* and setting $\beta_{01} = 0$ and $\beta_{11} = 1$. This leads to the simplified model

$$Y_1 = b + e_1, \quad Y_2 = \beta_0 + \beta_1 b + e_2, \tag{1.6}$$

where, for notational convenience, we have replaced (β_{02}, β_{12}) by (β_0, β_1). Note that it does not matter which method is tagged as the reference method; but if there is a gold standard, it makes sense to use it as the reference. The concept of a reference method is needed just to enforce identifiability.

This model offers a working definition of the true measurement as well. Since from (1.6), $E(Y_1|b) = b$, the true value is what the reference method measures on average. In other words, the true value is the error-free value of the reference method. However, we cannot say whether this method is accurate. Moreover, the intercept β_0 in the model (1.6) represents the difference in the fixed biases of the methods. When $\beta_0 = 0$, the methods have the same fixed bias. Similarly, a non-unit value of the slope β_1 indicates a difference in the proportional biases (or scales) of the methods.

The model (1.6) is an example of a *measurement error model*. It is also called an *errors-in-variable model* because the model for Y_2 can be interpreted as a linear regression model, where the covariate b on which Y_2 is regressed is not observed directly. Instead, b is measured with error as Y_1. In the parlance of measurement error models, (1.6) is a *structural model* or a *structural equation model*, as opposed to a *functional model*, because the true b is considered random.

To see how this model differs from the ordinary linear regression model of Y_2 on Y_1, substitute $b = Y_1 - e_1$ in the expression for Y_2 to get

$$Y_2 = \beta_0 + \beta_1 Y_1 + \tilde{e}_2, \quad \tilde{e}_2 = e_2 - \beta_1 e_1.$$

Despite a superficial similarity, this model is not the ordinary linear regression model because the explanatory variable Y_1 and the error $\tilde{e}_2$ are not independent in this model, unless of course, Y_1 is error free (i.e., $\sigma_{e1}^2 = 0$).

1.6.2   Model-Based Moments

The measurement error model (1.6) postulates that the paired measurements (Y_1, Y_2) follow a bivariate distribution with mean vector

$$\begin{pmatrix} \mu_1 \\ \mu_2 \end{pmatrix} = \begin{pmatrix} \mu_b \\ \beta_0 + \beta_1 \mu_b \end{pmatrix} \tag{1.7}$$

and covariance matrix

$$\begin{pmatrix} \sigma_1^2 & \sigma_{12} \\ \sigma_{12} & \sigma_2^2 \end{pmatrix} = \begin{pmatrix} \sigma_b^2 + \sigma_{e1}^2 & \beta_1 \sigma_b^2 \\ \beta_1 \sigma_b^2 & \beta_1^2 \sigma_b^2 + \sigma_{e2}^2 \end{pmatrix}, \tag{1.8}$$

see Exercise 1.3. Clearly, there are two factors that may lead to unequal means, viz., a nonzero β_0 and a non-unit β_1. Similarly, there are two factors that may cause unequal variances, viz., a non-unit β_1 and unequal error variances. Further, the dependence in the bivariate distribution is solely due to the sharing of the common true value b by the two methods.

It follows from (1.8) that the (Pearson) correlation between Y_1 and Y_2 is

$$\rho = \frac{\beta_1 \sigma_b^2}{(\sigma_b^2 + \sigma_{e1}^2)^{1/2} (\beta_1^2 \sigma_b^2 + \sigma_{e2}^2)^{1/2}}. \tag{1.9}$$

From (1.4), this correlation can be interpreted as the square root of the product of the reliabilities of methods 1 and 2, given by

$$\frac{\sigma_b^2}{\sigma_b^2 + \sigma_{e1}^2}, \quad \frac{\beta_1^2 \sigma_b^2}{\beta_1^2 \sigma_b^2 + \sigma_{e2}^2}.$$

Thus, the correlation also depends on the between-subject variation in the population being measured. If the same methods are used in two populations—one with greater heterogeneity than the other—the methods would exhibit higher correlation in the population with greater heterogeneity. Due to this property, comparisons of such correlations need to take the population variability into account.

From (1.7) and (1.8), simple algebra shows that the mean and variance of the difference $D = Y_2 - Y_1$ are

$$\xi = \beta_0 + (\beta_1 - 1)\mu_b, \quad \tau^2 = (\beta_1 - 1)^2 \sigma_b^2 + \sigma_{e1}^2 + \sigma_{e2}^2. \tag{1.10}$$

Thus, the effects of the difference in fixed biases and the difference in scales get confounded in the mean ξ. The difference in scales also contributes to the variance τ^2.

1.6.3   Conditions for Perfect Agreement

From the model-based expressions for the moments of (Y_1, Y_2) and D given by (1.7)–(1.10), and the definition of perfect agreement from Section 1.5, it follows that the methods can have perfect agreement only when

$$\beta_0 = 0, \ \beta_1 = 1, \ \sigma_{e1}^2 = \sigma_{e2}^2 = 0.$$

Hence for perfect agreement, not only must the methods have equal fixed and proportional biases, but they must also have no measurement errors. In other words, any imprecision in

Test Theory Term	Parameter Setting	Interpretation
essential tau-equivalence	$\beta_1 = 1$	equal proportional biases
tau-equivalence	$(\beta_0, \beta_1) = (0, 1)$	equal fixed and proportional biases
parallelism	$(\beta_0, \beta_1, \sigma_{e1}^2) = (0, 1, \sigma_{e2}^2)$	equal fixed and proportional biases, and equal precisions

Table 1.1 Interpretation of test theory terms in the context of method comparison studies under the measurement error model (1.6).

either method or any difference in the fixed or proportional biases of the methods is a source of disagreement. Therefore, when we say that some lack of agreement is acceptable, we essentially mean that we are willing to tolerate some imprecision in the methods and some differences in their fixed and proportional biases. For good agreement, the differences in these biases and the measurement errors of both methods must be small.

1.6.4 Link to Test Theory

If we refer to measurement methods as "tests" and measurements as "scores," then the model (1.6) is known in psychometry as a *test theory model*. The tests following this model are called *congeneric* as their error-free scores, b and $\beta_0 + \beta_1 b$, are linearly related. The tests are called *essentially tau-equivalent* if $\beta_1 = 1$. In this case, the error-free scores are measured on the same scale but they may differ by a constant. The tests are said to be *tau equivalent* if $(\beta_0, \beta_1) = (0, 1)$. In this case, the tests have the same error-free scores or accuracy, that is, they have the same fixed bias and the same scale, but their precisions may be different. Further, the tests are said to be *parallel* if they are tau equivalent and $\sigma_{e1}^2 = \sigma_{e2}^2$. In this case, the tests not only have the same accuracy, but they also have the same precision. These connections between the concepts in method comparison studies and test theory are summarized in Table 1.1.

1.7 SIMILARITY VERSUS AGREEMENT

1.7.1 Evaluation of Similarity

The measurement error model (1.6) suggests that the two methods can be compared on the following characteristics of their marginal distributions:

- *Fixed bias*: The intercept β_0 represents the difference in fixed biases of the methods. If $\beta_0 = 0$, the methods have the same fixed bias.

- *Scale* (or *proportional bias*): The slope β_1 indicates the difference in the scales of the methods. If $\beta_1 = 1$, the methods have the same scale.

- *Precision*: The difference in the precisions of the methods can be measured by the *precision ratio*, defined as

$$\lambda = \frac{\text{precision of method 2}}{\text{precision of method 1}} = \frac{1/\sigma_{e2}^2}{1/\sigma_{e1}^2} = \frac{\sigma_{e1}^2}{\sigma_{e2}^2}. \qquad (1.11)$$

If $\lambda = 1$, the methods are equally precise, whereas if $\lambda < 1$, method 1 is more precise than method 2, and the converse holds if $\lambda > 1$.

- *Sensitivity*: The sensitivities of the methods (Section 1.3.2) can be compared using the *squared sensitivity ratio*, defined as

$$\gamma^2 = \frac{(\text{sensitivity of method 2})^2}{(\text{sensitivity of method 1})^2} = \frac{\beta_1^2/\sigma_{e2}^2}{1/\sigma_{e1}^2} = \beta_1^2 \frac{\sigma_{e1}^2}{\sigma_{e2}^2} = \beta_1^2 \lambda. \qquad (1.12)$$

When $\gamma^2 < 1$, method 1 is more sensitive than method 2, and the converse is true if $\gamma^2 > 1$. The sensitivity metric γ^2 is the product of precision ratio and squared ratio of proportional biases. Thus, when the methods have the same scale (i.e., proportional bias) and precision, they also have equal sensitivity ($\gamma^2 = 1$).

The precisions of methods are comparable only when the methods have the same scale. For example, the precisions of two thermometers—one calibrated in Fahrenheit and another in Celsius—cannot be compared, unless one of them is transformed to have the same scale as the other. For methods following model (1.6), this transformation amounts to replacing Y_2 with Y_2/β_1, leading to σ_{e2}^2/β_1^2 as the new error variance. This error variance is comparable to σ_{e1}^2, and the precision ratio comparing them results in γ^2. Thus, γ^2 is actually the precision ratio after rescaling one of the methods to have the same scale as the other. For this reason, the squared sensitivity is often called the "precision" of a method and is unaffected by the intercept β_0.

To summarize, under model (1.6), the differences in the marginal characteristics of the methods are measured using β_0, β_1, λ, and γ^2. These quantities are collectively called the *measures of similarity*. None of these measures involve any parameters of b—the true quantity being measured. Therefore, the comparison of methods through these measures is unaffected by the properties of b such as its magnitude, variability, range, etc. This contrasts with measures of agreement that typically involve such parameters (see Section 1.5 and Chapter 2). Obviously, in the test theory language, parallelism is the best outcome we can expect when we evaluate similarity of two methods.

1.7.2 Evaluation of Agreement

Evaluation of similarity is essentially a comparison of marginal distributions of the methods. On the other hand, evaluation of agreement is an examination of joint distribution of the methods, which, of course, involves their marginal distributions as well. From Section 1.5, it is clear that the notion of perfect agreement is more restrictive than parallelism. In particular, perfect agreement implies parallelism, but the converse is not true in general. To understand this, note that parallel methods have the same accuracy and precision (see Table 1.1). As a result, they have the same mean ($\mu_1 = \mu_2$) and the same variance ($\sigma_1^2 = \sigma_2^2$), but their correlation given by (1.9) is not 1 unless both of them are error free ($\sigma_{e1}^2 = \sigma_{e2}^2 = 0$). Thus, simply an evaluation of similarity of methods is not enough to evaluate their agreement. The methods may have poor agreement despite having similar characteristics because their measurement errors may be significant. That said, it is often the case that if methods have very similar characteristics, they also have good agreement.

Although the agreement measures reflect the net effect of differences in marginal characteristics of the methods (see Chapter 2), the inference on them alone is not sufficient. This is because when methods do not agree well we would not know why they disagree and whether there is any method that is clearly superior to the other unless we examine the similarity measures. This shows that the inference on similarity measures is also necessary because it indicates which characteristics of methods are similar and which are different and by how much.

1.8 A TOY EXAMPLE

To get a better grasp on some of the concepts introduced thus far, consider a simple example of measuring weight using two digital scales (or instruments). The instruments are made by different manufacturers and both display results in grams. When b grams of true weight is measured, instrument 1 displays it as Y_1 grams and instrument 2 displays it as Y_2 grams, where

$$Y_1 = b + e_1, \quad Y_2 = 5 + 0.99b + e_2,$$

and e_1 and e_2 are measurement errors inherent in the two instruments. Assume also that $\sigma_{e1} = 0.01$ grams and $\sigma_{e2} = 1$ gram. This model is of the form (1.6).

Obviously these instruments have quite different characteristics and hence are not parallel. In fact, instrument 1 is much superior to instrument 2. In particular, it is correctly calibrated because its error-free measurement is identical to the true value, but this is not the case for instrument 2. There are two errors in the calibration of instrument 2—it has a fixed positive bias of 5 grams and a negative proportional bias of 1%. Instrument 1 has no bias of either kind and hence is *accurate*. These instruments have different measurement scales because what one measures as b is measured as $0.99b$ by the other. Note that the measurement scales are different despite the fact that the instruments have the same unit of measurement (grams). The scales would have been the same if either the b in the expression for Y_1 were $0.99b$ or the $0.99b$ in the expression for Y_2 were b. Furthermore, instrument 1 is much more precise than instrument 2. The measures of similarity, defined in Section 1.7.1, have the following values:

$$\beta_0 = 5, \ \beta_1 = 0.99, \ \lambda = 1 \times 10^{-4}, \ \gamma^2 = 9.8 \times 10^{-5}.$$

Clearly, these instruments do not have perfect agreement. There are four factors that contribute to disagreement—different fixed biases (zero versus 5), different scales (b versus $0.99b$), different error variances (0.01^2 versus 1), and nonzero measurement errors (positive error variances for both). Notwithstanding the fact that the instrument 1 is much superior to instrument 2, they may be considered to have sufficient agreement for interchangeable use in a home as kitchen scales. It, however, seems unlikely that they can be used interchangeably, for example, in a jewelry store. Thus, the same degree of agreement may be sufficient for one purpose but not for another.

Suppose now that instrument 1 is also miscalibrated in the same way as instrument 2. In this case, the instruments may have sufficient agreement—but they agree on the wrong thing. In fact, we are able to identify a method as miscalibrated just because we *assumed* that the true weight of b grams is measured. In practice, however, we may not be able to say whether a method is miscalibrated because we generally do not have access to true values in method comparison studies.

This example can also be used to demonstrate the effect of between-subject variation on correlation. For example, if $\sigma_b = 1$, the correlation between Y_1 and Y_2 from (1.9) is 0.70, whereas if $\sigma_b = 4$, the correlation increases to 0.97.

1.9   CONTROVERSIES AND OUR VIEW

The analysis of method comparison studies has generated controversies in the medical and clinical chemistry literature. The core questions include what really should be the goal of a method comparison study and how should the method comparison data be analyzed. Generally, only one of the two goals is put forward, albeit not always explicitly: (1) evaluation of agreement between the methods with the rationale that they can be used interchangeably if they agree well; and (2) evaluation of similarity by comparing characteristics such as biases, precisions, and scales of the methods to learn how the methods differ. In the first case, the data analysis typically consists of inference on agreement measures, whereas in the second, it consists of inference on measures of similarity such as the bias difference and precision ratio.

Some authors who believe in the goal of agreement evaluation forcefully reject the notion of correlation and correlation-type measures of agreement as irrelevant because they strongly depend on the between-subject variation of the population (Sections 1.6 and 1.8 and Chapter 2). It is argued that if correlation-type measures are used, then a high degree of agreement can simply be achieved by collecting data over a wide range of measurement. This is because a wide range effectively ensures large between-subject variation, which in turn leads to large values for the correlation-type measures. As an alternative, measures based on differences in measurements are suggested. In most cases, the popular approaches to inference on agreement measures do not emphasize explicit modeling of data, which is often considered unnecessary or too complicated to explain to practitioners who may be non-statisticians.

On the other hand, the authors who advocate comparing characteristics of methods criticize the goal of agreement evaluation as being too restrictive and often reject inference on agreement measures as serving a limited purpose. It is often asked: "What if the methods do not agree well?" Without comparing accuracies, precisions, and scales of the methods, we would not know why the methods disagree. Perhaps they disagree because one method is much better (e.g., much more precise) than the other or because they have different scales of measurement. But this analysis requires appropriate modeling of data, which often involves the correlation.

This book takes the view that both the aforementioned goals—evaluation of similarity and agreement—ought to be accomplished in the same method comparison study because the goals are interrelated and complementary (Sections 1.4 and 1.7.2). The key to accomplishing both goals is collecting data using sufficiently informative designs and appropriate modeling of data. There is universal agreement that the paired measurements design—which unfortunately is the most common design in practice—is completely inadequate for method comparison studies. The data from this design do not allow identifiability of the basic model parameters. Moreover, these data often do not even have sufficient information to reliably estimate precisions of the methods, making the comparison of precisions an unattainable goal (Section 1.12). At the very least, two measurements are needed from each method on every subject under identical conditions.

While the correlation-type agreement measures may mask important differences in the methods, there are other measures of agreement that do not have this drawback (see Chapter 2). We recommend examining more than one agreement measure because different measures quantify disagreement by looking at different aspects of the bivariate distribution of measurements from the two methods.

In this book, we espouse a model-based approach for the analysis of method comparison data. First, we fit an appropriate model to the data. Then, we use the fitted model to perform statistical inference on measures of similarity and agreement using standard tools of inference such as confidence intervals. This approach is illustrated in subsequent chapters of the book under various settings.

1.10 CONCEPTS RELATED TO AGREEMENT

The terms repeatability, reliability, and reproducibility are often used in the context of agreement evaluation. *Repeatability* of a measurement method refers to the variability in its repeated measurements made on the same subject under identical conditions. In this case, the true underlying value does not change, nor does the accuracy and precision of the method. Hence any variation in the repeated measurements is purely due to the inherent error in the measurement process. Thus, repeatability of a method refers to the size of its measurement errors. This explains why the error standard deviation is often called the repeatability standard deviation (Section 1.3.1). One can also think of this standard deviation as a measure of intra-method agreement.

Reliability, defined in (1.4), is also a characteristic of a measurement method that depends on the size of its measurement errors, but this size is measured relative to subject-to-subject variation in the true measurements.

Reproducibility is not a characteristic of a measurement method. It refers to the variation in the measurements made on the same subject under changing conditions. The "changing conditions" may be different instruments, different laboratories, or more generally, different measurement methods. The true value of the subject and the accuracy and precision of the measurement method may change between the conditions. If, however, the interest is in a small number of fixed and specified conditions, that is, the "condition" can be considered a *fixed effect* as opposed to a *random effect*, and the true value does not change between the conditions, then reproducibility is simply a synonym for agreement.

Equivalence is often used as a synonym for agreement, but it has a precise meaning in the statistical literature that differs from the notion of agreement. The concept of equivalence arises in the context of hypothesis testing. Equivalence hypothesis is used when the goal of the study is to demonstrate *practical equivalence* rather than a *significant difference*. For example, suppose ϕ is a scalar parameter of interest. In a typical significance testing problem, the null (H_0) and alternative (H_1) hypotheses are of the form

$$H_0 : \phi = \phi_0 \text{ and } H_1 : \phi \neq \phi_0,$$

where ϕ_0 is a specified reference value. In contrast, in an equivalence testing problem, the corresponding hypotheses are of the form

$$H_0 : \phi \leq \phi_0 - \epsilon_1 \text{ or } \phi \geq \phi_0 + \epsilon_2 \text{ and } H_1 : \phi_0 - \epsilon_1 < \phi < \phi_0 + \epsilon_2,$$

where $(\phi_0 - \epsilon_1, \phi_0 + \epsilon_2)$ is a specified "indifference zone" that consists of values of ϕ that are *practically the same as* ϕ_0. Equivalence testing is applied extensively in bioequivalence trials.

1.11   ROLE OF CONFIDENCE INTERVALS AND HYPOTHESES TESTING

1.11.1   Formulating the Agreement Hypotheses

Since agreement evaluation involves deducing whether two methods have sufficient agreement, it is natural to formulate this problem as a test of hypothesis. The question then becomes the following: Should the claim that "the methods have sufficient agreement" be formulated as the null hypothesis or the alternative hypothesis?

The answer to this question has important practical implications as statistical tests do not treat the null and alternative hypotheses in a symmetric manner. A test presumes that the null hypothesis is true and looks for evidence in the data against this hypothesis. If the data have strong evidence against the null, the test rejects the null in favor of the alternative; otherwise, the test accepts the null. Thus, the null hypothesis is treated like the default hypothesis—it is rejected only when the data strongly favor the alternative hypothesis.

A hypothesis test makes one of two types of errors. It makes a *type I error* if the test incorrectly rejects the null hypothesis (i.e., it incorrectly accepts the alternative hypothesis), and a *type II error* if it incorrectly accepts the null hypothesis. Ideally, we would like to have small probabilities for both the errors, but this is not possible for a test based on a fixed sample size. Therefore, a test is designed to ensure that its type I error probability is at most a prespecified small probability—also known as the *level of significance*. But the test has no control over its type II error probability, or its power, which is defined as 1 minus the probability of type II error. This is why the null and alternative hypotheses are formulated in a way that ensures that the more serious of the two errors becomes the type I error whose probability is guaranteed to be small. It is also expected that a power analysis is done prior to data collection and enough sample size is taken so that the test has adequate power to reject the null hypothesis when the alternative hypothesis is true.

The above arguments make it clear that whether "sufficient agreement" should be formulated as the null or the alternative hypothesis is determined by which of the two errors—the error of incorrectly declaring sufficient agreement or the error of incorrectly declaring insufficient agreement—is considered more serious. From the viewpoint of a user, clearly the former is the more serious error, and this should be the type I error. Therefore, the hypotheses for agreement evaluation should be formulated as

H_0 : The two methods *do not have* sufficient agreement, versus

H_1 : The two methods *have* sufficient agreement.   (1.13)

We refer to these hypotheses as the *agreement hypotheses*.

Suppose now that ϕ is a *scalar* measure of agreement. As mentioned in Section 1.5, this ϕ is a given function of parameters of the bivariate distribution of (Y_1, Y_2) (see also

Chapter 2). In some cases, a large value for ϕ implies good agreement, whereas in some other cases, a small value implies good agreement. Let ϕ_0 be the threshold for sufficient agreement specified by the practitioner. This threshold represents the value of ϕ beyond which the agreement is considered acceptable. When a small ϕ means good agreement, (1.13) becomes

$$H_0 : \phi \geq \phi_0 \text{ versus } H_1 : \phi < \phi_0. \tag{1.14}$$

Alternatively, when a large ϕ means good agreement, (1.13) becomes

$$H_0 : \phi \leq \phi_0 \text{ versus } H_1 : \phi > \phi_0. \tag{1.15}$$

In either case, the agreement hypotheses are one-sided and require the threshold ϕ_0. Statistical considerations alone cannot determine this threshold, or more generally, allow one to assess whether a given value of ϕ represents sufficient agreement. This is because a ϕ_0 that is sufficient for one application may not be so for another.

1.11.2 Testing Hypotheses Using Confidence Bounds

Although the agreement hypotheses can be tested directly, we prefer the use of the corresponding one-sided confidence bound for ϕ. This is because a confidence bound provides additional information about the magnitude of ϕ besides being useful for testing hypotheses.

In particular, when a small value for ϕ implies good agreement, we can compute a $100(1 - \alpha)\%$ *upper confidence bound* for ϕ, say U. This U can be interpreted as the largest plausible value of ϕ supported by the data and it represents the least plausible amount of agreement as suggested by the data. Further, U can be used for testing the agreement hypotheses at significance level α in the following way:

Reject H_0 in favor of H_1 if $U < \phi_0$, and accept H_0 otherwise.

This decision rule corresponds to the formulation in (1.14) (Exercise 1.4).

Similarly, when a large value for ϕ implies good agreement, we can compute a $100(1 - \alpha)\%$ *lower confidence bound* for ϕ, say L. This L leads to the following decision rule:

Reject H_0 in favor of H_1 if $L > \phi_0$, and accept H_0 otherwise,

and provides a level α test of the hypotheses in (1.15).

1.11.3 Evaluation of Agreement Using Confidence Bounds

The use of confidence bounds offers an important practical advantage over hypothesis tests. The test requires an advance specification of the threshold ϕ_0 for acceptable agreement, which may be a difficult task for the practitioner. On the other hand, the confidence bounds L or U can be computed without having to specify a ϕ_0. They can be directly used to evaluate agreement by assessing whether the magnitude of agreement that the bound represents can be considered sufficient. If the answer is yes, infer sufficient agreement; otherwise infer insufficient agreement. This way the agreement can be evaluated without resorting to an explicit test of hypothesis.

In agreement evaluation, sometimes one wonders whether to compute a one-sided confidence bound for the agreement measure ϕ or a two-sided confidence interval for it. The choice is guided by the use to which the result will be put. If the result will be used to infer whether the methods have sufficient agreement, which is generally the case, then an appropriate one-sided bound is the more relevant choice. This bound can be used either directly to infer sufficient agreement or it can be used to explicitly test the agreement hypotheses (1.13). If, however, the result will be used to examine the plausible values of ϕ supported by the data, then a two-sided interval is the more relevant choice.

It may be noted that a two-sided $100(1 - \alpha)\%$ confidence interval for ϕ can also be used to provide a level α test of the one-sided agreement hypotheses. But this test will be less powerful than the one based on the relevant one-sided bound (Exercise 1.4). We use confidence bounds for agreement measures throughout the book.

1.11.4   Evaluation of Similarity Using Confidence Intervals

Since the evaluation of similarity involves deducing whether two methods have similar characteristics, it is appropriate to consider the equivalence testing methodology described in Section 1.10. In particular, one can specify an indifference zone around each measure of similarity defined in Section 1.7.1 and test the resulting hypothesis of equivalence. The indifference zones, for example, may be taken as

$$-5 < \beta_0 < 5, \, 0.8 < \beta_1 \text{ (or } \lambda \text{ or } \gamma) < 1.2,$$

which essentially means that up to 5 units difference in fixed biases and up to 20% difference in measurement scales (or precisions or sensitivities) are acceptable.

We, nevertheless, eschew formal equivalence testing in this book in favor of two-sided confidence intervals for the similarity measures. This is because there is more than one measure of similarity and an indifference zone around each may lead to a substantial lack of overall agreement. We prefer to let the net effect of the differences in characteristics of methods be reflected in the values of agreement measures. These values can then be evaluated to see whether the extent of agreement may be considered sufficient. Besides, the confidence intervals of the similarity measures do reveal how much they differ from their ideal values. They can also be used to test equivalence hypothesis if needed.

1.12   COMMON MODELS FOR PAIRED MEASUREMENTS DATA

The paired measurements design is the most common design used for comparing two methods. It involves taking one measurement from each method on every subject in the study. Suppose there are n subjects. Let Y_{ij} denote the observed measurement from the jth method on the ith subject, $i = 1, \ldots, n$, $j = 1, 2$. For the purpose of modeling the data, we assume that the subjects are randomly selected from the population of interest, and treat the paired measurements (Y_{i1}, Y_{i2}) to be independently and identically distributed (i.i.d.) as (Y_1, Y_2). It follows that the measurement differences $D_i = Y_{i2} - Y_{i1}$ are i.i.d. as $D = Y_2 - Y_1$.

Often in practice, the subjects are selected deliberately rather than randomly so as to make the measurement range as wide as possible. The deliberate selection is reasonable from the viewpoint of experimenters as they would naturally like to compare the methods over the entire measurement range. But a model that takes such deliberate selection into account involves additional complications and is beyond the scope of this book.

Let $\overline{Y}_{\cdot j}$ and S_j^2, respectively, denote the mean and variance of the sample from the jth method. Further, let S_{12} and R, respectively, denote the sample covariance and sample correlation between the paired measurements. These statistics are defined as

$$\overline{Y}_{\cdot j} = \frac{1}{n}\sum_{i=1}^{n} Y_{ij}, \quad S_j^2 = \frac{1}{n-1}\sum_{i=1}^{n}(Y_{ij} - \overline{Y}_{\cdot j})^2,$$

$$S_{12} = \frac{1}{n-1}\sum_{i=1}^{n}(Y_{i1} - \overline{Y}_{\cdot 1})(Y_{i2} - \overline{Y}_{\cdot 2}),$$

$$R = \frac{S_{12}}{S_1 S_2} = \frac{\sum_{i=1}^{n}(Y_{i1} - \overline{Y}_{\cdot 1})(Y_{i2} - \overline{Y}_{\cdot 2})}{\left(\sum_{i=1}^{n}(Y_{i1} - \overline{Y}_{\cdot 1})^2 \sum_{i=1}^{n}(Y_{i2} - \overline{Y}_{\cdot 2})^2\right)^{1/2}}. \tag{1.16}$$

It is assumed that $S_1, S_2 > 0$, and $|R| < 1$. Let

$$\overline{D} = \frac{1}{n}\sum_{i=1}^{n} D_i, \quad S_D^2 = \frac{1}{n-1}\sum_{i=1}^{n}(D_i - \overline{D})^2 \tag{1.17}$$

denote the sample mean and sample variance of the differences. Clearly, $\overline{D} = \overline{Y}_{\cdot 1} - \overline{Y}_{\cdot 2}$ and $S_D^2 = S_1^2 + S_2^2 - 2S_{12}$. Except for the sample correlation R, all the above statistics are unbiased estimators of their population counterparts.

We now present three commonly used models for the paired measurements data. The first two are related to the measurement error model (1.6) introduced in Section 1.6, and the last is a simple bivariate normal model. All assume normality.

1.12.1   A Measurement Error Model

This model assumes that (Y_1, Y_2) follows the measurement error model presented in (1.6), which allows for potentially different measurement scales for the methods. Hence the model for the paired measurements (Y_{i1}, Y_{i2}) can be written as

$$Y_{i1} = b_i + e_{i1}, \quad Y_{i2} = \beta_0 + \beta_1 b_i + e_{i2}, \quad i = 1, \ldots, n, \tag{1.18}$$

where b_i is the true unobservable measurement for the ith subject and e_{ij} is the random error of the jth method ($j = 1, 2$). Further, b_i and e_{ij} are i.i.d. as b and e_j, respectively, where b and e_j are as defined in (1.6). In addition to the assumptions listed in Section 1.6, we assume that b and e_j are normally distributed, that is, $b \sim \mathcal{N}_1(\mu_b, \sigma_b^2)$ and $e_j \sim \mathcal{N}_1(0, \sigma_{ej}^2)$.

This model implies that the pairs (Y_{i1}, Y_{i2}) are i.i.d. as (Y_1, Y_2), which follows a bivariate normal distribution with mean vector given by (1.7) and covariance matrix given by (1.8). The measurement differences D_i and D can be written as

$$D_i = \beta_0 + (\beta_1 - 1)b_i + e_{i2} - e_{i1}, \quad D = \beta_0 + (\beta_1 - 1)b + e_2 - e_1.$$

They depend on the true measurement as well as the differences in fixed biases and the measurement errors. In particular, the D_i increase or decrease in proportion to the true values. This phenomenon is simply a consequence of unequal measurement scales. The D_i are i.i.d. as $D \sim \mathcal{N}_1(\xi, \tau^2)$, where ξ and τ^2 are given in (1.10).

Under the model (1.18), all four measures of similarity described in Section 1.7.1, viz., $\beta_0, \beta_1, \lambda$, and γ^2, can be used to compare characteristics of the methods.

Unfortunately, this measurement error model is not identifiable and hence its parameters cannot be estimated. The problem here is that there are six unrelated parameters in the model but we have only five sufficient statistics, namely, two sample means, two sample variances, and one sample covariance, under the bivariate normality of the data.

This problem of model non-identifiability can be resolved by making an assumption about one of the parameters, reducing the number of unknown parameters to five. Then, these parameters can be estimated using the *maximum likelihood* (ML) *method*. One possibility is to assume $\beta_1 = 1$, that is, the methods have the same scale. In this case, the model reduces to the mixed-effects model described in the next section. Another possibility is to assume that the precision ratio λ is known, that is, the precision of one method is a *known* multiple of the precision of the other. Under this assumption, the fitting of the model is known as *Deming regression* (see Section 1.14.2).

1.12.2   A Mixed-Effects Model

This is a special case of the measurement error model (1.18) obtained by taking $\beta_1 = 1$, thereby assuming that the two methods have the same measurement scale. Thus, we obtain

$$Y_{i1} = b_i + e_{i1}, \ \ Y_{i2} = \beta_0 + b_i + e_{i2}, \ \ i = 1, \ldots, n. \tag{1.19}$$

Interpretations of the terms in the model and assumptions regarding them are identical to those stated for the model (1.18).

This model is popularly known as the *Grubbs model*. It is a *variance components model* with three components of variance, namely, σ_b^2, σ_{e1}^2, and σ_{e2}^2. It can also be called a *mixed-effects* model because β_0 is a *fixed effect* and b_i is a subject-specific *random effect*. We can write this model in the familiar mixed-effects model form by assuming, without any loss of generality, that $E(b) = 0$ and writing $Y_{ij} = \mu_j + b_i + e_{ij}$, where $\mu_1 = \mu_b$ and $\mu_2 = \beta_0 + \mu_b$. This is also the form we use in the subsequent chapters of the book.

The model (1.19) implies that the measurement pairs (Y_{i1}, Y_{i2}) are i.i.d. as (Y_1, Y_2), which follows a bivariate normal distribution with mean vector

$$\begin{pmatrix} \mu_b \\ \beta_0 + \mu_b \end{pmatrix} \tag{1.20}$$

and covariance matrix

$$\begin{pmatrix} \sigma_b^2 + \sigma_{e1}^2 & \sigma_b^2 \\ \sigma_b^2 & \sigma_b^2 + \sigma_{e2}^2 \end{pmatrix}. \tag{1.21}$$

Further, the correlation between the methods is

$$\rho = \frac{\sigma_b^2}{(\sigma_b^2 + \sigma_{e1}^2)^{1/2}(\sigma_b^2 + \sigma_{e2}^2)^{1/2}}. \tag{1.22}$$

These expressions can also be obtained by setting $\beta_1 = 1$ in (1.7), (1.8), and (1.9). The correlation here is non-negative, and as noted in Section 1.6.2, warrants a careful interpretation because it depends on the between-subject variation.

The measurement differences D_i and D can be written as

$$D_i = \beta_0 + e_{i2} - e_{i1}, \ \ D = \beta_0 + e_1 - e_2. \tag{1.23}$$

They are just a sum of differences in the systematic biases of the methods and their measurement errors, and are free of the true measurement b_i. This contrasts with the case of measurement error model (1.18) where the differences depend on b_i. The D_i are i.i.d. as $D \sim \mathcal{N}_1(\xi, \tau^2)$, where

$$\xi = \beta_0, \ \tau^2 = \sigma_{e1}^2 + \sigma_{e2}^2. \tag{1.24}$$

Since the measurement methods following the mixed-effects model have the same scale, their error-free measurements differ only by a constant (b versus $\beta_0 + b$). As a result, the methods are assumed to be essentially tau equivalent (see Table 1.1). In other words, the methods may differ only on two characteristics—fixed bias and precision, and these differences can be measured by the similarity measures β_0 and λ (Section 1.7.1). Unlike the case of measurement error model (1.6), the measure β_0 for this mixed-effects model is actually the mean difference ξ.

The mixed-effects model (1.19) can be fit by the ML method. Any statistical software capable of fitting such models can provide the parameter estimates and their estimated covariance matrix. These estimates are used to perform inference on measures of agreement and similarity (see Chapter 2). Exercise 1.5 explores a simple *method of moments* approach for fitting this model. This method, however, may lead to negative estimates of error variances (see Exercise 1.6 for a real example). Besides, when the assumed model holds, the ML method is generally a more efficient method of estimation than the method of moments. Moreover, the latter does not generalize well for fitting more complicated models. For these reasons, we do not emphasize the method of moments in this book.

Although it is possible to get ML estimates of the error variances σ_{ej}^2 from the paired measurements, the estimates may be unreliable as they may have unrealistically large standard errors. In practice, it often happens that one estimate is zero (the smallest possible value for the variance) or near zero and the other is larger by several orders of magnitude (see Exercise 1.6). This gives the false impression that one method has near-perfect precision whereas the other is substantially worse. If we rule out the possibility that the precisions of the methods may truly differ by several orders of magnitude, then this phenomenon usually indicates one of two possibilities: either (1) an entirely wrong model is being fit to the data (e.g., the assumption of equal scales is incorrect), or (2) the model is reasonable, but the data do not have enough information to reliably estimate the error variances.

Often in practice, the mixed-effects models are fit by the method of restricted maximum likelihood (REML) instead of the ML method. Although a discussion of the REML method is outside the scope of this book (see Bibliographic Note), here we just note that this method, by design, only estimates the variance-covariance parameters and not the fixed-effect parameters. Since this method does not *jointly* estimate all model parameters, it does not provide a joint covariance matrix of all parameter estimates. This matrix, however, is needed for inference on agreement measures because they are functions of both fixed-effect and variance-covariance parameters. Therefore, we do not use the REML method in this book.

A limitation of the mixed-effects model is its assumption of a common scale of measurement for both methods. The methods may have different scales despite having the same nominal unit of measurement.

1.12.3 A Bivariate Normal Model

This model simply assumes that (Y_1, Y_2) follows a bivariate normal distribution with mean (μ_1, μ_2), variance (σ_1^2, σ_2^2), and covariance σ_{12} (or correlation ρ), and the paired measurements (Y_{i1}, Y_{i2}) form an i.i.d. sample of size n. Thus, the differences D_i are an i.i.d. sample from the distribution of $D \sim \mathcal{N}_1(\xi, \tau^2)$.

The paired measurements in the previous two models also follow a bivariate normal distribution. But these models make specific assumptions about how the observed measurements are related to the true measurements and the measurement errors. These assumptions induce some structure in the means and the variance-covariance parameters of the bivariate normal distribution that may be seen by examining the expressions for these parameters in (1.7), (1.8), (1.20), and (1.21).

In contrast, the bivariate model in this section does not make any such assumptions on its parameters. As a result, while the model is identifiable, unlike the previous two models, it does not allow inference on any measure of similarity. Of course, one can compare the means and variances of the methods by examining the mean difference $\mu_2 - \mu_1$ and variance ratio σ_2^2/σ_1^2. In fact, when the mean difference is close to zero and the variance ratio is close to one, we can validly conclude that the methods have similar characteristics. But we saw in Section 1.6.2 that the effects of difference in fixed biases and scale differences get confounded in $\mu_2 - \mu_1$, and the effects of scale differences and unequal precisions get confounded in σ_2^2/σ_1^2. Therefore, when the mean difference and the variance ratio are quite far from their respective ideal values of zero and one, we cannot be sure what the cause is in terms of the parameters of our interest. For example, it may be a difference in bias, scale, precision, or a combination thereof. Moreover, the variances σ_1^2 and σ_2^2 may be dominated by the between-subject variation. In such a case, the effect of unequal precisions may be missed by the variance ratio.

The bivariate normal model has five parameters—μ_1, μ_2, σ_1^2, σ_2^2, and ρ. Their ML estimators are simply their sample counterparts given in (1.16) with $n-1$ in the denominator replaced by n. The same is true for the ML estimators of ξ and τ^2, which are functions of the model parameters.

Which of the three models should be used? This is mostly a rhetorical question if paired measurements data are all we have. One would like to fit the measurement error model (1.18) as it offers the most flexibility, but this model is not identifiable without additional assumptions. The next best option is to fit the mixed-effects model (1.19), but often the error variances cannot be estimated in a reliable manner. This often makes the bivariate normal model the only viable option. This model makes the fewest assumptions but is also the least informative among the three models for our purposes.

1.12.4   Limitations of the Paired Measurements Design

The paired measurements design is wholly inadequate for method comparison studies because the resulting data do not have sufficient information to allow estimation of all model parameters of interest. In particular, the measurement error model (1.18) is not identifiable on the basis of paired measurements alone, unless one is willing to make a potentially restrictive assumption (e.g., identical measurement scales or known precision ratio). Thus, the assumption that needs to be made a priori is unfortunately one of the issues that must be investigated in a method comparison study. To make matters worse, even if the model (1.19) with common measurement scale is assumed, we have seen in Section 1.12.2 that the data may not have enough information to reliably estimate such key parameters as the precisions of the methods. These serious difficulties show that the data need to be collected using designs that are more informative than the paired measurements design. A particularly attractive option is to use a repeated measurements design, where the measurements are replicated from each method on every subject. Modeling and analysis of such repeated measurements data are discussed in Chapter 5.

1.13   THE BLAND-ALTMAN PLOT

Consider the paired measurements data (Y_{i1}, Y_{i2}), $i = 1, \ldots, n$. Their differences are $D_i = Y_{i2} - Y_{i1}$ and let their averages be $A_i = (Y_{i1} + Y_{i2})/2$. The Bland-Altman plot is a plot of the difference D_i on the vertical axis against the average A_i on the horizontal axis. Although the *limits of agreement* are superimposed on this plot, we defer their discussion to the next chapter. The average A_i serves as a proxy for the true unobservable measurement b_i. This plot is an invaluable supplement to the usual scatterplot of the paired measurements. There is much empty space in a typical scatterplot as the points tend to tightly cluster around a line, making it hard to see any patterns that may be present. But the plot of difference against average magnifies key features of disagreement such as fixed and proportional biases, and also helps in diagnosing common departures from assumptions regarding data such as the presence of outliers and heteroscedasticity.

As an illustration, Figure 1.2 shows scatterplots and Bland-Altman plots for two simulated datasets, each with $n = 100$. The first dataset is simulated from the measurement error model (1.18) with the following parameter values:

$$(\beta_0, \beta_1) = (0, 1.15), (\mu_b, \sigma_b) = (100, 16), (\sigma_{e1}, \sigma_{e2}) = (4, 4).$$

In this case, the methods have a 15% difference in proportional biases. Although the scatterplot of these data in panel (a) shows a systematic difference in the methods, it may be hard to see that the difference is in proportional biases and not in fixed biases. However, as explained in Section 1.13.2 below, the linear trend in the Bland-Altman plot in panel (b) does suggest that the difference may be in proportional biases.

The second dataset is simulated from the mixed-effects model (1.19) with the following parameter values:

$$\beta_0 = 0, (\mu_b, \sigma_b) = (100, 16), (\sigma_{e1}, \sigma_{e2}) = (4, 12).$$

In this case, the precision ratio λ, given by (1.11), is $1/9$, meaning that method 1 is nine times more precise than method 2. But this difference is difficult to discern in the scatterplot in panel (c), whereas the upward linear trend in the Bland-Altman plot in panel (d) indicates this possibility, see Section 1.13.2.

1.13.1   The Ideal Plot

The ideal Bland-Altman plot results in the case when the mixed-effects model (1.19) holds and the two methods have equal fixed biases and error variances. To see how this plot should look, note that if the model (1.19) holds, then from (1.23), the distribution of differences does not depend on the true values. Next, if the fixed biases are equal, then from (1.24), the differences have mean zero. Further, if the error variances are equal, then from Exercise 1.7, the differences are uncorrelated with the averages. It, therefore, follows that the points in the ideal Bland-Altman plot are scattered around zero in a random manner. Such a plot

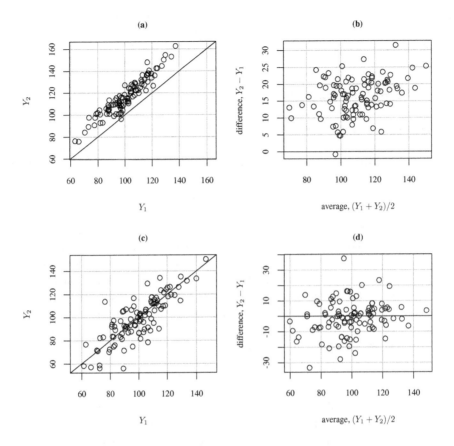

Figure 1.2   Scatterplots (panels (a) and (c)) and Bland-Altman plots (panels (b) and (d)) for two simulated datasets. The line of equality and the zero line are, respectively, superimposed on the two plots.

resembles the ideal plot of residuals versus fitted values in a regression analysis. If the points in the plot are not centered at zero, this suggests a difference in the fixed biases of the methods. Moreover, any pattern in this plot, such as a trend, nonconstant spread, or presence of outliers may suggest a potential failure of the model (1.19).

For a real example of the ideal situation, consider the oxygen saturation data. In this dataset, percent saturation of hemoglobin with oxygen is measured in 72 adult patients receiving general anesthesia or intensive care with two instruments. One is an oxygen saturation monitor (OSM) that uses arterial blood to take measurements, and the other is a pulse oximetry screener (POS) that is noninvasive and easy to use. Figure 1.3 displays these data. The Bland-Altman plot represents an ideal situation as the points are centered at zero and do not exhibit any pattern. Thus, we may conclude that the methods have similar fixed and proportional biases, and equal variances. The latter implies equal error variances for the methods unless they are dominated by the between-subject variation (see the next section). The scatterplot too does not show any evidence of unequal biases. Hence there is indication that the model (1.19) holds well. We return to these data in Chapter 4.

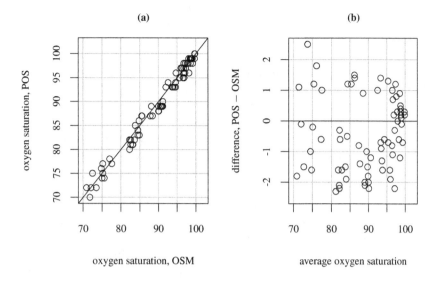

Figure 1.3 Plots for oxygen saturation data. Panel (a): Scatterplot with line of equality. Panel (b): Bland-Altman plot with zero line.

1.13.2   A Linear Trend in the Bland-Altman Plot

A departure from the assumptions behind the ideal Bland-Altman plot results in patterns in the plot. Two frequently seen patterns are a linear trend and heteroscedasticity. A linear trend indicates a correlation between differences and averages. A formal test for this trend is discussed later in Section 1.15.3. Since the averages serve as a proxy for the true measurements, this trend may suggest a relation between differences and true values. But from (1.23), such a relation is a violation of the equal proportional biases (or scales) assumption of the mixed-effects model (1.19). Nevertheless, it may also be that this model holds well for the data and the trend simply indicates a difference in precisions of the methods. These phenomena can be seen in Figure 1.2 where both Bland-Altman plots exhibit a trend. But the cause of the trend in panel (b) is unequal proportional biases, whereas it is unequal precisions in panel (d).

To understand the causes behind the trend, consider the measurement error model (1.18). Under this model, we have (Exercise 1.7)

$$\operatorname{cov}(D, A) = \frac{\sigma_{e1}^2}{2} \left\{ (\beta_1^2 - 1) \frac{\sigma_b^2}{\sigma_{e1}^2} + \frac{\sigma_{e2}^2}{\sigma_{e1}^2} - 1 \right\}.$$

This covariance is nonzero when the Bland-Altman plot exhibits a linear trend. It is zero when $\beta_1 = 1$ and $\sigma_{e1}^2 = \sigma_{e2}^2$, and when the covariance is nonzero, at least one of these two conditions fails to hold. Thus, in explaining a linear trend, the effect of unequal proportional biases (i.e., $\beta_1 \neq 1$) gets confounded with the effect of unequal precisions (i.e., $\sigma_{e1}^2 \neq \sigma_{e2}^2$). Hence, on the basis of the plot alone, we cannot be sure whether the presence of a trend is due to unequal proportional biases, meaning that the mixed-effects model does not hold; or whether this model holds but the methods have unequal precisions. That said, if a trend is seen, it is most likely due to unequal proportional biases because the between-subject variance σ_b^2 dominates the error variances. Therefore, we generally take the lack of a trend to imply equal proportional biases. It is also a good idea to use this plot together with the scatterplot of data, which may confirm the presence of a systematic difference between the methods (see, e.g., Figure 1.2, panel (a)).

One way to deal with the linear trend in the Bland-Altman plot is to remove it by a suitable transformation of measurements. The (natural) log transformation is often successful for this purpose. This transformation has the additional advantage that differences of log-scale measurements can be interpreted as logs of ratios of original measurements. No other transformation is generally suggested because the differences on transformed scale are difficult to interpret in terms of original measurements. If the log transformation fails or a curvilinear trend is seen in the plot, explicit modeling of the trend using a regression model may be called for.

As an illustrative example, consider the plasma volume data displayed in Figure 1.4. These data consist of measurements of plasma volume expressed as a percentage of normal in 99 subjects, using two sets of normal values—one due to Nadler and the other due to Hurley. The Bland-Altman plot in panel (b) clearly shows a linear trend, and the point cloud in the scatterplot in panel (a) is not parallel to the line of equality, confirming that the methods have unequal proportional biases. It is also clear from the plot in panel (c) that the log transformation is successful in removing the trend. But this plot is not centered at zero, meaning that after the transformation, there is a difference in the fixed biases of the methods. The scatterplot in panel (c) essentially confirms this observation. The impact of log transformation is highly visible in the Bland-Altman plots whereas it is less noticeable in the scatterplots. We return to these data in Chapter 4.

1.13.3   Heteroscedasticity in the Bland-Altman Plot

Heteroscedasticity refers to a change in the vertical scatter of the plot as the average increases. It indicates that the variability of the difference changes with the magnitude of measurement. This pattern is generally caused by dependence of the error variation of one or both methods on the magnitude of measurement. One of the most common patterns of heteroscedasticity is a fan shape, which typically occurs when the error variation increases in a constant proportion to the magnitude of measurement. Often, a log transformation of data removes this kind of heteroscedasticity. Potentially other transformations may stabilize the variance as well. But they are generally not used because of the difficulty in interpreting the transformed scale differences. If the log transformation does not succeed or the plot exhibits a complex pattern of heteroscedasticity, modeling of the variation may be necessary (see Chapter 6).

Figure 1.5 shows scatterplots and Bland-Altman plots of vitamin D data. This dataset consists of vitamin D concentrations (ng/mL) in 34 samples measured using two assays. There are two noteworthy features of these data. First, the Bland-Altman plot in panel (b) shows a fan-shaped heteroscedasticity, which is impossible to see in the scatterplot in panel (a). Further, as panel (d) shows, the log transformation of the data successfully removes this heteroscedasticity. Second, there are three outliers in the data, with values that are much larger than the rest. But these outliers play a special role as they allow the comparison of assays over the range of 0–250, whereas without them, the assays may only be compared over the range of 0–50. Notice also an additional outlier in the top left corner of panel (d), which is difficult to see in other plots. This outlier may be the result of an

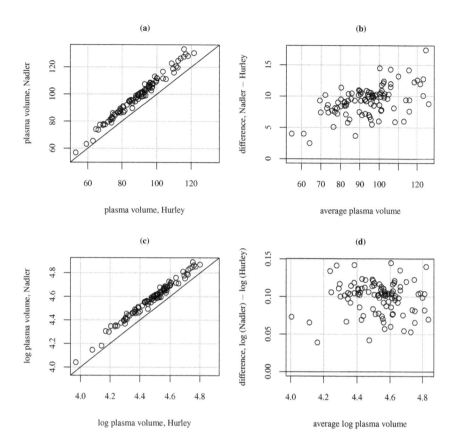

Figure 1.4 Scatterplots and Bland-Altman plots for plasma volume data. Panels (a) and (b) show measurements on original scale (%); panels (c) and (d) show log-scale measurements. The line of equality and the zero line are, respectively, superimposed on the two plots.

error in conducting the experiment or in recording of data, or it may be a bona fide value. Regardless of its origin, this outlier is likely to exert considerable influence on results due its location in the point cloud. Hence it is necessary to assess its impact on overall conclusions by doing the analysis with and without it. We consider this in Chapter 4.

1.13.4 Variations of the Bland-Altman Plot

Three variations of the Bland-Altman plot are often considered in practice. The first one is suggested when one method in the comparison is a reference or gold standard. In this case, the measurements Y_{i1} from the reference method are plotted on the horizontal axis because the Y_{i1} are thought to be a better proxy for the true measurements than the average measurements. Assuming the measurement error model (1.18) for the data, it can be seen that

$$\text{cov}(D, Y_1) = (\beta_1 - 1)\sigma_b^2 - \sigma_{e1}^2.$$

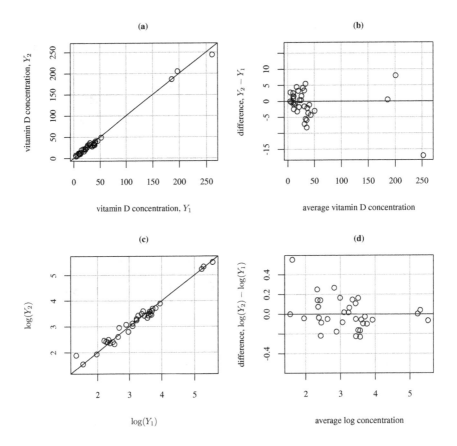

Figure 1.5 Scatterplots and Bland-Altman plots for vitamin D data. Panels (a) and (b) show measurements on original scale (ng/mL); panels (c) and (d) show log-scale measurements. The line of equality and the zero line are, respectively, superimposed on the two plots.

This covariance is zero if and only if $\beta_1 = 1 + (\sigma_{e1}^2/\sigma_b^2)$. When $\beta_1 \neq 1$, it is highly unlikely that β_1 precisely equals $1 + (\sigma_{e1}^2/\sigma_b^2)$. On the other hand, when $\beta_1 = 1$, this covariance is negative unless the reference method is error-free, in which case the covariance is zero. Combining the two cases, it is clear that the plot of differences against the reference measurements generally exhibits a trend, regardless of whether methods have equal proportional biases or not, unless, of course, the reference method is error-free. But since an error-free method is not available in method comparison studies, this plot is of limited use in detecting a difference in proportional biases of two methods. Nevertheless, it remains useful for diagnosing heteroscedasticity and detecting presence of outliers.

In the second variation, the Y_{i2}/Y_{i1} ratio is plotted on the vertical axis. In yet another variation, the difference between two methods expressed as a percentage of their average, that is, $100(D_i/A_i)\%$, is plotted on the vertical axis. Just like the Bland-Altman plot, these are often better than the usual scatterplot at revealing key features of interest in a method comparison study. These alternatives are typically considered when the Bland-Altman plot shows either a trend or a nonconstant scatter.

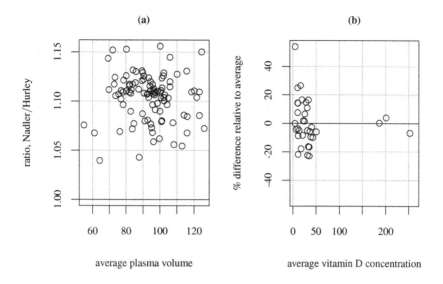

Figure 1.6 Variations of the usual Bland-Altman plot. Panel (a): Plot of ratio versus average for plasma volume data. Panel (b): Plot of relative difference versus average for vitamin D data. The horizontal lines in the plots, respectively, mark the points 1 and 0.

Sometimes when the differences are proportional to the true values, it may be that the ratios are free of the true values. So if the Bland-Altman plot has a trend, the ratio plot may not have it. This can be seen for plasma volume data in Figures 1.4 (panel (b)) and 1.6 (panel (a)). The ratio plot can also be used to get a rough estimate of β_1 when $\beta_0 = 0$, that is, the data in the usual scatterplot of Y_{i2} versus Y_{i1} are clustered around a line that has zero intercept. Further, if the Bland-Altman plot shows a fan-shaped pattern of heteroscedasticity implying that the variation in differences may be proportional to true values, the percent difference plot may show a constant scatter. This can be seen for vitamin D data by comparing panel (b) of Figures 1.5 and 1.6.

1.14 COMMON REGRESSION APPROACHES

1.14.1 Ordinary Linear Regression

The ordinary linear regression of a new method (Y_2) on a reference method (Y_1) is often suggested to study the relation between the two methods. Since Y_2 is regressed on Y_1, we say Y_2 is a *response variable* and Y_1 is an *explanatory variable* or a *covariate*. The ordinary linear regression presumes that the explanatory variable is error-free and only the response variable is measured with error. It posits that the paired measurements (Y_{i1}, Y_{i2}) follow the model

$$Y_{i2} = \tilde{\beta}_0 + \tilde{\beta}_1 Y_{i1} + e_{i2}, \ i = 1, \ldots, n, \tag{1.25}$$

where the intercept $\tilde{\beta}_0$ and slope $\tilde{\beta}_1$ are fixed unknown coefficients; and e_{i2} is the random error of the new method. These errors are i.i.d. with mean zero and variance σ_{e2}^2, and are independent of reference method measurements. This model has the same form as the measurement error model (1.18) except for the important assumption that $e_{i1} = 0$, that is, there is no random error in the reference method. In other words, the observed Y_1 is also the true measurement of the reference method. It may be noted that Y_1 is still being treated as a random quantity rather than a fixed quantity, but Y_1 inherits its variability solely from the variability in the true values. This contrasts with Y_2, which has two sources of variability—the variability in the true value and the variability in the errors.

The model (1.25) can also be written as

$$Y_{i2} = E(Y_{i2}|Y_{i1}) + e_{i2}, \text{ where } E(Y_{i2}|Y_{i1}) = \tilde{\beta}_0 + \tilde{\beta}_1 Y_{i1}.$$

This form makes it clear that the conditional mean of Y_2 given Y_1 is being modeled as a linear function of Y_1. The function that describes the relation between $E(Y_2|Y_1)$ and Y_1 is called the *true regression function* of Y_2 on Y_1. In ordinary linear regression, this function is linear and hence is referred to as the *true regression line*.

The regression coefficients $\tilde{\beta}_0$ and $\tilde{\beta}_1$ are commonly estimated using the *method of least squares*. The least squares estimators are those values of $\tilde{\beta}_0$ and $\tilde{\beta}_1$ that minimize the sum of squares of errors in the response variable, which from (1.25) is

$$\sum_{i=1}^{n} e_{i2}^2 = \sum_{i=1}^{n} (Y_{i2} - \tilde{\beta}_0 - \tilde{\beta}_1 Y_{i1})^2.$$

If the paired data are plotted in a scatterplot with response variable on the vertical axis and explanatory variable on the horizontal axis, the error e_{i2} represents the *vertical* distance of the point (Y_{i1}, Y_{i2}) from the true regression line. Therefore, the error sum of squares can be interpreted as the sum of squares of vertical distances between the observed data points and the regression line. Minimization of this sum of squares leads to the following least squares estimators (Exercise 1.11):

$$\hat{\tilde{\beta}}_1 = R \cdot S_2/S_1, \ \hat{\tilde{\beta}}_0 = \overline{Y}_{\cdot 2} - \hat{\tilde{\beta}}_1 \overline{Y}_{\cdot 1}, \tag{1.26}$$

where $R, \overline{Y}_{\cdot j}$, and S_j are given in (1.16). The estimators in (1.26) are unbiased for their population counterparts. The line $\hat{Y}_2 = \hat{\tilde{\beta}}_0 + \hat{\tilde{\beta}}_1 Y_1$ is called the *fitted* regression line of Y_2 on Y_1. Here $\hat{Y}_2$, known as the *predicted value* or the *fitted value* of Y_2, represents an unbiased estimator of the conditional mean $E(Y_2|Y_1)$.

The assumptions underlying the ordinary regression model (1.25) need to be expanded in order to perform inference on the model parameters. It is common to assume that the data follow the bivariate normal model described in Section 1.12.3. The bivariate normality of (Y_1, Y_2) implies that the conditional distribution of $Y_2|Y_1$ is normal with mean

$$E(Y_2|Y_1) = \mu_2 + (\rho\sigma_2/\sigma_1)(Y_1 - \mu_1)$$
$$= \{\mu_2 - (\rho\sigma_2/\sigma_1)\mu_1\} + (\rho\sigma_2/\sigma_1)Y_1,$$

which is a linear function of Y_1. Thus, the linearity of the true regression function is not an additional assumption as it follows from the assumed bivariate normality. We can write this regression line in the form $E(Y_2|Y_1) = \tilde{\beta}_0 + \tilde{\beta}_1 Y_1$ by taking

$$\tilde{\beta}_0 = \mu_2 - (\rho\sigma_2/\sigma_1)\mu_1, \ \tilde{\beta}_1 = \rho\sigma_2/\sigma_1. \tag{1.27}$$

Under the bivariate normal model, the least squares estimators of $\tilde{\beta}_0$ and $\tilde{\beta}_1$ in (1.26) are also their ML estimators (Exercise 1.11).

The assumption of an error-free reference method in (1.25) is quite important. If it is violated, the least squares estimators in (1.26) do not estimate the intercept and slope of the true line around which the data are scattered. To see this, assume that the reference method also measures with error and the data follow the measurement error model (1.18). This model assumes that the data are scattered around a line with intercept β_0 and slope β_1. However, under this model, the regression line of Y_2 on Y_1 has coefficients $\tilde{\beta}_0$ and $\tilde{\beta}_1$ that can be obtained by substituting the expressions of moments from (1.7) and (1.8) in (1.27). This substitution yields

$$\tilde{\beta}_0 = \beta_0 + \left(\frac{\sigma_{e1}^2}{\sigma_b^2 + \sigma_{e1}^2} \right) \beta_1 \mu_b, \ \tilde{\beta}_1 = \left(\frac{\sigma_b^2}{\sigma_b^2 + \sigma_{e1}^2} \right) \beta_1. \tag{1.28}$$

Obviously, the coefficients $(\tilde{\beta}_0, \tilde{\beta}_1)$ of the regression line differ from the coefficients (β_0, β_1) of the true line unless $\sigma_{e1}^2 = 0$, implying an error-free reference method. In particular, $|\tilde{\beta}_1|$ shrinks $|\beta_1|$ by the factor $\sigma_b^2/(\sigma_b^2 + \sigma_{e1}^2)$, which represents the reliability (Section 1.6.2) of the reference method. This shrinkage phenomenon where the slope of the regression line is less than the true slope, in absolute value terms, is called the *attenuation of slope* caused by the error in the explanatory variable. The higher the reliability of the explanatory variable, the less severe is the attenuation. It also causes $\tilde{\beta}_0$ to differ from β_0 by the amount $\tilde{\beta}_1 \mu_b$.

In summary, if the reference method is error-prone, the true regression line is not the line around which the data are scattered. In particular, if β_1 and μ_b are both positive, the regression line tilts towards the horizontal axis resulting in reduced slope and increased intercept when compared to the true line. The difference between the two lines decreases as the reliability of the reference method increases, and the lines become identical when the reference is error-free. Note that there is nothing wrong per se with the least squares estimators (1.26), which correctly estimate the regression coefficients given by (1.28). It is just that these coefficients themselves do not represent the intercept and slope of the true line.

Figure 1.7 shows an example of difference between the two lines. It displays a scatterplot of $n = 100$ pairs of observations simulated from the model (1.18) with the following parameter values:

$$(\beta_0, \beta_1) = (0, 1), (\mu_b, \sigma_b) = (100, 16), (\sigma_{e1}, \sigma_{e2}) = (8, 8).$$

The data here are truly scattered around the line of equality. But, from (1.28), the true regression line of Y_2 on Y_1 has increased intercept $\tilde{\beta}_0 = 22$ and decreased slope $\tilde{\beta}_1 = 0.8$. The least squares estimates of these coefficients, 22.9 and 0.77, are close to their respective true values.

1.14.2 Deming Regression

Deming regression is a popular approach for fitting a line through the paired measurements $(Y_{i1}, Y_{i2}), i = 1, \ldots, n$, when both the response variable Y_2 and the explanatory variable Y_1 are measured with error. This contrasts with ordinary regression where only the response variable is measured with error and the explanatory variable is error-free. In Deming regression, we assume that the data follow the measurement error model (1.18) and the ratio of error variances, $\lambda = \sigma_{e1}^2/\sigma_{e2}^2$, is known. The line $\hat{Y}_2 = \hat{\beta}_0 + \hat{\beta}_1 Y_1$ is called the

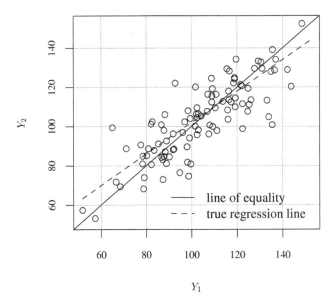

Figure 1.7 A scatterplot of simulated data superimposed with the line of equality, around which the data are truly scattered, and the true regression line of Y_2 on Y_1.

Deming regression line and also the *orthogonal regression line*. Here $(\hat{\beta}_0, \hat{\beta}_1)$ is an estimate of (β_0, β_1) in the model (1.18) and $\hat{Y}_2$ is the value of Y_2 predicted by the line when the other variable is Y_1. Despite being called a regression line, this line does not estimate the true regression of Y_2 on Y_1, that is, $E(Y_2|Y_1) = \tilde{\beta}_0 + \tilde{\beta}_1 Y_1$, with coefficients given by (1.27).

The coefficients in Deming regression are estimated using the method of *orthogonal least squares*. Assume for now that $\lambda = 1$ so that the two variables are measured with equal precision. It is then natural to estimate the coefficients by minimizing the sum of squares of perpendicular (or orthogonal) distances of the points (Y_{i1}, Y_{i2}) from the line $Y_2 = \beta_0 + \beta_1 Y_1$. This is the method of orthogonal least squares. It is a generalization of the least squares method used in ordinary regression wherein the sum of squares of vertical distances is minimized because only the response variable, plotted on the vertical axis, is measured with error. Figure 1.8 displays the vertical and perpendicular distances from a point to a line. The latter is also the shortest distance between a point and a line.

The perpendicular from (Y_{i1}, Y_{i2}) intersects the line $Y_2 = \beta_0 + \beta_1 Y_1$ at the point $(\tilde{Y}_{i1}, \tilde{Y}_{i2})$, where

$$\tilde{Y}_{i1} = (\beta_1 Y_{i2} + Y_{i1} - \beta_0 \beta_1)/(1 + \beta_1^2), \quad \tilde{Y}_{i2} = \beta_0 + \beta_1 \tilde{Y}_{i1}.$$

The perpendicular distance between the point (Y_{i1}, Y_{i2}) and the line $Y_2 = \beta_0 + \beta_1 Y_1$ equals the Euclidean distance between the points (Y_{i1}, Y_{i2}) and $(\tilde{Y}_{i1}, \tilde{Y}_{i2})$—see Figure 1.8. The square of this distance is

$$(Y_{i1} - \tilde{Y}_{i1})^2 + (Y_{i2} - \tilde{Y}_{i2})^2,$$

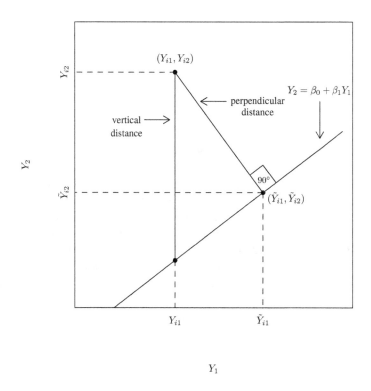

Figure 1.8   Vertical and perpendicular distances of a data point from a line. The former is used in ordinary least squares whereas the latter is used in orthogonal least squares.

which simplifies to

$$(Y_{i2} - \beta_0 - \beta_1 Y_{i1})^2 / (1 + \beta_1^2).$$

The orthogonal least squares estimators of coefficients in the Deming regression line are obtained by minimizing the sum of these squared perpendicular distances,

$$\sum_{i=1}^{n} (Y_{i2} - \beta_0 - \beta_1 Y_{i1})^2 / (1 + \beta_1^2), \tag{1.29}$$

with respect to (β_0, β_1). This sum is a weighted sum where the weight given to each data point is $1/(1 + \beta_1^2)$. Without the weights, this sum is simply the sum of squares of vertical distances, which is minimized in ordinary least squares.

Consider now the general case when λ may be any known value, not necessarily one. In this case, it is not appropriate to minimize the sum of squares of perpendicular distances because the two variables are not measured with equal precision. Therefore, orthogonal least squares is applied after rescaling one of the variables, say Y_1, by dividing it with $\sqrt{\lambda}$ to make the two error variances equal. This method leads to the following estimates of coefficients in the Deming regression line (Exercise 1.12):

$$\hat{\beta}_0 = \overline{Y}_{.2} - \hat{\beta}_1 \overline{Y}_{.1}, \quad \hat{\beta}_1 = W + \sqrt{W^2 + (1/\lambda)}, \tag{1.30}$$

where

$$W = \frac{\sum_{i=1}^n (Y_{i2} - \overline{Y}_{.2})^2 - (1/\lambda) \sum_{i=1}^n (Y_{i1} - \overline{Y}_{.1})^2}{2 \sum_{i=1}^n (Y_{i1} - \overline{Y}_{.1})(Y_{i2} - \overline{Y}_{.2})} = \frac{S_2^2 - (1/\lambda) S_1^2}{2 R S_1 S_2}.$$

These estimators are also the ML estimators of (β_0, β_1) in model (1.18) with known λ.

It follows that Deming regression is equivalent to orthogonal regression only when $\lambda = 1$. If $\lambda \neq 1$, Deming regression minimizes the sum of squared distances at an angle other than $90°$.

There is just one Deming regression line irrespective of whether Y_1 or Y_2 is used as the explanatory variable (Exercise 1.13). In other words, if $\hat{Y}_2 = \hat{\beta}_0 + \hat{\beta}_1 Y_1$ is the Deming regression line for predicting Y_2 from Y_1, then the same line, written as $\hat{Y}_1 = -(\hat{\beta}_0/\hat{\beta}_1) + (1/\hat{\beta}_1)Y_2$, is the Deming regression line for predicting Y_1 from Y_2. This is intuitive as the perpendicular distance of a point from a line does not depend on the choice of explanatory and response variables. This contrasts with ordinary least squares where there are two different lines—one for the regression of Y_2 on Y_1, obtained by minimizing the sum of squares of vertical distances, and the other for the regression of Y_1 on Y_2, obtained by minimizing the sum of squares of horizontal distances. These two least squares lines are special cases of the Deming regression line, respectively, when one takes $\lambda \to 0$, or Y_1 is error-free, and when $\lambda \to \infty$, or Y_2 is error-free (Exercise 1.14). It can also be seen that the Deming regression line falls between the two least squares lines. However, all three lines pass through the point $(\overline{Y}_{.1}, \overline{Y}_{.2})$. This phenomenon is illustrated in Figure 1.9 using the data displayed in Figure 1.7.

1.15   INAPPROPRIATE USE OF COMMON TESTS IN METHOD COMPARISON STUDIES

We now describe some commonly used hypothesis tests that have limited value in method comparison studies. There is nothing wrong with these tests, but the resulting conclusions are not in line with the stated goals of the method comparison studies. All the tests discussed here are based on the paired measurements data and bivariate normality (Section 1.12.3) is assumed for them. Some tests additionally assume a measurement error model (Section 1.12.1) or a mixed-effects model (Section 1.12.2). We will also suggest appropriate modifications to these tests in order to address issues of direct concern in method comparison studies.

1.15.1   Test of Zero Correlation

To perform a test of significance for correlation ρ between Y_1 and Y_2 in a bivariate normal setup, one formulates the null and alternative hypotheses as

$$H_0 : \rho = 0 \text{ and } H_1 : \rho \neq 0,$$

and computes the test statistic

$$T = \sqrt{n-2} \, R / \sqrt{1 - R^2},$$

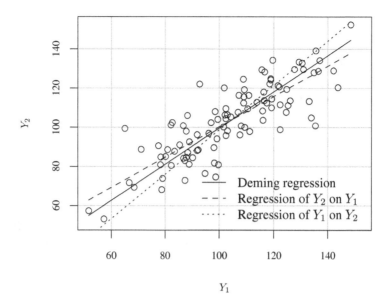

Figure 1.9   Deming regression line and the two ordinary least squares regression lines for the data displayed in Figure 1.7.

where R is the sample correlation defined in (1.16). This statistic follows a t distribution with $n - 2$ degrees of freedom when the null hypothesis is true. The test rejects the null hypothesis at level α if $|T| > t_{n-2,1-\alpha/2}$.

Sometimes in practice a significant result of this test is taken as evidence of "agreement" between two methods. This, however, is clearly inadequate since correlation is a measure of linear relationship and not of agreement. Besides, two methods designed to measure the same quantity will rarely be uncorrelated. To determine the strength of correlation, a better alternative is to use a lower confidence bound for ρ. This bound indicates the worst case (i.e., the smallest) value of ρ that is plausible with the data. An approximate $100(1 - \alpha)\%$ lower bound for ρ is

$$\tanh\left(\tanh^{-1}(R) - z_{1-\alpha}/\sqrt{n-3}\right). \tag{1.31}$$

This formula works well when n is large. To understand how it is derived, consider the *Fisher's z-transformation* of R, defined as

$$z(R) = \frac{1}{2}\log\left(\frac{1+R}{1-R}\right), \tag{1.32}$$

which represents $\tanh^{-1}(R)$. When n is large, $z(R)$ approximately follows a normal distribution with mean $z(\rho)$ and variance $1/(n-3)$. From this result, an approximate $100(1 - \alpha)\%$ lower confidence bound for $z(\rho)$ is

$$z(R) - z_{1-\alpha}/\sqrt{n-3}.$$

The formula (1.31) now follows by transforming back this bound to the original scale by applying the inverse of the Fisher's z-transformation.

1.15.2 Paired t-test

The paired t-test is a test of equality of means of the paired measurements (Y_1, Y_2). It is essentially the usual one-sample t-test of zero mean applied to the differences D_i in the paired measurements. One sets up the null and alternative hypotheses as

$$H_0 : \xi = 0 \text{ and } H_1 : \xi \neq 0,$$

and computes $T = \sqrt{n}\overline{D}/S_D$, where $\overline{D}$ and S_D are defined in (1.17). The test statistic T follows a t distribution with $n - 1$ degrees of freedom under H_0. The level α paired t-test rejects the null hypothesis if $|T| > t_{n-1,1-\alpha/2}$.

If in addition to bivariate normality, the data also follow the mixed-effects model (1.19), then from (1.24), ξ equals β_0—the difference in fixed biases of the methods. Therefore, a test of $\xi = 0$ is also a test of $\beta_0 = 0$. This correspondence, however, fails to hold if the methods have unequal proportional biases. To see this, suppose now that the data follow the measurement error model (1.18). Then from (1.10), $\xi = \beta_0 + (\beta_1 - 1)\mu_b$. As a result, testing for $\xi = 0$ does not amount to testing for $\beta_0 = 0$.

Being a test of equality of means, the paired t-test has limited value in method comparison studies (Section 1.11.4). If the null hypothesis of no difference in means is accepted, it may not be because $\overline{D}$ is small (implying that its mean ξ may be small), but because S_D^2/n is large (implying that ξ is not estimated precisely either due to large variability in the differences or due to a small sample size). In other words, the test may simply have a low power. To examine the mean difference in paired measurements, a better alternative is to use a $100(1 - \alpha)\%$ confidence interval for ξ, given as

$$\overline{D} \pm t_{n-1,1-\alpha/2}S_D/\sqrt{n},$$

where S_D is the sample standard deviation of the paired differences. The interval gives the plausible values of ξ that are supported by the data.

1.15.3 Pitman-Morgan and Bradley-Blackwood Tests

The Pitman-Morgan test is a test for equality of variances of the paired measurements (Y_1, Y_2). It exploits a useful fact about the covariance between difference D and average A of the paired measurements. Since

$$\text{cov}(D, A) = \text{cov}(Y_2 - Y_1, (Y_1 + Y_2)/2) = (\sigma_2^2 - \sigma_1^2)/2,$$

the null hypothesis of equality of variances is equivalent to assuming zero correlation between D and A. Thus, to test

$$H_0 : \sigma_1^2 = \sigma_2^2 \text{ versus } H_1 : \sigma_1^2 \neq \sigma_2^2,$$

it actually tests the following hypotheses:

$$H_0 : \text{cor}(D, A) = 0 \text{ versus } H_1 : \text{cor}(D, A) \neq 0.$$

Since (Y_1, Y_2) and hence (D, A) follow a bivariate normal distribution, this null hypothesis can be tested by applying the test of zero correlation in Section 1.15.1 to (D, A) instead of (Y_1, Y_2). Thus, the test statistic is

$$T = \sqrt{n - 2}\, R_1 / \sqrt{1 - R_1^2},$$

where R_1 is the sample correlation of the observed (D, A) values. The level α Pitman-Morgan test rejects the null hypothesis of equal variances if $|T| > t_{n-2, 1-\alpha/2}$.

If in addition to bivariate normality, the paired measurements also follow the mixed-effects model (1.19), then it can be seen that

$$\text{cov}(D, A) = (\sigma_{e2}^2 - \sigma_{e1}^2)/2.$$

This way the Pitman-Morgan test provides a test of equality of precisions of the methods. This test is also known as the Maloney-Rastogi test.

The Bradley-Blackwood test is a generalization of the Pitman-Morgan test as it simultaneously tests for equality of means and equality of variances of the paired measurements (Y_1, Y_2). Since (D, A) is bivariate normal, the conditional distribution of D given A is normal with mean

$$E(D|A) = E(D) + \{\text{cov}(D, A)/\text{var}(A)\}\{A - E(A)\} = \tilde{\beta}_0 + \tilde{\beta}_1 A,$$

where

$$\tilde{\beta}_0 = E(D) - \{\text{cov}(D, A)/\text{var}(A)\}E(A), \quad \tilde{\beta}_1 = \text{cov}(D, A)/\text{var}(A).$$

These $\tilde{\beta}_0$ and $\tilde{\beta}_1$ represent the intercept and slope of the linear regression of D on A. Moreover, since $E(D) = \mu_2 - \mu_1$ and $\text{cov}(D, A) = (\sigma_2^2 - \sigma_1^2)/2$, the hypothesis $\{\mu_1 = \mu_2, \sigma_1^2 = \sigma_2^2\}$ is equivalent to $\{\tilde{\beta}_0 = \tilde{\beta}_1 = 0\}$. Exploiting this equivalence, the Bradley-Blackwood test simultaneously tests the hypotheses

$$H_0 : \mu_1 = \mu_2 \text{ and } \sigma_1^2 = \sigma_2^2 \text{ versus } H_1 : \mu_1 \neq \mu_2 \text{ or } \sigma_1^2 \neq \sigma_2^2$$

by actually testing the hypotheses

$$H_0 : \tilde{\beta}_0 = 0 \text{ and } \tilde{\beta}_1 = 0 \text{ versus } H_1 : \tilde{\beta}_0 \neq 0 \text{ or } \tilde{\beta}_1 \neq 0$$

using an F-test of zero intercept and zero slope in the regression of D on A. From the standard linear regression analysis, this F-test is based on the statistic

$$F = \frac{(\sum_{i=1}^n D_i^2 - \text{RSS})/2}{\text{RSS}/(n - 2)},$$

where RSS represents the residual sum of squares from the regression of D on A, and can be written as

$$\text{RSS} = (1 - R_1^2) \sum_{i=1}^n (D_i - \overline{D})^2 = (n - 1)(1 - R_1^2) S_D^2.$$

When the null hypothesis is true, the statistic follows an F distribution with numerator and denominator degrees of freedom 2 and $n - 2$, respectively. The level α Bradley-Blackwood test rejects the simultaneous null hypothesis of equality of means and equality of variances when $F > f_{2,n-2,1-\alpha}$.

If the paired measurements actually follow the mixed-effects model (1.19), the Bradley-Blackwood test provides a simultaneous test of equality of fixed biases ($\beta_0 = 0$) and equality of error variances ($\sigma_{e1}^2 = \sigma_{e2}^2$) of the two methods. Thus, it is a test of parallelism (Section 1.6.4) of the methods under the assumption of equal proportional biases for the methods.

Moreover, just like the paired t-test, these tests are also of limited value in method comparison studies because the hypotheses being tested are not the right ones (Section 1.11.4). To determine the extent of difference in variances of the paired measurements, one may use the following $100(1 - \alpha)\%$ confidence interval for σ_2^2/σ_1^2 (Exercise 1.15):

$$\left[\frac{S_2^2}{S_1^2} \frac{\left(t_1\sqrt{1 - R^2} - \sqrt{1 - t_1^2 R^2}\right)^2}{1 - t_1^2}, \frac{S_2^2}{S_1^2} \frac{\left(t_1\sqrt{1 - R^2} + \sqrt{1 - t_1^2 R^2}\right)^2}{1 - t_1^2} \right], \quad (1.33)$$

where $t_1 = t_{n-2,1-\alpha/2}/\sqrt{n - 2 + t_{n-2,1-\alpha/2}^2}$.

In a Bland-Altman plot (Section 1.13), we were interested in checking for a linear trend in D versus A. The null hypothesis of $\text{cor}(D, A) = 0$ is equivalent to equality of variances of Y_1 and Y_2. Further, the simultaneous null hypothesis of $(\tilde{\beta}_0, \tilde{\beta}_1) = (0, 0)$ is equivalent to equality of means of Y_1 and Y_2 in addition to equality of their variances. Although these hypotheses may be tested using Pitman-Morgan and Bradley-Blackwood tests, we do not use them in the book as they test for significance, not for agreement.

1.15.4   Test of Zero Intercept and Unit Slope

The test for zero intercept and unit slope is suggested in two contexts—the ordinary linear regression (Section 1.14.1) and Deming regression (Section 1.14.2) of Y_2 on Y_1. In either case, one generally sets up separate hypotheses for intercept and slope, namely,

$$H_0 : \text{intercept} = 0 \text{ versus } H_1 : \text{intercept} \neq 0,$$
$$H_0 : \text{slope} = 1 \text{ versus } H_1 : \text{slope} \neq 1.$$

These hypotheses are tested individually.

In the case of ordinary regression, zero intercept and unit slope means $E(Y_2|Y_1) = Y_1$. Upon taking expectation on both sides with respect to Y_1, we get $\mu_2 = \mu_1$—the equality of means of the methods. For the Deming regression, zero intercept and unit slope means tau-equivalence (Section 1.6.4) of the methods. In other words, the methods have equal fixed and proportional biases. Thus, in both cases, the sole concern is with differences in biases of the two methods. However, just like the other tests of equality in this section, these tests have rather limited usefulness as the null hypotheses may be accepted due to low power of the tests. Instead of testing for zero intercept and unit slope, a better alternative is to use confidence intervals for these parameters to examine their magnitudes.

Since the equality of means (or even tau-equivalence) of methods is not enough by itself for good agreement between them (Section 1.7.2), the testing for zero intercept and unit slope is often suggested only when the methods have high correlation. But this raises the question of how high the correlation should be before one can proceed to the regression step. Unfortunately, any answer to this question is likely to be arbitrary, especially since the correlation depends heavily on the range of the true values in the population.

The above discussion on the value of testing for zero intercept and unit slope tacitly assumes that the regression is fit appropriately. However, the ordinary regression is not appropriate for method comparison studies because it requires the explanatory variable Y_1 to be error-free, which is generally not the case in practice. Further, the Deming regression requires the precision ratio λ to be known, which too is generally not the case. So λ is often replaced by an estimate based on error variances estimated from replicate measurements. But the use of an estimated λ as a known λ invalidates the use of original expressions for the standard errors of the estimates. Thus, the typical fitting of Deming regression in practice is also inappropriate. Moreover, if replications are available, it is more efficient to model all the data together and jointly estimate all the parameters to carry out inference on parametric functions of interest.

1.16 KEY STEPS IN THE ANALYSIS OF METHOD COMPARISON DATA

The key steps in the analysis of method comparison data are given below. These steps are illustrated throughout the book.

1. *Perform exploratory analysis of data by displaying them graphically.* Make both scatterplot and Bland-Altman plot. Superimpose the equality line in the scatterplot and the zero line in the Bland-Altman plot. Use the two plots in a complementary manner. Look for patterns in the plots. Look especially for evidence of outliers, fixed and proportional biases, and heteroscedasticity.

   Other plots may also be useful such as the *trellis plot*. It is constructed as follows. The subjects are sorted in ascending order according to their average measurement. The vertical axis is divided into rows, one for each sorted subject, and each row displays all measurements for the corresponding subject. Different symbols are used for different methods. The vertical axis is labeled "sorted subject ID," with ID $= 1$ referring to the subject with the smallest average, and so on. A key feature of this plot is that it shows within-subject variation. Figure 1.10 shows a trellis plot of log-scale plasma volume data. The Nadler measurements are higher than Hurley's by an almost a constant amount. The data appear homoscedastic. The plots in Figure 1.4 led to the same conclusions.

2. *Model the data.* Come up with a plausible model for the data. To the extent the model and the information in the data allow, let the model have method-specific parameters. Be sure to check goodness of fit and perform model diagnostics to verify the underlying assumptions.

3. *Evaluate similarity of methods by examining the confidence intervals for relevant measures of similarity.* Use the fitted model to compute these confidence intervals.

4. *Evaluate agreement between the methods by examining confidence bounds for measures of agreement.* Use a variety of agreement measures. Use the fitted model to compute the confidence bounds.

5. *Decide whether the methods agree sufficiently well to be used interchangeably.* Identify causes of disagreement and see whether a simple recalibration of one of the

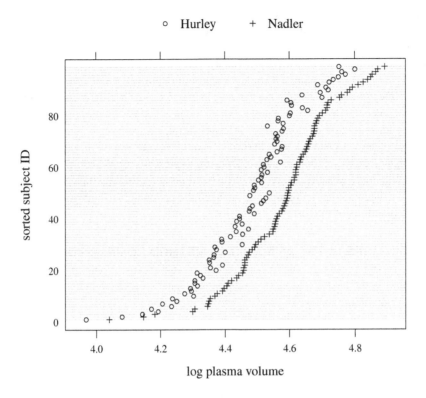

Figure 1.10 Trellis plot of log-scale plasma volume data. The subjects are sorted according to their average measurement.

methods may improve its agreement with the other. Be sure to check whether one method is clearly superior to the other.

1.17 CHAPTER SUMMARY

1. A method comparison study has two complementary goals—evaluation of similarity and evaluation of agreement. The latter is the primary goal.

2. Having similar characteristics is not enough for good agreement between methods.

3. Finding an adequate model for data is a necessary step in the analysis of method comparison data.

4. Agreement between methods is evaluated by performing model-based inference on measures of agreement. Generally, one-sided confidence bounds for agreement measures are more relevant for this purpose than their two-sided counterparts.

5. Characteristics of methods are compared by performing model-based inference on measures of similarity. Generally, two-sided confidence intervals for similarity measures are appropriate for this purpose.

6. The widely used paired measurement design is wholly inadequate for collecting data for method comparison studies. The measurements should be replicated by each method on every subject.

7. Ordinary regression of a new method on a reference method is appropriate only when the reference method measures without error.

8. Deming regression is appropriate only when the ratio of precisions of methods is known.

9. Testing null hypothesis of equality should be avoided in favor of appropriate confidence intervals.

10. In general, testing whether the regression line of one method on the other coincides with the 45° line does not amount to checking for good agreement.

1.18   BIBLIOGRAPHIC NOTE

Models for Measurements

The classical model (1.1) for measurements of a method is studied in detail in Fleiss (1986, Chapter 1) and Dunn (2004, Chapter 1). These authors, together with Barnhart et al. (2007a) and Bartlett and Frost (2008), provide a good discussion of the notions of accuracy, precision, repeatability, and reliability of a method.

Grubbs (1948) is one of the earliest articles devoted to comparison of methods. It essentially assumes the mixed-effects model (1.19) and estimates its parameters using the method of moments. The model (1.19) is also called the *Grubbs model* after this article. In the clinical chemistry literature, Westgard and Hunt (1973) use the measurement error model (1.18) for paired measurements. These authors call attention to pitfalls in interpretation of correlation coefficients and t-tests. But they also advocate the classical least squares regression as "potentially the most useful statistical technique" for analysis of method comparison data, provided a scatterplot of the data does not show nonlinearity and outliers. Cornbleet and Gochman (1979) point out that the classical least squares estimators of slope and intercept are incorrect if the independent variable is measured with error. To fit the model (1.18), they suggest the regression method of Deming (1943)—popularly known as *Deming regression* even though the method is originally due to Kummell (1879). See Finney (1996) for an interesting historical account of regression when both independent and dependent variables are measured with error.

Two assumptions in the model (1.18) are often violated in practice. The first is that the methods have uncorrelated measurement errors. Rifkin (1995) gives examples of clinical diagnostic methods with potentially correlated measurement errors and discusses the effect of this correlation on inference regarding the slope parameter. The second is that the error variances remain constant throughout the measurement range. Nix and Dunstan (1991) assume that the error variances are known, but they are free to vary from subject to subject in an unstructured manner. They propose an ML method to estimate the regression coefficients. The usual Deming regression is a special case of this method when the error variances do not change with subjects. Linnet (1990) lets the error standard deviations be proportional to the average of the true values of the subjects. He proposes an iteratively reweighted modification of Deming regression to estimate the regression coefficients. See Rubin (1983) for an introduction to the iteratively reweighted least squares technique. Martin (2000) describes an approach similar to Linnet (1990) but with different assumptions on error variances.

One may refer to the books by Searle et al. (1992), Vonesh and Chinchilli (1997), Pinheiro and Bates (2000), and Gelman and Hill (2007) for an introduction to mixed-effects models and their applications. These books also describe the ML and REML methods for fitting such models. The book by Cheng and Van Ness (1999) contains a comprehensive treatment of measurement error models. Kutner et al. (2004) provide a good introduction to linear regression models. A rigorous introduction to statistical inference is provided by Casella and Berger (2001). It also provides (in Chapters 11 and 12) a succinct account of the ordinary regression model and the measurement error model. Graybill (2001) is a handy reference on matrix algebra.

Deming Regression and Alternatives

Dunn (2007) notes that Deming regression has limited application in practice because it requires the error variance ratio to be known, which is generally not the case. It is common to deal with this issue by simply replacing the unknown ratio with the ratio of error variances estimated using replications from the present experiment or from previous experiments (see, e.g., Cornbleet and Gochman, 1979; and Linnet, 1993). No account is taken of the sampling variability in the estimated ratio and its consequences. As a result, the standard errors of the estimated parameters are incorrect. Besides, if replications are available from the present experiment, it is more efficient to analyze all the data together rather than using the replications just for estimating the error variances. Dunn and Roberts (1999) prefer modeling all the data together as it allows simultaneous estimation of error variances and regression coefficients. Carroll and Ruppert (1996) also criticize Deming regression for being unable to account for a potential *equation error* in the measurement error model (see also pages 71–77 of Dunn, 2004; Sections 1.8 and 2.2 of Cheng and Van Ness, 1999; and page 120 of this book). The equation error is also known as a random subject-specific bias or a random matrix effect. Edland (1996) discusses the impact of equation error on slope estimates obtained using Deming regression. Dunn (2004, Section 4.10) shows how the equation error can be taken into account when replications are available.

When an estimated error variance ratio is used in Deming regression, authors like Kelly (1985) and Lewis et al. (1991) try to assess the robustness of the estimated slope to misspecification of the variance ratio. A theoretical investigation by Lakshminarayanan and Gunst (1984) shows that the slope estimate is not robust unless the error variance of the independent variable is small relative to the variance of the true values and the error variance of the dependent variable. In practice, this condition typically holds when the correlation between the variables is nearly one. In fact, this is also the case when both least squares regression and Deming regression tend to produce close estimates. Thus, the case when Deming regression differs from least squares regression is also the case when the former is sensitive to the choice of the variance ratio. Simulation studies by Linnet (1998) essentially confirm these observations. Lakshminarayanan and Gunst also note that to realize full benefits of Deming regression over least squares, the selected variance ratio must be relatively close to the true ratio and the sample size should be large. Dunn (2004, page 72) notes that the choice of the variance ratio probably has more impact on the sensitivity ratio, defined in (1.12), than the slope parameter.

A nonparametric rank-based alternative to Deming regression—also known as *Passing-Bablok regression*—and the associated tests of zero intercept and unit slope are provided by Passing and Bablok (1983, 1984) and Bablok et al. (1988). This approach assumes that the square of the slope in the model (1.18) is equal to the ratio of error variances of method 2 over method 1. Linnet (1998) considers this assumption to be potentially more restrictive than the assumption of known error variance ratio needed in Deming regression. A number of articles have compared the estimates from classical least squares, Deming, and Passing-Bablok regressions using simulated as well as real data, see, for example, Linnet, (1993), Stöckl et al. (1998), and the references therein.

Evaluation of Similarity

Statistical procedures for comparing characteristics of methods such as biases and precisions based on paired measurements data have been available at least since the paper by Grubbs (1948). Evaluation of similarity has also long been a goal of method comparison studies in the clinical chemistry literature—see, for example, the detailed schemes of Barnett (1965) and Barnett and Youden (1970) for collection and analysis of method comparison data. Dunn (2004) and Barnhart et al. (2007a) use the test theory terminology (Section 1.6.4) for method comparison studies.

Assuming the mixed-effects model (1.19), Maloney and Rastogi (1970) use the test of equality of variances of paired measurements—developed independently by Pitman (1939) and Morgan (1939)—to test for equality of precisions of two methods. Jaech (1971) provides tests of additional hypotheses involving these precisions. Bradley and Blackwood (1989) generalize the Pitman-Morgan test to provide a simultaneous test of equality of means and equality of variances of paired measurements. Under the model (1.19), this test is a simultaneous test of equality of biases and equality of precisions (Blackwood and Bradley, 1991). Proponents of these tests include Bartko (1994), Krummenauer (1999), and Krummenauer et al. (2000).

Mandel and Stiehler (1954) argue that the usual two criteria of accuracy and precision may not be enough to evaluate a measurement method. Accuracy is applicable only when comparisons with a reference can be a made. Moreover, a method may appear to be highly precise just because it is not sensitive enough to detect small changes in the true quantity being measured. They propose the criterion of sensitivity as this takes into account not only the repeatability of a method but also its ability to detect small changes in the true value (see also Mandel, 1978). The square of sensitivity (β_1^2/σ_e^2) is sometimes called the precision of a method (see, e.g., Shyr and Gleser, 1986). These articles also discuss tests of hypotheses involving ratio of sensitivities of two methods.

Tan and Iglewicz (1999) provide confidence interval and equivalence tests for the slope parameter assuming that the measurement error model (1.18) is fit using Deming regression. Dunn (2004, 2007) discuss inference on measures of similarity defined in Section 1.7.1 based on this model.

Evaluation of Agreement

The articles of Bland and Altman (1986) and Lin (1989) are the two classic references on the topic of measuring agreement in two methods of quantitative measurement. The Bland

and Altman paper is known for the *limits of agreement* approach (see Chapter 2) and the companion plot of difference against average, which is also known as the Bland-Altman plot. It is among the most-cited statistical papers of all time (Ryan and Woodall, 2005). The methodology was actually proposed in Altman and Bland (1983), but Bland and Altman (1986) popularized it among medical researchers. It is currently the de facto standard technique for analysis of method comparison studies in health-related disciplines. The article of Lin (1989) is known for introducing the *concordance correlation coefficient* as a measure of agreement; it will be discussed in Chapter 2. Incidentally, while Bland and Altman (1986) is the most popular method in practice, Lin (1989) has received the most attention in the statistical literature.

The statistical literature on measuring agreement has grown steadily since the appearance of the above two articles. Reviews of the literature can be found in Barnhart et al. (2007a), Lin (2008), and Choudhary (2009). This topic is also covered in the books by Dunn (2004), Broemeling (2009), Shoukri (2010), Carstensen (2010), and Lin et al. (2011).

Lewis et al. (1991) describe how the problem of agreement evaluation differs from calibration and scale conversion problems even though all three involve comparison of methods. See Osborne (1991) for an introduction to calibration problems and Lewis et al. (1991) for scale conversion problems. The evaluation of agreement is also called the evaluation of *substantial equivalence* in the terminology of the US Food and Drug Administration (Lin et al., 1998). Tan and Iglewicz (1999) and Hawkins (2002) present various notions of equivalence that may be relevant for method comparison studies. See the book of Wellek (2010) for a comprehensive account of equivalence testing problems. Chow and Liu (2008) provide a good introduction to bioequivalence studies.

Controversies

Bland and Altman (1986) and Lin (1989) espouse evaluation of agreement as the goal of method comparison studies. These authors deem Pearson correlation, paired t-test of equality of means, and the test of zero intercept and unit slope using classical least squares regression as inadequate for the task of agreement evaluation. Lin (1992) also contends that any test of hypothesis for evaluating agreement must have sufficient agreement as the alternative hypothesis. In a letter to the editor regarding Kelly (1985), Altman and Bland (1987) point out that even though fitting the measurement error model (1.18) leads to more accurate estimates than the classical least squares regression, the resulting test of zero intercept and unit slope is not adequate for evaluation of agreement (see also Kelly, 1987, for the author's reply). In addition to providing a test with low power, the approach of comparing the fitted line with the line of equality only focuses on bias between the methods and totally ignores the variability around the line of equality.

In a series of papers (Bland and Altman, 1990, 1995a, 1999, 2003; and Altman and Bland, 2002), Bland and Altman not only forcefully reject correlation-type measures but also consider explicit modeling of data (e.g., using a measurement error model) as unnecessary or too complicated to explain to practitioners. Instead, they offer their limits of agreement and the plot of difference against average, commonly known as the Bland-Altman plot, proposed in Altman and Bland (1983) and Bland and Altman (1986) as a simple approach for agreement evaluation. This method of analysis is preferred by several health-related journals over the analysis using scatterplot together with correlation and even appropriately fitted regression (see, e.g., Hollis, 1996a; Dewitte et al., 2002; and Twomey, 2006).

On the other hand, Dunn and Roberts (1999) lament the limited use of statistical models in method comparison studies as explicit modeling of data is sidelined by the widespread use of the Bland-Altman method that does not make many demands on the design of the study (see also Marshall et al., 1994; and Dunn, 2004, Chapters 3–4). The authors such as Linnet (1999), Dunn and Roberts (1999), Dunn (2007), and Alanen (2010) favor explicit modeling of data through a measurement error model. This is because the fitted model clearly shows the extent of fixed and proportional biases and the differences in precisions of the measurement methods. Ludbrook (2010) also suggests an appropriately fit regression if the goal is to detect bias between the methods. If the goal is to determine whether one method can be substituted for another, he suggests the Bland-Altman approach.

Although Bland and Altman recommend replicating the measurements instead of simply using a paired measurements design (see, e.g., Bland and Altman, 1999, 2007), the papers of Dunn show that only when one tries to model the data does the inadequacy of the paired design become apparent. He emphasizes collecting data using sufficiently informative designs that include replicating the measurements so as to allow estimation of all model parameters. He also suggests estimating parameters by jointly modeling all the data together, and highlights the importance of large sample sizes.

Bland-Altman Plot

While the plot of difference versus average is popularized by Altman and Bland (1983) and Bland and Altman (1986), a similar plot of ratio versus average was proposed earlier by Eksborg (1981). He shows that the ratio plot is better than a scatterplot of data overlaid with the Deming regression line at revealing key features of method comparison data such as fixed and proportional biases and nonconstant precision. However, Eksborg does not propose any measures to indicate limits of agreement as done by Bland and Altman. Pollock et al. (1992) reach the same conclusion as Eksborg by using a plot that has relative difference, that is, difference expressed as a percentage of average, on the vertical axis. Stöckl (1996) also concurs that these two difference plots are superior to a scatterplot for graphical presentation of method comparison data (see also Hollis, 1996b). Twomey (2006) compares the two plots and discusses when one should be used in place of the other.

Hawkins (2002) shows that the Bland-Altman plot can be used to diagnose departures from the assumptions of the measurement error model (1.18). He argues that if there is a linear trend in this plot, it is more likely to be due to a proportional bias between the methods than due to unequal precisions. Assuming equal precisions for the methods, Hawkins supplements this plot with diagnostic checks of the simple linear regression of difference on average to formally verify whether the fixed and the proportional biases between the methods are equal.

Bartko (1994) and Stöckl et al. (2004) propose further embellishments to the Bland-Altman plot to show the magnitude of the between-subject variation relative to the within-subject variations and the effect of the sample size. Oftentimes, authors use the reference method measurements on the horizontal axis of the difference plot instead of the average measurement. But Bland and Altman (1995b) argue against this practice as this may incorrectly suggest the presence of unequal proportional biases (see also Section 1.13; Krouwer, 2008; and Woodman, 2010).

Data Sources

The oxygen saturation data used in this chapter come from Bland and Altman (1986). Hawkins (2002) is the source of the vitamin D data. The plasma volume data are from Bland and Altman (1999), and are presented in Table 1.2. All three datasets can be obtained from the book's website.

ID	Method Hurley	Method Nadler	ID	Method Hurley	Method Nadler	ID	Method Hurley	Method Nadler
1	52.9	56.9	34	86.0	93.5	67	97.1	104.8
2	59.2	63.2	35	84.3	94.5	68	97.3	105.1
3	63.0	65.5	36	87.6	94.6	69	95.1	105.5
4	66.2	73.6	37	84.0	95.0	70	95.8	105.7
5	64.8	74.1	38	85.9	95.2	71	95.5	106.1
6	69.0	77.1	39	84.4	95.3	72	95.9	106.8
7	67.1	77.3	40	85.2	95.6	73	95.4	107.2
8	70.1	77.5	41	85.2	95.9	74	97.3	107.4
9	69.2	77.8	42	89.2	96.4	75	97.7	107.5
10	73.8	78.9	43	87.8	97.2	76	93.0	107.5
11	71.8	79.5	44	88.0	97.5	77	97.6	108.0
12	73.3	80.8	45	88.7	97.9	78	96.1	108.2
13	73.1	81.2	46	91.2	98.2	79	96.2	108.6
14	74.7	81.9	47	91.8	98.5	80	99.5	109.1
15	74.1	82.2	48	92.5	98.8	81	99.8	110.1
16	74.1	83.1	49	88.0	98.9	82	105.3	111.2
17	76.0	84.4	50	93.5	99.0	83	103.6	111.7
18	75.4	84.9	51	89.0	99.3	84	100.2	111.7
19	74.6	86.0	52	89.4	99.3	85	100.0	112.0
20	79.2	86.3	53	89.2	99.9	86	98.8	113.1
21	77.8	86.3	54	91.3	100.1	87	110.0	116.0
22	80.8	86.6	55	90.4	101.0	88	103.5	116.7
23	77.6	86.6	56	91.2	101.0	89	109.4	118.8
24	77.5	86.6	57	91.4	101.5	90	112.1	119.7
25	78.6	87.1	58	93.0	101.5	91	111.3	120.7
26	78.7	87.5	59	91.2	101.5	92	108.6	122.8
27	81.5	87.8	60	92.0	101.8	93	112.4	124.7
28	79.3	88.6	61	91.8	101.8	94	113.8	126.4
29	78.9	89.3	62	96.8	102.8	95	115.6	127.6
30	85.9	89.6	63	92.8	102.9	96	118.1	128.2
31	80.7	90.3	64	94.0	103.2	97	116.8	129.6
32	80.6	91.1	65	93.5	103.8	98	121.6	130.4
33	82.8	92.1	66	95.8	104.4	99	115.8	133.2

Reprinted from Bland and Altman (1999) with permission from SAGE.

Table 1.2   Plasma volume measurements expressed as a percentage of normal values due to Hurley and Nadler (data originally provided by C. Doré, see Cotes et al., 1986).

EXERCISES

1.1 Consider the classical linear model (1.1).

(a) Show that $E(Y|b) = \beta_0 + \beta_1 b$ and $\text{var}(Y|b) = \sigma_e^2$.

(b) Show that $E(Y) = \beta_0 + \beta_1 \mu_b$ and $\text{var}(Y) = \beta_1^2 \sigma_b^2 + \sigma_e^2$.

(c) Let $\tilde{Y}_1$ and $\tilde{Y}_2$ be two replications of Y following model (1.1). That is,

$$\tilde{Y}_1 = \beta_0 + \beta_1 b + \tilde{e}_1, \ \tilde{Y}_2 = \beta_0 + \beta_1 b + \tilde{e}_2,$$

where $\tilde{e}_1$ and $\tilde{e}_2$ are independently distributed as e. Show that the correlation between $\tilde{Y}_1$ and $\tilde{Y}_2$ is $(\beta_1^2 \sigma_b^2)/(\beta_1^2 \sigma_b^2 + \sigma_e^2)$. (This is the expression for reliability given in (1.4).)

1.2 Show that the following conditions are equivalent for perfect agreement in the paired measurements (Y_1, Y_2) under the assumption that $\sigma_1^2, \sigma_2^2 > 0$:

(a) $P(Y_1 = Y_2) = 1$.

(b) $\{\mu_1 = \mu_2, \sigma_1^2 = \sigma_2^2, \rho = 1\}$.

(c) $\{\xi = 0, \tau^2 = 0\}$.

1.3 Suppose (Y_1, Y_2) follow the measurement error model (1.6).

(a) Verify the expressions (1.7) and (1.8) for the mean vector and covariance matrix of (Y_1, Y_2).

(b) Verify the expressions for mean and variance of D given in (1.10).

1.4 Suppose for a scalar parameter ϕ we have two tests for the hypotheses

$$H_0 : \phi \geq \phi_0 \text{ versus } H_1 : \phi < \phi_0.$$

The first test rejects H_0 if a $100(1 - \alpha)\%$ upper confidence bound for ϕ of the form $\hat{\phi} + c_{1-\alpha} \text{SE}(\hat{\phi})$ is less than ϕ_0. The second test rejects H_0 if the upper limit of a $100(1 - \alpha)\%$ two-sided confidence interval for ϕ of the form $\hat{\phi} \pm c_{1-\alpha/2} \text{SE}(\hat{\phi})$ is less than ϕ_0. Here it is assumed that $(\hat{\phi} - \phi)/\text{SE}(\hat{\phi})$ has a known distribution that is symmetric about zero for all ϕ, and c_α is the αth percentile of this distribution.

(a) Prove that both tests have level of significance α.

(b) Prove that the first test is uniformly more powerful than the second test.

1.5 Consider the Grubbs model given in (1.19).

(a) Show that the method of moments provides the following estimators of its parameters:

$$\hat{\mu}_b = \overline{Y}_{.1}, \ \hat{\beta}_0 = \overline{Y}_{.2} - \overline{Y}_{.1}, \ \hat{\sigma}_b^2 = S_{12}, \ \hat{\sigma}_{e1}^2 = S_1^2 - S_{12}, \ \hat{\sigma}_{e2}^2 = S_2^2 - S_{12}.$$

These estimators do not require the normality assumption and are called *Grubbs estimators*.

[*Hint*: Equate the mean vector and covariance matrix of (Y_1, Y_2), given by (1.20) and (1.21), to their sample counterparts, and solve.]

(b) Under what conditions are the error variance estimators positive? Do these conditions always hold?

1.6 Table 1.3 presents a dataset containing weights (grams) of 15 packets of potatoes measured using two kitchen scales, A and B.

Packet	Scale A	Scale B	Packet	Scale A	Scale B
1	135	165	9	650	630
2	940	910	10	1380	1370
3	1075	1060	11	970	1000
4	925	925	12	1000	1000
5	2330	2290	13	1640	1575
6	2870	2850	14	345	345
7	1490	1425	15	310	320
8	2110	2050			

Reprinted from Dunn (2004, page 51), ©2004 Wiley, with permission from Wiley.

Table 1.3   Potato weights (grams) data for Exercise 1.6.

(a) Use Exercise 1.5 formulas to compute the Grubbs estimates for these data. What do you notice about the error variance estimates?

(b) Use a statistical software to fit the mixed-effects model (1.19) to these data using the ML method. What do you notice about the error variance estimates?

(c) Comment on the results.

1.7 Assuming that the paired measurements follow the measurement error model (1.18), show that the joint distribution of (D, A) is bivariate normal with mean vector

$$\begin{pmatrix} \beta_0 + (\beta_1 - 1)\mu_b \\ \{\beta_0 + (\beta_1 + 1)\mu_b\}/2 \end{pmatrix}$$

and covariance matrix

$$\begin{pmatrix} (\beta_1 - 1)^2\sigma_b^2 + \sigma_{e1}^2 + \sigma_{e2}^2 & \{(\beta_1^2 - 1)\sigma_b^2 - \sigma_{e1}^2 + \sigma_{e2}^2\}/2 \\ \{(\beta_1^2 - 1)\sigma_b^2 - \sigma_{e1}^2 + \sigma_{e2}^2\}/2 & \{(\beta_1 + 1)^2\sigma_b^2 + \sigma_{e1}^2 + \sigma_{e2}^2\}/4 \end{pmatrix}.$$

1.8 Table 1.4 contains measurements of inferior pelvic infundibular (IPI) angle in degrees taken from 52 kidneys using computerized tomography (method 1) and urography (method 2). Urography offers a cheaper alternative to tomography for diagnosis and treatment of kidney stones (renal lithiasis).

(a) Make a scatterplot and a Bland-Altman plot.

(b) Do these plots show any evidence of differences in fixed and proportional biases and precisions of the two methods?

(c) Is there any evidence of heteroscedasticity or of outliers?

Kidney	Method 1	Method 2	Kidney	Method 1	Method 2	Kidney	Method 1	Method 2
1	97	100	19	95	85	37	105	90
2	77	58	20	78	105	38	65	60
3	74	95	21	70	80	39	80	80
4	59	55	22	80	85	40	90	96
5	79	79	23	78	82	41	58	54
6	85	95	24	102	102	42	75	80
7	78	60	25	102	100	43	83	88
8	78	88	26	77	75	44	78	70
9	68	68	27	45	40	45	85	90
10	96	94	28	60	70	46	65	79
11	74	60	29	50	63	47	90	100
12	64	64	30	94	103	48	76	85
13	76	88	31	91	95	49	100	108
14	60	57	32	66	80	50	65	53
15	78	66	33	63	72	51	40	58
16	71	67	34	65	68	52	53	49
17	67	76	35	58	48			
18	103	95	36	75	70			

Reprinted from Luiz et al. (2003), ©2003 Elsevier, with permission from Elsevier.

Table 1.4   IPI angle (°) data for Exercise 1.8.

1.9 Table 1.5 shows the estimated fat content (g/100 ml) of human milk measured using the standard Gerber method (method 1) and a procedure that measures the amount of glycerol released by enzymic hydrolysis of triglycerides (method 2). The second method requires only 10–50 microliters of milk and is suitable for use with autoanalyzers, permitting rapid sample throughput.

(a) Make a scatterplot and the Bland-Altman plot for these data.

(b) Do these plots show any evidence of differences in fixed and proportional biases and precisions of the two methods? Explain.

(c) Is there any evidence of heteroscedasticity or of outliers? Explain.

(d) You should notice a linear trend in the Bland-Altman plot. Discuss whether the trend may be due to a difference in proportional biases or precisions or both.

(e) Make a ratio plot of these data. Does this plot also show a linear trend? If yes, explain what this may suggest about the cause of the trend.

(f) Make a Bland-Altman plot of log-transformed data. Does this plot also show a linear trend? Explain.

1.10 Consider the dataset presented in Bland and Altman (1986) consisting of measurements of mean velocity of circumferential fiber shortening (VCF) obtained in 100 cases by M-mode echocardiography using two methods: the standard left ventricular

Sample	Method 1	2	Sample	Method 1	2	Sample	Method 1	2
1	0.85	0.96	16	2.17	2.28	31	3.15	3.19
2	1.00	1.16	17	2.20	2.15	32	3.15	3.12
3	1.00	0.97	18	2.28	2.29	33	3.40	3.33
4	1.00	1.01	19	2.43	2.45	34	3.42	3.51
5	1.20	1.25	20	2.55	2.40	35	3.62	3.66
6	1.20	1.22	21	2.60	2.79	36	3.95	3.95
7	1.38	1.46	22	2.65	2.77	37	4.27	4.20
8	1.65	1.66	23	2.67	2.64	38	4.30	4.05
9	1.68	1.75	24	2.70	2.73	39	4.35	4.30
10	1.70	1.72	25	2.70	2.67	40	4.75	4.74
11	1.70	1.67	26	2.70	2.61	41	4.79	4.71
12	1.70	1.67	27	3.00	3.01	42	4.80	4.71
13	1.88	1.93	28	3.02	2.93	43	4.80	4.74
14	2.00	1.99	29	3.03	3.18	44	5.42	5.23
15	2.05	2.01	30	3.11	3.18	45	6.20	6.21

Reprinted from Bland and Altman (1999) with permission from SAGE.

Table 1.5   Fat content (g/100ml) data for Exercise 1.9.

long axis recordings and the left ventricular short axis recordings. These data can be obtained from the book's website.

(a) Construct a scatterplot and the Bland-Altman plot.

(b) Do these plots show any evidence of differences in fixed and proportional biases and precisions of the two methods?

(c) Is there any evidence of heteroscedasticity or outliers?

(d) If you see any evidence of heteroscedasticity, make a Bland-Altman plot of log-transformed data. Does the transformation remove heteroscedasticity? Explain.

1.11 Consider the estimation of intercept $\tilde{\beta}_0$ and slope $\tilde{\beta}_1$ in the ordinary regression model (1.25).

(a) Show that the estimators given in (1.26) are the least squares estimators of $\tilde{\beta}_0$ and $\tilde{\beta}_1$.

(b) Assuming that the paired measurements follow the bivariate normal model (Section 1.12.3) and using the expressions for $(\tilde{\beta}_0, \tilde{\beta}_1)$ given in (1.27), show that the least squares estimators in (a) are also the ML estimators of their respective parameters.

1.12 Consider the problem of fitting the line $Y_2 = \beta_0 + \beta_1 Y_1$ to the paired measurements using the Deming regression.

(a) Assume that the error variance ratio $\lambda = 1$. Show that the orthogonal least squares estimators of (β_0, β_1) obtained by minimizing (1.29) are $(\hat{\beta}_0, \hat{\beta}_1)$ given in (1.30) with $\lambda = 1$.

(b) Suppose λ is known and transform Y_1 as $\tilde{Y}_1 = Y_1/\sqrt{\lambda}$. Use part (a) to show that the orthogonal least squares estimators of the coefficients $\tilde{\beta}_0$ and $\tilde{\beta}_1$ in the line $Y_2 = \tilde{\beta}_0 + \tilde{\beta}_1 \tilde{Y}_1$ corresponding to the transformed data $(\tilde{Y}_{i1}, Y_{i2})$ are, respectively, $\hat{\beta}_0$ and $\sqrt{\lambda}\hat{\beta}_1$.

(c) Use part (b) to show that the Deming regression line fit to the transformed data is $\hat{Y}_2 = \hat{\beta}_0 + \sqrt{\lambda}\hat{\beta}_1 \tilde{Y}_1$. Deduce that the Deming regression line fit to the original data is $\hat{Y}_2 = \hat{\beta}_0 + \hat{\beta}_1 Y_1$.

1.13 Consider the Deming regression line of Y_2 on Y_1, namely, $\hat{Y}_2 = \hat{\beta}_0 + \hat{\beta}_1 Y_1$, where the coefficients are given by (1.30).

(a) Show that the Deming regression line of Y_1 on Y_2 is $\hat{Y}_1 = (-\hat{\beta}_0/\hat{\beta}_1) + (1/\hat{\beta}_1)Y_2$.

(b) Deduce that there is only one Deming regression line regardless of whether Y_1 or Y_2 is treated as the explanatory variable.

1.14 (Casella and Berger, 2001, Exercise 12.4) Let $\hat{\beta}_1$, given by (1.30), be the estimator of the slope in the Deming regression line. It can be expressed as

$$\hat{\beta}_1(\lambda) = \frac{(\lambda S_2^2 - S_1^2) + \sqrt{(\lambda S_2^2 - S_1^2)^2 + 4\lambda S_{12}^2}}{2\lambda S_{12}},$$

where $\lambda = \sigma_{e1}^2/\sigma_{e2}^2$ is assumed to be known.

(a) Show that $\hat{\beta}_1(\lambda)$ is an increasing function of λ if $S_{12} > 0$ and a decreasing function if $S_{12} < 0$.

(b) Show that $\lim_{\lambda \to 0} \hat{\beta}_1(\lambda) = S_{12}/S_1^2$, the slope of the ordinary regression line of Y_2 on Y_1.

(c) Show that $\lim_{\lambda \to \infty} \hat{\beta}_1(\lambda) = S_2^2/S_{12}$, the reciprocal of the slope of the ordinary regression line of Y_1 on Y_2.

1.15 Assume that the paired measurements represent a random sample from a bivariate normal distribution (Section 1.12.3). The goal of this exercise is to derive the formula (1.33) for a $100(1 - \alpha)\%$ confidence interval for σ_2^2/σ_1^2. We will do so by inverting the acceptance region of a level α test of hypotheses

$$H_0 : \sigma_2^2/\sigma_1^2 = c \text{ versus } H_1 : \sigma_2^2/\sigma_1^2 \neq c,$$

where c is a specified positive constant.

(a) Define $U = Y_2 + \sqrt{c}Y_1$ and $V = Y_2 - \sqrt{c}Y_1$. Show that the above hypotheses are equivalent to

$$H_0 : \text{cor}(U, V) = 0 \text{ versus } H_1 : \text{cor}(U, V) \neq 0,$$

where the correlation between U and V is given by

$$\frac{(\sigma_2^2/\sigma_1^2) - c}{\sqrt{(\sigma_2^2/\sigma_1^2) + c + 2\rho\sqrt{c}(\sigma_2/\sigma_1)}\sqrt{(\sigma_2^2/\sigma_1^2) + c - 2\rho\sqrt{c}(\sigma_2/\sigma_1)}}.$$

(b) Show that the sample (product-moment) correlation based on the (U, V) sample can be expressed as

$$R_2 = \frac{(S_2^2/S_1^2) - c}{\sqrt{(S_2^2/S_1^2) + c + 2R\sqrt{c}(S_2/S_1)}\sqrt{(S_2^2/S_1^2) + c - 2R\sqrt{c}(S_2/S_1)}}.$$

(c) Show that rejecting H_0 if

$$\sqrt{n-2}|R_2|/\sqrt{1 - R_2^2} > t_{n-2,1-\alpha/2}$$

provides a level α test.

(d) Show that the acceptance region of the test in part (c) can be written as

$$R_2^2 \le t_1^2, \ \ t_1 = \frac{t_{n-2,1-\alpha/2}}{\sqrt{n - 2 + t_{n-2,1-\alpha/2}^2}}.$$

(e) Show that the confidence interval for σ_2^2/σ_1^2 obtained by inverting the acceptance region in part (d) consists of values of w that satisfy

$$(1 - t_1^2)w^2 - 2(\sigma_2^2/\sigma_1^2)\{t_1^2(1 - R^2) + (1 - t_1^2 R^2)\}w + (1 - t_1^2)(\sigma_2^4/\sigma_1^4) \le 0.$$

(f) Show that the values of w that satisfy the condition in part (e) form the interval

$$\left[\frac{S_2^2}{S_1^2}\frac{\left(t_1\sqrt{1 - R^2} - \sqrt{1 - t_1^2 R^2}\right)^2}{1 - t_1^2}, \frac{S_2^2}{S_1^2}\frac{\left(t_1\sqrt{1 - R^2} + \sqrt{1 - t_1^2 R^2}\right)^2}{1 - t_1^2}\right].$$

(See Wang (1999) and Choudhary and Nagaraja (2005a) for related confidence intervals.)

CHAPTER 2

COMMON APPROACHES FOR MEASURING AGREEMENT

2.1 PREVIEW

The notion of agreement between two methods of measurement of a continuous response variable was introduced in Section 1.5. This chapter describes some common measures of agreement and discusses approaches for agreement evaluation based on those measures. The specific ones considered include concordance correlation coefficient, total deviation index, and limits of agreement. These are used throughout the book.

2.2 INTRODUCTION

As in Chapter 1, we use (Y_1, Y_2) to denote a pair of measurements by the two methods on a randomly selected subject from a population of interest. The pair follows a continuous bivariate distribution with mean (μ_1, μ_2), variance (σ_1^2, σ_2^2), covariance σ_{12}, and correlation ρ. Let $D = Y_1 - Y_2$ denote the difference in measurements. It follows a continuous distribution with mean $\xi = \mu_1 - \mu_2$ and variance $\tau^2 = \sigma_1^2 + \sigma_2^2 - 2\sigma_{12}$. The distributions of Y_1, Y_2, and D need not be normal, although we often make such an assumption for inference purposes.

From Section 1.5, when the methods have perfect agreement, that is, $P(Y_1 = Y_2) = 1$, the bivariate distribution of Y_1 and Y_2 is concentrated on the 45° line. The deviation from this ideal are quantified by agreement measures, which are functions of parameters of the bivariate distribution. Different measures quantify the deviation differently. For example,

Measuring Agreement: Models, Methods, and Applications. By P. K. Choudhary and H. N. Nagaraja
Copyright © 2017 John Wiley & Sons, Inc.

some are based on the joint properties of Y_1 and Y_2 while others are based directly on the difference. Likewise, some are defined in terms of moments of a distribution and others are defined in terms of quantiles. Nevertheless, the agreement measures generally tend to be scalar quantities, with either small or large values implying good agreement between the methods. Perfect agreement is implied by specific boundary values of the measures. We now define some commonly used measures and explain how they are used to evaluate agreement. The estimation of these measures is discussed in subsequent chapters.

2.3 MEAN SQUARED DEVIATION

The mean squared deviation (MSD) is based on the difference D. It is defined as

$$\text{MSD} = E(D^2) = \xi^2 + \tau^2 = (\mu_1 - \mu_2)^2 + \sigma_1^2 + \sigma_2^2 - 2\sigma_{12}, \tag{2.1}$$

where the second equality follows from the fact that

$$E(D^2) = \{E(D)\}^2 + \text{var}(D). \tag{2.2}$$

This measure quantifies the average size of the squared differences in measurements. Clearly, MSD ≥ 0, with small values implying good agreement. It depends on the parameters of the bivariate distribution of (Y_1, Y_2) through the mean ξ and variance τ^2 of D. For this measure to be small, both $|\xi|$ and τ must be small. Perfect agreement corresponds to MSD $= 0$.

To evaluate agreement using MSD, we can construct its upper confidence bound U from the data and judge whether the extent of agreement represented by the value U for MSD may be considered acceptable (Section 1.11). Alternatively, letting ϕ denote the MSD and ϕ_0 denote a specified threshold below which MSD is considered small enough for sufficient agreement, we can test the agreement hypotheses (1.14). Sufficient agreement is inferred if $U < \phi_0$. However, judging whether a given value of MSD represents acceptable agreement is generally a difficult task for practitioners. The same holds for specifying the cutoff ϕ_0. This difficulty in interpretation of an MSD limits its practical utility. But due to its intuitively appealing properties, MSD often serves as a starting point for defining other measures of agreement.

The notion of MSD can be generalized to get an entire class of MSD-like measures. For this, we replace D^2 in (2.1) with a *distance function* $g(Y_1, Y_2)$ to get

$$E\{g(Y_1, Y_2)\} \tag{2.3}$$

as the generalized measure. In particular, taking $g(y_1, y_2) = (y_1 - y_2)^2$, the squared distance function, leads to the usual MSD. Additional choices for g, for example, $g(y_1, y_2) = |y_1 - y_2|$, the absolute distance function, lead to other MSD-like measures (see Bibliographic Note).

2.4 CONCORDANCE CORRELATION COEFFICIENT

To define the concordance correlation coefficient (CCC), we start with the MSD measure and rescale it to lie between -1 to 1. Formally,

$$\text{CCC} = 1 - \frac{\text{MSD}}{\text{MSD}_0}, \tag{2.4}$$

where MSD_0 is the MSD value assuming Y_1 and Y_2 are independent. Under independence, the covariance $\sigma_{12} = 0$, implying

$$\text{var}(D) = \text{var}(Y_1) + \text{var}(Y_2).$$

Therefore, it follows from (2.2) that

$$\text{MSD}_0 = (\mu_1 - \mu_2)^2 + \sigma_1^2 + \sigma_2^2. \tag{2.5}$$

Substituting (2.1) and (2.5) in (2.4) and simplifying, we get the CCC as (Exercise 2.1)

$$\text{CCC} = \frac{2\sigma_{12}}{(\mu_1 - \mu_2)^2 + \sigma_1^2 + \sigma_2^2} = \frac{2\rho\sigma_1\sigma_2}{(\mu_1 - \mu_2)^2 + \sigma_1^2 + \sigma_2^2}. \tag{2.6}$$

This measure is a function of the first- and second-order moments of (Y_1, Y_2).

An alternative form for CCC is obtained by dividing both numerator and denominator in (2.6) by $\sigma_1\sigma_2$ to get

$$\text{CCC} = \rho \left\{ 2 \left/ \left(\frac{(\mu_1 - \mu_2)^2}{\sigma_1\sigma_2} + \frac{\sigma_1}{\sigma_2} + \frac{\sigma_2}{\sigma_1} \right) \right. \right\}. \tag{2.7}$$

This form decomposes CCC as a product of two factors. The first factor is simply the correlation ρ, which measures how tightly concentrated the bivariate distribution is around a straight line. The second factor measures how close the two marginal distributions are with respect to their means and variances, and itself is made up of two components. The first component measures squared difference in the means standardized by the product of the standard deviations. The second component, consisting of the sum of ratios of the standard deviations, measures difference in the standard deviations. It is smallest (with a value of 2) when the standard deviations are equal. Taken together, the second factor lies between zero and one, with the value of one corresponding to $\{\mu_1 = \mu_2, \sigma_1 = \sigma_2\}$. Thus, it shrinks the first factor ρ towards zero.

The CCC has the following properties (Exercise 2.1):

(*i*) CCC has the same sign as ρ.

(*ii*) $0 \leq |\text{CCC}| \leq |\rho| \leq 1$.

(*iii*) $\text{CCC} = \rho \iff \{\mu_1 = \mu_2, \sigma_1 = \sigma_2\}$.

(*iv*) $|\text{CCC}| = $ second factor in (2.7) $\iff |\rho| = 1$.

(*v*) $\text{CCC} = 0 \iff \rho = 0$, implying uncorrelated measurements.

(*vi*) $\text{CCC} = 1 \iff \{\mu_1 = \mu_2, \sigma_1 = \sigma_2, \rho = 1\}$, implying perfect agreement.

(*vii*) $\text{CCC} = -1 \iff \{\mu_1 = \mu_2, \sigma_1 = \sigma_2, \rho = -1\}$, implying perfect *negative* agreement, that is, $P(Y_1 = -Y_2) = 1$.

Clearly, large positive values of CCC indicate good agreement. Since the CCC cannot exceed ρ in absolute value, a weak correlation always implies a low agreement. The converse, however, is not true in general because CCC may be small even when $\rho = 1$ due to a large value for the denominator of the second factor in (2.7), see *(iv)* above. Although the CCC may be negative, it is rarely so in practice because two methods designed to measure the same underlying quantity tend to be positively correlated. The interpretation of a negative CCC is problematic in view of the fact that a larger difference in the means of the methods, implying worse agreement, leads to a higher value for the CCC (Exercise 2.2).

We may think of MSD_0 in (2.5) as a measure of *chance agreement* in that it reflects the extent of agreement expected when the measurements from the two methods are independent. Therefore, from (2.4), the CCC may be viewed as a *chance-corrected measure*, reflecting the extent of agreement in excess of what is expected by chance alone. Such measures have a history dating back to at least 1960 when the *kappa statistic*—a popular chance-corrected measure of agreement for categorical data—became available. Agreement measures for categorical data are presented in Chapter 12, where we will explore this connection further.

The CCC has an important limitation that needs to be considered while interpreting it. Just like any correlation-type measure, CCC is highly sensitive to the between-subject variation in the data (Section 1.6.2). If this variation is large, the estimated CCC may be high regardless of how large or small the differences in measurements are. The converse would be true if this variation is small. Exercise 2.3 illustrates this point with two datasets that have identical differences in measurements, and hence exhibit the same level of agreement in a sense, but have substantially different estimates of CCC simply because one dataset is more heterogeneous than the other. Thus, it follows that the CCCs estimated from two different datasets are not comparable unless the data have similar levels of heterogeneity. This behavior of CCC can be explained by its expression in (2.7). Therein the CCC is shown as a product of correlation ρ, which from (1.9) in Section 1.6.2 is known to be sensitive to heterogeneity of true values expressed through σ_b^2, and a term that is relatively unaffected by σ_b^2 (see Exercise 2.3).

As large (positive) values for CCC imply good agreement, we can evaluate agreement based on CCC by constructing its lower confidence bound L from the data, and assessing whether the value L for CCC represents acceptable agreement. Alternatively, letting ϕ denote the CCC and ϕ_0 denote a threshold above which the CCC represents acceptable agreement, we can test the agreement hypotheses (1.15). Sufficient agreement is inferred if $L > \phi_0$. In the light of the drawback of CCC, this assessment should be cognizant of the between-subject variation in the data. An assessment based on arbitrary cutoffs, such as "high agreement if L exceeds 0.90," may be misleading and therefore should be avoided. Besides, any analysis based on CCC should be supplemented by an analysis based on another measure that is not as sensitive to the between-subject variation as the CCC. Examples are provided in subsequent chapters.

Note that the assumption of independence is not necessary to define the MSD_0 in (2.4) and hence the CCC. The weaker assumption of uncorrelated Y_1 and Y_2 leads to the same expression. However, the independence assumption is useful in generalizing CCC to a class of CCC-like measures. The generalization is accomplished by simply replacing the MSD in (2.4) by its generalized version (2.3), yielding

$$1 - \frac{E\{g(Y_1, Y_2)\}}{E_0\{g(Y_1, Y_2)\}}, \tag{2.8}$$

as the generalized CCC. Here g is a distance function and E_0 denotes expectation under the assumption that Y_1 and Y_2 are independent. Taking $g(y_1, y_2) = (y_1 - y_2)^2$ in (2.8) gives the usual CCC. A version that is more robust to outliers in the data can be obtained by taking $g(y_1, y_2) = |y_1 - y_2|$ (see Bibliographic Note). The generalization (2.8) also allows unifying the treatment of chance-corrected measures for both continuous and categorical data in a single framework (see Chapter 12).

2.5 A DIGRESSION: TOLERANCE AND PREDICTION INTERVALS

In this section, we briefly digress to present an overview of tolerance and prediction intervals. These intervals provide interval estimates of a range containing a specified proportion of the population being sampled. They play a prominent role in agreement evaluation and are used in subsequent sections. They are distinct from a confidence interval, which provides an interval estimate for a population parameter.

2.5.1 Definitions

Let X denote a continuous random variable, and f_X and F_X be its probability density function (pdf) and cumulative distribution function (cdf), respectively. In practice, we will have some data from the population of X, but to define the intervals there is no need to make assumptions about the data design. Let $I = (L, U)$ be a random interval computed from the sample data. Define the *probability content* of the interval I as

$$C(I) = \int_L^U f_X(y)dy = F_X(U) - F_X(L). \tag{2.9}$$

This probability content, also called the *coverage* of the interval I, is a random variable representing the proportion of the population of X values contained in I. It can also be interpreted as the proportion of *all* future observations from the population of X, sampled independently of the observed data, that is contained in I.

Definition (Tolerance interval) A random interval $I = (L, U)$ is a *tolerance interval* containing $100p\%$ of the distribution of X with $100(1 - \alpha)\%$ confidence if

$$P(C(I) \geq p) \geq 1 - \alpha, \tag{2.10}$$

where $C(I)$ is the probability content given by (2.9).

The probability in (2.10) is computed using the sampling distribution of the data. The endpoints of a tolerance interval are called *tolerance limits*. There are two equivalent interpretations of this interval. One, it contains at least p proportion of the sampled population with confidence $1 - \alpha$. Two, it covers at least p proportion of all future observations from the population of X with confidence $1 - \alpha$.

Let X_f denote a single future observation from the population of X, sampled independently of the observed data. By definition, X and X_f are identically distributed.

Definition (Prediction interval) A random interval $I = (L, U)$ is a *prediction interval* for X with $100p\%$ confidence if

$$P(L \leq X_f \leq U) \geq p. \tag{2.11}$$

The probability in (2.11) is computed using the joint distribution of the sample data and X_f. The endpoints of a prediction interval are called *prediction limits*. There are two equivalent interpretations of a prediction interval as well. The first follows directly from its definition: the interval contains a *single* future observation from the sampled population with confidence p. The second is due to the fact that

$$P(L \leq X_f \leq U) = E\{C(I)\}, \tag{2.12}$$

where the expectation on the right is with respect to the sampling distribution of the data (Exercise 2.4). Thus, a $100p\%$ prediction interval contains, on average, at least p proportion of the sampled population.

A comparison of (2.10), (2.11), and (2.12) shows that, for a specified p, the probability content of a prediction interval is at least p on average, whereas that of a tolerance interval is at least p with probability $1 - \alpha$. Since $1 - \alpha$ in practice is close to 1, we may say that what a prediction interval does merely *on average* is done by a tolerance interval with a *large probability* $1 - \alpha$. As a result, a tolerance interval is generally wider than the corresponding prediction interval. These intervals are said to be *conservative* if the probabilities in their definitions (2.10) and (2.11) are strictly greater than the specified lower bounds.

Prediction and tolerance intervals are not unique. Two such intervals may contain the same overall proportion of the population, but the specific regions they contain may be located in different parts of the distribution, for example, in the center or in the tails. In particular, the intervals can be one-sided (if either $L = -\infty$ or $U = \infty$) or two-sided. Here we focus only on two-sided intervals.

2.5.2 Normally Distributed Data

We now describe a methodology for computing two-sided tolerance and prediction intervals that contain $100p\%$ of the population of X, assuming that $X \sim \mathcal{N}_1(\mu, \sigma^2)$ with both parameters unknown. For simplicity, we also assume that the data consist of a random sample $X_1, \ldots, X_n$ from this population. The methodology can be generalized to handle data from more complex designs. We also focus on the intervals of the form

$$I = (\overline{X} - kS, \overline{X} + kS), \tag{2.13}$$

where $\overline{X} = \sum_{i=1}^{n} X_i/n$ is the sample mean, $S^2 = \sum_{i=1}^{n} (X_i - \overline{X})^2/(n-1)$ is the sample variance, and k—a positive quantity—is an appropriately chosen factor. The probability content of this interval can be expressed as

$$C(I) = \Phi\left\{(\overline{X} + kS - \mu)/\sigma\right\} - \Phi\left\{(\overline{X} - kS - \mu)/\sigma\right\},$$

where Φ is the cdf of a $\mathcal{N}_1(0, 1)$ distribution. Note that $C(I)$ is a function of k as well as unknown (μ, σ^2) and their estimates. But it is a *pivotal quantity* whose distribution is completely known and is free of the unknown parameters.

By definition, the factor k for a tolerance interval is obtained by solving the equation

$$P(C(I) \geq p) = 1 - \alpha$$

for k. Let $k_{\text{tol}} = k_{\text{tol}}(n, p, \alpha)$ be the solution, implying

$$\overline{X} \pm k_{\text{tol}} S \tag{2.14}$$

forms a $100p\%$ tolerance interval with $100(1 - \alpha)\%$ confidence. The factor k_{tol} is not available in a closed form and must be computed numerically. A good approximation is given by (see Bibliographic Note)

$$k_{\text{tol}} \approx \sqrt{\frac{(n - 1)\chi^2_{1,p}(1/n)}{\chi^2_{n-1,\alpha}}}. \tag{2.15}$$

It is worth noting that the interval (2.14), although centered at $\overline{X}$, does not guarantee to contain the interval

$$(\mu - z_{(1+p)/2}\,\sigma, \mu + z_{(1+p)/2}\,\sigma), \tag{2.16}$$

holding the *middle* $100p\%$ of the population. The interval (2.14) merely guarantees to contain a two-sided region of the distribution that holds $100p\%$ of the population. It is possible to compute the factor k so that the resulting interval does contain the middle $100p\%$ of the population (Exercise 2.7).

To determine the factor k for a prediction interval, first we see that (Exercise 2.5)

$$E\{C(I)\} = 2P\big(T_{n-1} \le (1 + 1/n)^{-1/2}k\big) - 1, \tag{2.17}$$

where the random variable T_ν follows a t distribution with ν degrees of freedom. Next, we set (2.17) equal to p and explicitly solve for k. This leads to a $100p\%$ prediction interval of the form (Exercise 2.5)

$$\overline{X} \pm k_{\text{pred}}\,S, \ k_{\text{pred}} = (1 + 1/n)^{1/2}t_{n-1,(1+p)/2}. \tag{2.18}$$

2.6 LIN'S PROBABILITY CRITERION AND BLAND-ALTMAN CRITERION

In this section, we present an intuitively appealing premise that lies at the heart of three approaches for agreement evaluation that will be described in the next two sections. These are limits of agreement, total deviation index, and coverage probability. The premise is that two measurement methods may be considered to have sufficient agreement if a large proportion of their differences is small. To state the underlying criterion more precisely, let p be a specified large proportion, and $\pm\delta$, for $\delta > 0$, be a specified acceptable margin for the differences in that a difference falling within $\pm\delta$ is acceptably small (or practically insignificant). The choices of p and δ are subjective and depend on the application. The criterion can now be stated as follows: the two methods have sufficient agreement if

$$P(|D| \le \delta) > p. \tag{2.19}$$

We call it the *Lin's probability criterion* after L. I. Lin, who developed the total deviation index and was involved in the development of the coverage probability approach. It simply asks for more than $100p\%$ of the distribution of D to be contained within the acceptable margin, without being specific about the location of the differences. A more stringent variant of it requires the *middle* $100p\%$ of the distribution of D to be contained within $\pm\delta$. We refer to it as the *Bland-Altman criterion* after J. M. Bland and D. G. Altman, who developed the limits of agreement approach. This criterion may be appropriate when D has a symmetric distribution. For example, when $D \sim \mathcal{N}_1(\xi, \tau^2)$, from (2.16), the criterion requires

$$(\xi - z_{(1+p)/2}\,\tau, \ \xi + z_{(1+p)/2}\,\tau) \subset (-\delta, \delta). \tag{2.20}$$

If two measurement methods satisfy the Bland-Altman criterion, then they necessarily satisfy the Lin's probability criterion, but the converse is not true.

To evaluate agreement using these criteria, three statistical approaches seem natural. The first approach is to compute a tolerance interval for D and compare it with the margin $\pm\delta$. Sufficient agreement can be inferred if the interval falls within the margin. As see in Section 2.5, the interval guarantees to contain at least $100p\%$ of differences in all future measurements with $100(1 - \alpha)\%$ confidence. Therefore, for sufficient agreement, this decision rule requires more than $100p\%$ of differences in measurements to be acceptable with $100(1-\alpha)\%$ confidence. This rule may be useful for a regulator in charge of approving measurement methods for interchangeable use, who needs to ensure that the differences in a large proportion of all future measurements from the two methods are acceptably small.

The second approach is to perform a test of agreement hypotheses of the form (1.13) where either the Lin's probability criterion (2.19) or the Bland-Altman criterion (2.20) forms the alternative hypothesis. The former is pursued later in Section 2.8, where we will also see that testing the relevant hypotheses is equivalent to employing a tolerance interval. Exercise 2.9 provides an example of the latter.

The third approach is to compute a prediction interval for D and compare it with the margin $\pm\delta$. It may seem that sufficient agreement can be inferred if the interval falls within the margin. However, from Section 2.5, a prediction interval for D merely guarantees to contain the difference in a single future measurement from the two methods with $100p\%$ confidence. Therefore, this decision rule is only useful for an individual who just needs to make a single measurement and is trying to decide which method to use. It is not useful if the individual desires to select a method and use it for making several measurements because the prediction interval offers no guarantees for containing more than one future difference. Thus, a prediction interval is of limited value in the usual agreement evaluation problems where one would like to infer whether two methods agree sufficiently well for interchangeable use of the methods, not just for making a single future measurement, but for making at least a large proportion of all future measurements. When both p and $1 - \alpha$ are close to 1, as is typically the case, a prediction interval is completely contained within the corresponding tolerance interval. As a result, whenever the tolerance interval lies within the margin, so does the prediction interval.

2.7 LIMITS OF AGREEMENT

2.7.1 The Approach

The limits of agreement approach is presently the most popular approach for agreement evaluation in biomedical disciplines. It works with the difference D, and assumes that $D \sim \mathcal{N}_1(\xi, \tau^2)$. Then, it takes the interval $(\xi - 1.96\,\tau, \xi + 1.96\,\tau)$ covering the middle 95% of the population of D as the measure of agreement. The endpoints of this interval represent the 2.5th and the 97.5th percentiles of D. This population interval is estimated by the interval $(\hat{\xi} - 1.96\,\hat{\tau}, \hat{\xi} + 1.96\,\hat{\tau})$, whose endpoints are called the 95% *limits of agreement*. In the case of paired measurements data, the estimator $(\hat{\xi}, \hat{\tau}^2)$ of (ξ, τ^2) is taken as $(\overline{D}, S_D^2)$, where the sample mean $\overline{D}$ and the sample variance S_D^2 of the differences are given by (1.17).

If the limits of agreement fall within a specified margin $\pm\delta$, that is,

$$(\hat{\xi} - 1.96\,\hat{\tau}, \hat{\xi} + 1.96\,\hat{\tau}) \subset (-\delta, \delta), \tag{2.21}$$

the methods are inferred to have sufficient agreement for interchangeable use. Although δ is recommended to be specified in advance, it is rarely done so in practice. Instead, the practitioners typically evaluate agreement by judging whether or not the endpoints of the region $\hat{\xi} \pm 1.96\,\hat{\tau}$ may be considered unacceptably large.

An integral component of this approach is the use of the Bland-Altman plot (Section 1.13) to display the data. Further, to provide a graphical summary of the results, three horizontal lines—one for the mean difference $\hat{\xi}$ and one each for the two limits—are superimposed on this plot. It is also necessary to verify the normality assumption for D because the 95% limits may not estimate a 95% population range if the distribution is not normal.

Although this approach uses 95% limits by default, the limits for some other specified large percentage, say $100p\%$, may be used as well. The general approach takes the interval $(\xi - z_{(1+p)/2}\,\tau, \xi + z_{(1+p)/2}\,\tau)$ covering the middle $100p\%$ of the differences in the population as the measure of agreement. The corresponding $100p\%$ limits of agreement are defined as $\hat{\xi} \pm z_{(1+p)/2}\,\hat{\tau}$. With the $100p\%$ limits, the analog of the decision rule (2.21) infers sufficient agreement between two methods if

$$(\hat{\xi} - z_{(1+p)/2}\,\hat{\tau}, \hat{\xi} + z_{(1+p)/2}\,\hat{\tau}) \subset (-\delta, \delta). \tag{2.22}$$

This rule may be thought of as an implementation of the Bland-Altman criterion (2.20).

The limits of agreement have sampling variability because they are estimators of the population percentiles. It is recommended to examine this variability by computing separate two-sided confidence intervals for the two percentiles. Wide confidence intervals reflect low precision for the estimates. These intervals, however, are not used in practice very often, probably because of the difficulty inherent in simultaneous interpretation of separate two-sided confidence intervals for the two percentiles. The interpretation might be easier if an appropriate upper (lower) confidence bound for the upper (lower) percentile is used (see, e.g., Exercise 2.9).

2.7.2 Why Ignore the Variability?

The simplicity and the intuitive appeal of the decision rule (2.21) explain why the limits of agreement approach is so popular among the practitioners. But there is a serious issue with this decision rule because it simply compares the limits of agreement—the estimates of the percentiles—with the acceptable margin and completely ignores the uncertainty in these estimates. Without taking this uncertainty into account, the limits provide an optimistic assessment of the extent of agreement. A post hoc examination of the variability in the limits to see how precise they are does not remedy this problem. From a statistical point of view, comparing the limits with the acceptable margin to deduce whether the methods agree sufficiently well is akin to deducing whether a population mean is near zero by comparing the sample mean with zero, without taking the standard error of the sample mean into account. It is universally accepted that to deduce whether a population mean is near zero, one must use either an appropriate confidence interval or an appropriate test of hypothesis. Therefore, in line with the traditional statistical inference methods, what is needed for the evaluation of agreement using Bland-Altman criterion is either a comparison of an appropriate interval estimate of the percentile interval $(\xi - z_{(1+p)/2}\,\tau,\ \xi + z_{(1+p)/2}\,\tau)$ with $(-\delta, \delta)$ or a test of agreement hypotheses of the form (1.13) with (2.20) as the alternative hypothesis. Both these approaches do take the variability of the limits of agreement into account. To this end, some authors adopt a decision rule of the form (2.22) but replace the limits of agreement with either prediction limits or tolerance limits for D (see the next subsection), while others take a testing route (Exercise 2.9).

2.7.3   Limits of Agreement versus Prediction and Tolerance Intervals

For paired measurements data, the $100p\%$ limits of agreement $\hat{\xi} \pm z_{(1+p)/2}\,\hat{\tau}$ are of the same form as the prediction interval (2.18) for D, except that the latter uses the factor

$$k_{\text{pred}} = (1 + 1/n)^{1/2}\,t_{n-1,(1+p)/2}$$

in place of $z_{(1+p)/2}$. The factor k_{pred} decreases to $z_{(1+p)/2}$ as $n \to \infty$ (Exercise 2.5). Therefore, when n is large, the interval within the limits of agreement can be interpreted as an approximate $100p\%$ prediction interval for D. But this interval overestimates the extent of agreement because it is completely contained within the corresponding exact interval. This is an issue unless n is quite large. Besides, since the exact interval is not much harder to compute than the approximate one, the exact approach is preferred if a prediction interval is indeed desired. However, we have already argued in Section 2.6 that a prediction interval for D has limited usefulness in agreement evaluation because it only guarantees to cover the difference of a single future pair of measurements from the two methods. A tolerance interval for D is generally more suitable for this task. Of the two tolerance intervals discussed in Section 2.5—the ordinary interval (2.14) covering $100p\%$ of the population and the interval from Exercise 2.7 covering the *middle* $100p\%$ of the population—the latter appears more consistent with the Bland-Altman criterion.

2.8   TOTAL DEVIATION INDEX AND COVERAGE PROBABILITY

2.8.1   The Approaches

The measures total deviation index (TDI) and coverage probability (CP) provide two equivalent approaches for agreement evaluation using the Lin's probability criterion presented in Section 2.6. Both are based on the statistical properties of the difference D. However, unlike the limits of agreement, they do not require the normality assumption for D (see, e.g., Chapter 10), although such an assumption is often made in practice.

For a specified large proportion p, the TDI measure is defined as:

$$\text{TDI}(p) = 100p\text{th percentile of } |D|. \tag{2.23}$$

It is a non-negative measure, and a small value implies high agreement between the methods and the converse is true for a large value. When $\text{TDI}(p) = 0$ for all p, the methods have perfect agreement. By definition, the interval $(-\text{TDI}(p), \text{TDI}(p))$ represents a population range centered at zero that contains $100p\%$ of the distribution of D.

For a specified small positive margin δ, the CP measure is defined as:

$$\text{CP}(\delta) = P(|D| \leq \delta). \tag{2.24}$$

It represents the proportion of the population of D contained within the margin $\pm\delta$. It lies between zero and one, and a large value indicates high agreement. When $\text{CP}(\delta) = 1$ for all δ, the methods have perfect agreement.

For specified (δ, p), Lin's criterion (2.19) for sufficient agreement can be expressed in terms of the CP measure as $\text{CP}(\delta) > p$. It can also be equivalently expressed in terms of the TDI measure as $\text{TDI}(p) < \delta$ because (Exercise 2.10)

$$\text{CP}(\delta) > p \iff \text{TDI}(p) < \delta. \tag{2.25}$$

This equivalence implies that agreement can be evaluated using either of the two measures. In particular, with Lin's criterion in the alternative, the agreement hypotheses (1.13) can be formulated in terms of either TDI or CP. Further, since the resulting alternative hypotheses are one-sided, they can be tested using appropriate one-sided confidence bounds (Section 1.11.2). The hypotheses (1.13) can be expressed in terms of TDI as

$$H_0 : \text{TDI}(p) \geq \delta \quad \text{and} \quad H_1 : \text{TDI}(p) < \delta. \tag{2.26}$$

These can be tested by computing an *upper* $100(1 - \alpha)\%$ confidence bound U for $\text{TDI}(p)$ and comparing it with δ. Sufficient agreement is inferred if $U < \delta$. Similarly, the hypotheses (1.13) can be expressed in terms of CP as

$$H_0 : \text{CP}(\delta) \leq p \quad \text{and} \quad H_1 : \text{CP}(\delta) > p. \tag{2.27}$$

These can be tested by computing a *lower* $100(1 - \alpha)\%$ confidence bound L for $\text{CP}(\delta)$ and comparing it with p. Sufficient agreement is inferred if $L > p$.

There is an interesting connection between performing the test based on TDI and employing a tolerance interval to evaluate agreement. It can be seen that if U is a $100(1 - \alpha)\%$ upper confidence bound for $\text{TDI}(p)$, the interval $(-U, U)$ is a tolerance interval containing $100p\%$ of the distribution of D with $100(1 - \alpha)\%$ confidence (Exercise 2.11). By design, this tolerance interval is centered at zero. From Section 2.6, the decision rule based on a tolerance interval infers sufficient agreement if $(-U, U) \subset (-\delta, \delta)$. Obviously, this rule is equivalent to inferring sufficient agreement on the basis of the test of hypotheses in (2.26). Thus, there is a one-to-one correspondence between a test of hypothesis and a tolerance interval for evaluating agreement using the Lin's probability criterion.

Although the TDI and CP measures provide equivalent approaches for agreement evaluation, the TDI has one practical advantage. This has to do with the fact that the practitioners generally find it easier to specify p, which is commonly chosen to be one of $\{0.80, 0.90, 0.95\}$, than δ, whose value depends on the application. Of course, advance specification of both δ and p is necessary to formally test the agreement hypotheses. However, only p is needed in advance to compute the upper bound U for $\text{TDI}(p)$. The practitioner can then evaluate agreement by examining whether the tolerance interval $(-U, U)$ contains any unacceptably large differences, without having to explicitly provide a δ. On the other hand, advance specification of δ is necessary to perform inference using the CP measure. Because of this practical advantage, we only use TDI (with $p = 0.90$) in this book.

2.8.2 Normally Distributed Differences

If $D \sim \mathcal{N}_1(\xi, \tau^2)$, the TDI defined by (2.23) can be obtained as the solution of the equation (Exercise 2.12)

$$p = P\{|D| \leq \text{TDI}(p)\} = \Phi\{(\text{TDI}(p) - \xi)/\tau\} - \Phi\{(-\text{TDI}(p) - \xi)/\tau\}. \tag{2.28}$$

Alternatively, since

$$P\{|D| \leq \text{TDI}(p)\} = P(D^2/\tau^2 \leq \text{TDI}^2(p)/\tau^2),$$

and D^2/τ^2 follows a noncentral χ^2 distribution with 1 degree of freedom and noncentrality parameter ξ^2/τ^2, $\text{TDI}(p)$ can be explicitly expressed as (Exercise 2.12)

$$\text{TDI}(p) = \tau \left\{ \chi^2_{1,p}(\xi^2/\tau^2) \right\}^{1/2}. \tag{2.29}$$

Generally it is easier to compute TDI using (2.29) than (2.28) because major statistical software packages have built-in functions for computing noncentral χ^2 percentiles.

If $D \sim \mathcal{N}_1(\xi, \tau^2)$, the CP defined by (2.24) can be determined as

$$\text{CP}(\delta) = P(|D| \leq \delta) = \Phi\{(\delta - \xi)/\tau\} - \Phi\{(-\delta - \xi)/\tau\}. \tag{2.30}$$

Following the approach that led to (2.29), $\text{CP}(\delta)$ can also be determined as a noncentral χ^2 probability (Exercise 2.13).

2.9   INFERENCE ON AGREEMENT MEASURES

In this chapter, we have generally refrained from discussing point and interval estimation of agreement measures. The data may come from a variety of designs, for example, a paired design or a repeated measurements design. Once we have settled on a model for the data, the measures can be written as functions of the model parameters and can be estimated by simply plugging in the corresponding estimates. The standard errors of the estimates and the confidence intervals or bounds for the measures can be approximated using large-sample theory. When the sample size is not large enough for the standard approximations to be accurate, one can resort to bootstrap. These ideas are discussed in detail in the next chapter.

The measures like MSD, CCC, TDI, and CP are scalar functions of parameters. An exception is the limits of agreement approach in which two population percentiles are used to define the measure of agreement. Among the scalar measures, only CCC and TDI are used in this book. We also use the 95% of limits of agreement as a summary of the data, but do not use them for inference for the reasons explained in Section 2.7.

As argued in Section 1.11, we use confidence bounds instead of hypothesis tests for evaluating measures of agreement. Our emphasis is on lower bound for CCC and upper bound for TDI. However, we do use hypothesis tests for model comparison.

2.10   CHAPTER SUMMARY

1. Different agreement measures quantify the extent of agreement differently, but all are functions of parameters of the bivariate distribution of (Y_1, Y_2).

2. CCC is defined in terms of first- and second-order moments of (Y_1, Y_2). Its large positive values (nearing 1) imply high agreement.

3. The measures MSD, TDI, and CP are based on the difference D. For MSD and TDI, small values (nearing zero) imply high agreement, whereas the converse is true for CP.

4. For measures whose large values imply good agreement, for example, CCC and CP, a lower confidence bound can be used for evaluating agreement.

5. For measures whose small values imply good agreement, for example, MSD and TDI, an upper confidence bound can be used for assessing the extent of agreement.

6. TDI and CP provide equivalent metrics for agreement evaluation.

7. Using an upper confidence bound for TDI is equivalent to using a tolerance interval for inference purposes.

8. The limits of agreement are also based on the difference D. They are useful as an estimated summary measure of the data, but they should not be directly compared with the acceptable margin to infer sufficient agreement.

2.11 BIBLIOGRAPHIC NOTE

This chapter focuses only on common approaches for measuring agreement. Review of the literature on these and additional approaches can be found in Barnhart et al. (2007a) and Choudhary (2009). The MSD measure has been used by Hutson et al. (1998) and Choudhary and Nagaraja (2005b, c) for comparing extent of agreement in pairs of methods. The scaled versions of MSD, including CCC, have been considered by Lin (1989, 2000), Lin et al. (2002, 2007), Barnhart et al. (2007b), and Haber and Barnhart (2008).

The CCC was proposed by Lin (1989). However, the same measure, although not by the same name, appeared much earlier in Krippendorff (1970) in the psychology literature. The Krippendorff article, together with those of Fay (2005) and Haber and Barnhart (2006), discusses the issue of chance correction in the measure. Its connection and equivalence with intraclass correlation (McGraw and Wong, 1996) has been discussed in Lin (1989), Nickerson (1997), and Carrasco and Jover (2003). Undue influence of between-subject variation on the CCC and similar correlation-type measures has been pointed out by a number of authors, including Bland and Altman (1990), Müller and Büttner (1994), Atkinson and Nevill (1997), and Barnhart et al. (2007c). Lin and Chinchilli (1997) suggest comparing measurement ranges of datasets before comparing CCC estimates based on them. King and Chinchilli (2001a, b) present the generalized CCC, given by (2.8), in which MSD is replaced by $E\{g(Y_1, Y_2)\}$, where g is a distance function. Robust versions of CCC can be obtained by choosing appropriate g functions. King and Chinchilli (2001a) unify the treatment of chance-corrected agreement measures for continuous as well as categorical data by showing that, for some particular g functions, CCC reduces to kappa statistics (Cohen, 1960, 1968), which are popular measures of agreement for categorical data (see Chapter 12 for an introduction). The CCC has been generalized to deal with a variety of data types, summary of which can be found in Barnhart et al. (2007a) and Lin et al. (2011).

While the CCC has received the most attention in the statistical literature, the limits of agreement approach is the most popular approach in biomedical literature. It is proposed by Bland and Altman (1986). This article also recommends examining two-sided confidence intervals for the population percentiles that these limits estimate, and provides expressions for them. To evaluate agreement using the Bland-Altman criterion, Lin et al. (1998) formulate the problem as a test of agreement hypotheses (1.13) and provide an approximate test. This test employs two approximate one-sided confidence bounds, an upper bound for the upper percentile and a lower bound for the lower percentile. Liu and Chow (1997) provide an exact test for the same hypotheses (see Exercise 2.9), although the test was developed in a different context than ours. Instead of the limits of agreement, Carstensen et al. (2008) use a prediction interval for D and Ludbrook (2010) uses a tolerance interval for D. Ludbrook also recognizes that for agreement evaluation a tolerance interval is more appropriate than a prediction interval. Bland and Altman (1999) describe a nonparametric analog of the limits of agreement for the scenario when the normality assumption for D cannot be justified.

The TDI measure was proposed by Lin (2000). This article argues that directly testing (2.26) based on the TDI is difficult. Therefore, the TDI is approximated by a multiple of MSD, and a large-sample test is proposed. The CP measure was introduced by Lin et al. (2002). They provide a large-sample test for the hypothesis (2.27) based on CP. Wang and Hwang (2001) also present a test of (2.27), although in a different context. All these tests assume a random sample of differences. Choudhary and Nagaraja (2007) evaluate properties of these tests, and provide alternatives, including an exact test, that generally work better. This article also discusses the equivalence of the TDI and CP approaches and the connection between testing (2.26) and using a tolerance interval. Escaramis et al. (2010) provide another approach for inference on the TDI measure.

Guttman (1988) and Vardeman (1992) provide good introductions to prediction and tolerance intervals. See Krishnamoorthy and Mathew (2009) and Meeker et al. (2017) for book-length treatments. The former book also describes the tolerance factor approximation (2.15). The `tolerance` package of Young (2010) for the statistical software R provides additional methods for computing tolerance intervals.

EXERCISES

2.1 (a) Verify the expression for CCC given in (2.6).

   (b) Show that the second term on the right-hand side in (2.7) lies between zero and one, and the latter value corresponds to $\{\xi = 0, \sigma_1 = \sigma_2\}$.

   (c) Verify the properties of CCC listed on page 55.

2.2 Consider two bivariate distributions for (Y_1, Y_2), both with $(\sigma_1^2, \sigma_2^2) = (1, 1)$ and $\rho = -0.1$. The first distribution has $(\mu_1, \mu_2) = (0, 0)$, and the second distribution has $(\mu_1, \mu_2) = (-2, 2)$.

   (a) Which distribution exhibits worse agreement between Y_1 and Y_2? Why?

   (b) Calculate CCC for both distributions. Which CCC is higher?

   (c) Do you see any contradiction in the results in (a) and (b)? If yes, what explains the contradiction?

   (This example is from Fay (2005).)

2.3 Suppose, based on paired measurements data, the CCC is estimated by replacing the population moments in its definition by their sample counterparts from (1.16). Consider two datasets presented in Table 2.1. Dataset A presents paired test-retest measurements of predicted maximal oxygen consumption (ml/kg/min) in 30 subjects using the Fitech test. Dataset B shows the same data as A but manipulated to get a less heterogeneous sample.

Subject	Dataset A		Dataset B	
	Test	Retest	Test	Retest
1	31	27	41	37
2	33	35	43	45
3	42	47	42	47
4	40	44	40	44
5	63	63	43	43
6	28	31	48	51
7	43	54	43	54
8	44	54	44	54
9	68	68	48	48
10	47	58	47	58
11	47	48	47	48
12	40	43	40	43
13	43	45	43	45
14	47	52	47	52
15	58	48	58	48
16	61	61	41	41
17	45	52	45	52
18	43	44	43	44
19	58	48	58	48
20	40	44	40	44
21	48	47	48	47
22	42	52	42	52
23	61	45	61	45
24	48	43	48	43
25	43	52	43	52
26	50	52	50	52
27	39	40	39	40
28	52	58	52	58
29	42	45	42	45
30	77	67	57	47

Reprinted from Atkinson and Nevill (1997), ©1997 Wiley, with permission from Wiley.

Table 2.1 Oxygen consumption (ml/kg/min) data for Exercise 2.3.

(a) Verify that both datasets have exactly the same differences in test-retest measurements and Dataset A has larger between-subject variation than B.

(b) Estimate the correlation ρ from both data. Which estimate is higher? Why?

(c) Estimate the second factor on the right side in (2.7) from both data. How do the estimates compare?

(d) Estimate CCC for both data. Which estimate is higher?

(e) What do you conclude about the dependence of CCC on between-subject variation?

(This example is from Atkinson and Nevill (1997).)

2.4 Verify the relation (2.12) between the probability of covering one future observation and the expected probability content of a prediction interval.

2.5 Consider a $100p\%$ prediction interval of the form (2.13) for a single observation from a normal distribution using a random sample from this distribution.

  (a) Verify the expression (2.17) for expected probability content of the interval.

  (b) Show that the interval in (2.18) is a $100p\%$ prediction interval.

  (c) Show that the factor k_{pred} in (2.18) is greater than $z_{(1+p)/2}$ and decreases to $z_{(1+p)/2}$ as $n \to \infty$.

2.6 Perform a Monte Carlo simulation study to evaluate the accuracy of the approximation (2.15) for the tolerance factor k_{tol}. You can examine how close the probability on the left in the definition (2.10) is to the nominal confidence level as a function of p, α, and n.

2.7 Consider a tolerance interval of the form (2.13) using a random sample from a normal distribution that contains the middle $100p\%$ of the population.

  (a) Show that this interval is $\overline{X} \pm k_{mid}S$, where $k_{mid} = k_{mid}(n, p, \alpha)$ solves for k the equation

$$P\{(\mu - z_{(1+p)/2}\,\sigma, \mu + z_{(1+p)/2}\,\sigma) \subset (\overline{X} - kS, \overline{X} + kS)\} = 1 - \alpha.$$

  Obtain an expression for the probability on the left.

  (b) Show that $k_{mid} > k_{tol}$, where k_{tol} is the tolerance factor for the usual interval (2.14). This implies that the new interval is wider than the usual interval. Does this seem intuitively reasonable? Explain.

2.8 Compute tolerance and prediction intervals with $(p, 1 - \alpha) = (0.90, 0.95)$ for the difference in test-retest measurements of Exercise 2.3, and interpret them. Assume normality for the differences. Can you justify this assumption?

2.9 The evaluation of agreement using Bland-Altman criterion can be performed by testing the following hypotheses which are of the general form (1.13):

$$H_0 : \left(\xi - z_{(1+p)/2}\,\tau,\ \xi + z_{(1+p)/2}\,\tau\right) \not\subset (-\delta, \delta) \text{ versus}$$
$$H_1 : \left(\xi - z_{(1+p)/2}\,\tau,\ \xi + z_{(1+p)/2}\,\tau\right) \subset (-\delta, \delta). \tag{2.31}$$

This exercise derives an *intersection-union test* (Casella and Berger, 2001, Chapter 8) of these hypotheses assuming we have a random sample $D_1, \ldots, D_n$ from the population of $D \sim \mathcal{N}_1(\xi, \tau^2)$. This test was proposed by Liu and Chow (1997) in a context different from agreement evaluation.

  (a) Argue that the hypotheses in (2.31) can be divided into two subhypotheses involving the lower and the upper percentiles,

$$H_{01} : \xi - z_{(1+p)/2}\,\tau \le -\delta \ \text{ and } \ H_{11} : \xi - z_{(1+p)/2}\,\tau > -\delta,$$

and

$$H_{02} : \xi + z_{(1+p)/2}\tau \geq \delta \quad \text{and} \quad H_{12} : \xi + z_{(1+p)/2}\tau < \delta,$$

respectively, so that H_0 is a union of H_{01} and H_{02}, and H_1 is an intersection of H_{11} and H_{12}. The intersection-union test rejects H_0 when *both* H_{01} and H_{02} are rejected. Show that if a level α test is used for each subhypothesis, then the level of the intersection-union test is also α.

(b) Show that rejecting H_{01} in favor of H_{11} if $\overline{D} - k_0 S_D > -\delta$ provides a level α test, where

$$k_0 = n^{-1/2}t_{n-1,1-\alpha}\left(n^{1/2}z_{(1+p)/2}\right).$$

(c) Similarly, show that rejecting H_{02} in favor of H_{12} if $\overline{D} + k_0 S_D < \delta$ provides a level α test.

(d) Deduce that rejecting H_0 in favor of H_1 if

$$(\overline{D} - k_0 S_D, \overline{D} + k_0 S_D) \subset (-\delta, \delta)$$

provides the desired intersection-union test with level α.

(e) Can the interval $\overline{D} \pm k_0 S_D$ be interpreted as a tolerance interval? Explain.

2.10 For specified (δ, p), establish the equivalence (2.25) of TDI and CP criteria for sufficient agreement.

2.11 Show that if U is a $100(1 - \alpha)\%$ upper confidence bound for $\text{TDI}(p)$, the interval $(-U, U)$ is a tolerance interval containing $100p\%$ of the distribution of D with $100(1 - \alpha)\%$ confidence.

2.12 Show that if $D \sim \mathcal{N}_1(\xi, \tau^2)$, $\text{TDI}(p)$ can be obtained by solving

$$p = \Phi\{(t - \xi)/\tau\} - \Phi\{(-t - \xi)/\tau\}$$

with respect to t for $t > 0$. Further, verify the expression (2.29) for $\text{TDI}(p)$.

2.13 Show that if $D \sim \mathcal{N}_1(\xi, \tau^2)$, $\text{CP}(\delta)$ can be written as (2.30). Also express $\text{CP}(\delta)$ as a noncentral χ^2 probability.

CHAPTER 3

A GENERAL APPROACH FOR MODELING AND INFERENCE

3.1 PREVIEW

This chapter is concerned with a general discussion that is relevant for much of the book. First, we provide an introduction to linear mixed-effects models. This includes a discussion of prediction, model fitting, and model diagnostics. Next, we present the large-sample methodology for statistical inference based on ML estimators. Special attention is paid to construction of confidence intervals and bounds using both the standard large-sample theory and bootstrap. Finally, we present a general framework for modeling method comparison data using mixed-effects models and doing inference on measures of similarity and agreement. This framework is followed in subsequent chapters in the analysis of various types of data. Readers familiar with mixed-effects modeling and large-sample inference may just skim through this chapter. Those not interested in technical details may skip it entirely.

3.2 MIXED-EFFECTS MODELS

Suppose there are n subjects in the study. Let $\mathbf{Y}_i$ be an $M_i \times 1$ vector of observations on the ith subject, $i = 1, \ldots, n$. The M_i need not be equal for all i. The total number of observations in the data is $N = \sum_{i=1}^{n} M_i$. The observations from different subjects are independent, whereas those from the same subject are assumed to be dependent.

Measuring Agreement: Models, Methods, and Applications. By P. K. Choudhary and H. N. Nagaraja
Copyright © 2017 John Wiley & Sons, Inc.

3.2.1 The Model

A general mixed-effects model for the data $\mathbf{Y}_1, \ldots, \mathbf{Y}_n$ can be written as

$$\mathbf{Y}_i = \mathbf{X}_i\boldsymbol{\beta} + \mathbf{Z}_i\mathbf{u}_i + \mathbf{e}_i, \ \ i = 1, \ldots, n, \tag{3.1}$$

where

- $\boldsymbol{\beta}$ is a $p \times 1$ vector of *fixed effects*,

- $\mathbf{X}_i$ is an $M_i \times p$ *design* (or *regression*) *matrix* associated with the fixed effects,

- $\mathbf{u}_i$ is a $q \times 1$ vector of *random effects* of subject i,

- $\mathbf{Z}_i$ is an $M_i \times q$ design matrix associated with the random effects, and

- $\mathbf{e}_i$ is an $M_i \times 1$ vector of within-subject random errors.

Both $\mathbf{X}_i$ and $\mathbf{Z}_i$ are assumed to have full rank. It is further assumed that

- $\mathbf{u}_i \sim$ independent $\mathcal{N}_q(\mathbf{0}, \mathbf{G})$ distributions,

- $\mathbf{e}_i \sim$ independent $\mathcal{N}_{M_i}(\mathbf{0}, \mathbf{R}_i)$ distributions, and

- $\mathbf{u}_i$ and $\mathbf{e}_i$ are mutually independent.

The $q \times q$ matrix $\mathbf{G}$ and the $M_i \times M_i$ matrix $\mathbf{R}_i$ are unknown *positive definite* covariance matrices. This formulation allows the random effects of a subject as well as the within-subject errors to be correlated and to have nonconstant variances. These matrices are usually assumed to have some structure among their elements and are parameterized in terms of a small number of unknown parameters. For example, the matrices may have a diagonal structure with unequal diagonal elements, or a *compound symmetric* structure wherein all diagonal elements are equal and all off-diagonal elements are equal.

The model assumptions imply that the conditional distribution of the observation vector given the random effects is

$$\mathbf{Y}_i | \mathbf{u}_i \sim \text{ independent } \mathcal{N}_{M_i}(\mathbf{X}_i\boldsymbol{\beta} + \mathbf{Z}_i\mathbf{u}_i, \mathbf{R}_i), \ \ i = 1, \ldots, n.$$

Thus, the marginal distribution of the observation vector is (Exercise 3.1)

$$\mathbf{Y}_i \sim \text{ independent } \mathcal{N}_{M_i}(\mathbf{X}_i\boldsymbol{\beta}, \mathbf{V}_i), \ \ \mathbf{V}_i = \mathbf{Z}_i\mathbf{G}\mathbf{Z}_i^T + \mathbf{R}_i, \ \ i = 1, \ldots, n. \tag{3.2}$$

Notice that the covariance structure of the observations is induced by the covariance structures of the random effects and errors and the design matrix of the random effects. One can also deduce that (Exercise 3.2)

$$\begin{pmatrix} \mathbf{u}_i \\ \mathbf{Y}_i \end{pmatrix} \sim \mathcal{N}_{q+M_i}\left(\begin{pmatrix} \mathbf{0} \\ \mathbf{X}_i\boldsymbol{\beta} \end{pmatrix}, \begin{pmatrix} \mathbf{G} & \mathbf{G}\mathbf{Z}_i^T \\ \mathbf{Z}_i\mathbf{G} & \mathbf{V}_i \end{pmatrix} \right), \tag{3.3}$$

from which it follows that

$$\mathbf{u}_i | \mathbf{Y}_i \sim \mathcal{N}_q\left(\mathbf{G}\mathbf{Z}_i^T\mathbf{V}_i^{-1}(\mathbf{Y}_i - \mathbf{X}_i\boldsymbol{\beta}), \mathbf{G} - \mathbf{G}\mathbf{Z}_i^T\mathbf{V}_i^{-1}\mathbf{Z}_i\mathbf{G} \right). \tag{3.4}$$

3.2.2 Prediction

In classical statistics, estimation of random quantities is called "prediction" to distinguish it from estimation of parameters that are fixed quantities. To discuss prediction of the random $\mathbf{u}_i$ based on the data $\mathbf{Y}_1, \ldots, \mathbf{Y}_n$, we begin by ignoring the model (3.1), but retaining the independence assumptions and further assuming that the joint distribution of $\mathbf{u}_i$ and the data is known. This, in particular, implies that the first- and second-order moments of the distribution are known.

Suppose $\tilde{\mathbf{u}}_i$ is a predictor of $\mathbf{u}_i$. Obviously, the difference $\tilde{\mathbf{u}}_i - \mathbf{u}_i$ represents the error in prediction. A predictor $\tilde{\mathbf{u}}_i$ of $\mathbf{u}_i$ is *unbiased* if its prediction error is zero on average, that is,

$$E(\tilde{\mathbf{u}}_i - \mathbf{u}_i) = \mathbf{0}. \tag{3.5}$$

The notion of an unbiased predictor is similar to that of an unbiased estimator. An overall measure of error of a predictor $\tilde{\mathbf{u}}_i$ is given by the *mean squared prediction error*,

$$E\big\{(\tilde{\mathbf{u}}_i - \mathbf{u}_i)^T(\tilde{\mathbf{u}}_i - \mathbf{u}_i)\big\} = \sum_{j=1}^{q} E\big\{(\tilde{u}_{ij} - u_{ij})^2\big\}. \tag{3.6}$$

It represents the sum of mean squares of errors in predicting each element of $\mathbf{u}_i$. See Exercise 3.6 for a generalization of this measure.

Our interest is in finding a predictor that is the best in that it minimizes (3.6) over certain classes of predictors. First we consider the class of all predictors. It is well known that the best member of this class—the *best predictor* of $\mathbf{u}_i$—based on the data $\mathbf{Y}_1, \ldots, \mathbf{Y}_n$ is the conditional mean $E(\mathbf{u}_i|\mathbf{Y}_1, \ldots, \mathbf{Y}_n)$ (Exercise 3.6). The mean actually equals $E(\mathbf{u}_i|\mathbf{Y}_i)$ because the random effects and data from different subjects are independent. This predictor is unbiased since $E(E(\mathbf{u}_i|\mathbf{Y}_i)) = E(\mathbf{u}_i)$, implying that (3.5) holds.

In practice, however, an explicit expression for the best predictor is generally not available. Besides, it is not necessarily *linear* in $\mathbf{Y}_i$, that is, of the form

$$\tilde{\mathbf{u}}_i = \mathbf{A}\mathbf{Y}_i + \mathbf{b} \tag{3.7}$$

for some matrix $\mathbf{A}$ and vector $\mathbf{b}$ that may both depend on i. To simplify the prediction problem, one alternative is to reduce the class of predictors to only the predictors that are linear in $\mathbf{Y}_i$ and find the best member in the smaller class. This leads to the *best linear predictor* of $\mathbf{u}_i$, which can be explicitly obtained as (Exercise 3.7)

$$E(\mathbf{u}_i) + \mathrm{cov}(\mathbf{u}_i, \mathbf{Y}_i)\,\mathrm{var}(\mathbf{Y}_i)^{-1}\{\mathbf{Y}_i - E(\mathbf{Y}_i)\}.$$

This predictor requires knowing only the first- and second-order moments of $(\mathbf{u}_i, \mathbf{Y}_i)$. It is also unbiased as its expectation equals that of $\mathbf{u}_i$.

We now return to the mixed-effects model (3.1) but without the normality assumption. However, we still assume that all the model parameters are known. Using the moments in (3.3), the best linear predictor of $\mathbf{u}_i$ under this model can be written as

$$\mathbf{G}\mathbf{Z}_i^T\mathbf{V}_i^{-1}(\mathbf{Y}_i - \mathbf{X}_i\boldsymbol{\beta}). \tag{3.8}$$

Next, we allow $\boldsymbol{\beta}$ in (3.1) to be unknown, while still assuming that the matrices $\mathbf{G}$ and $\mathbf{R}_i$ are known. The task now is to jointly estimate $\boldsymbol{\beta}$ and $\mathbf{u}_1, \ldots, \mathbf{u}_n$ from the data. For this, it is common to take the approach of *best linear unbiased predictor* (BLUP), see Exercise 3.8

for the details. It shows that the BLUP of $\mathbf{u}_i$ has the same form as (3.8) but with β replaced by its best linear unbiased estimator (BLUE).

Finally, we consider the mixed-effects model (3.1) that already incorporates the normality assumption. If all parameters are known, we have from (3.4) that the best predictor of $\mathbf{u}_i$ is

$$E(\mathbf{u}_i|\mathbf{Y}_i) = \mathbf{GZ}_i^T\mathbf{V}_i^{-1}(\mathbf{Y}_i - \mathbf{X}_i\beta). \tag{3.9}$$

The right-hand side of (3.9) is nothing but the expression in (3.8), implying that the best linear predictor of $\mathbf{u}_i$ under normality is also its best predictor. In case β is unknown but $\mathbf{G}$ and $\mathbf{R}_i$ are known, this predictor is also the BLUP provided β is replaced by its BLUE. To further compare the three predictors of $\mathbf{u}_i$—the best predictor, the best linear predictor, and the BLUP—assume now that all parameters in (3.1) are unknown. In this case, one can replace the unknown parameters appearing in the expressions of these predictors by the corresponding ML estimators to get the *estimated* versions of the predictors. It can be seen that the BLUE of β appearing in the BLUP of $\mathbf{u}_i$ is actually its ML estimator under (3.1). It then follows that the estimated BLUP of $\mathbf{u}_i$ is identical to the estimated versions of the other two predictors. Thus, we have the remarkable conclusion that the estimated versions of all three predictors of $\mathbf{u}_i$ are identical under model (3.1).

3.2.3 Model Fitting

Let θ be a $K \times 1$ vector denoting the unknown parameters in the mixed-effects model (3.1). Letting $\mu_i = \mathbf{X}_i\beta$ in (3.2), the joint pdf of the observations $\mathbf{Y}_1, \ldots, \mathbf{Y}_n$ can be written as

$$
\begin{aligned}
f_\theta(\mathbf{y}_1, \ldots, \mathbf{y}_n) &= \prod_{i=1}^{n} f_\theta(\mathbf{y}_i) \\
&= \prod_{i=1}^{n} (2\pi)^{-M_i/2}|\mathbf{V}_i|^{-1/2} \exp\left\{-\frac{1}{2}(\mathbf{y}_i - \mu_i)^T\mathbf{V}_i^{-1}(\mathbf{y}_i - \mu_i)\right\} \\
&= (2\pi)^{-N/2}\Big(\prod_{i=1}^{n}|\mathbf{V}_i|\Big)^{-1/2} \exp\left\{-\frac{1}{2}\sum_{i=1}^{n}(\mathbf{y}_i - \mu_i)^T\mathbf{V}_i^{-1}(\mathbf{y}_i - \mu_i)\right\}.
\end{aligned}
$$

Considering this pdf as a function of θ while keeping the observed data fixed gives the likelihood function $L(\theta)$. Taking its log yields the log-likelihood function as

$$\log\{L(\theta)\} = -\frac{N}{2}\log(2\pi) - \frac{1}{2}\sum_{i=1}^{n}\log(|\mathbf{V}_i|) - \frac{1}{2}\sum_{i=1}^{n}(\mathbf{y}_i - \mu_i)^T\mathbf{V}_i^{-1}(\mathbf{y}_i - \mu_i).$$

The value of θ that maximizes this function is the ML estimator $\hat{\theta}$ of θ. In principle, the function in its present form can be given to an optimization routine for numerical maximization. However, this computation is often quite involved as one has to resolve a number of issues before employing the optimization routine to make the computations feasible, reliable, and fast. This is best left to a good statistical software package for fitting mixed-effects models. A reference is provided in Section 3.6 for the reader interested in the computational details.

Replacing θ by $\hat{\theta}$ in β, $\mathbf{G}$, $\mathbf{R}_i$, and $\mathbf{V}_i$ gives their ML estimators $\hat{\beta}$, $\hat{\mathbf{G}}$, $\hat{\mathbf{R}}_i$, and $\hat{\mathbf{V}}_i$, respectively. Similar substitution in (3.9) gives $\hat{\mathbf{u}}_i$—the estimated BLUP of $\mathbf{u}_i$—as

$$\hat{\mathbf{u}}_i = \hat{\mathbf{G}}\mathbf{Z}_i^T\hat{\mathbf{V}}_i^{-1}(\mathbf{Y}_i - \mathbf{X}_i\hat{\beta}). \tag{3.10}$$

These can be used to get the fitted values and the residuals, respectively, as

$$\hat{\mathbf{Y}}_i = \mathbf{X}_i\hat{\boldsymbol{\beta}} + \mathbf{Z}_i\hat{\mathbf{u}}_i, \ \ \hat{\mathbf{e}}_i = \mathbf{Y}_i - \hat{\mathbf{Y}}_i, \ \ i = 1,\ldots,n.$$

We can also get the *standardized residuals*

$$\hat{\mathbf{R}}_i^{-1/2}\,\hat{\mathbf{e}}_i, \tag{3.11}$$

where $\hat{\mathbf{R}}_i^{-1/2}$ is a *matrix inverse square root* of $\hat{\mathbf{R}}_i$. These residuals play a key role in checking model adequacy. The predicted random effects, the fitted values, and the residuals are automatically computed by a model fitting software.

When the within-subject errors are independent, $\mathbf{R}_i$ is a diagonal matrix, and the standardized residuals in (3.11) are simply the residuals divided by the corresponding estimated error standard deviations. Such residuals are often called *studentized residuals*. If, however, there is dependence in the within-subject errors, the residuals standardized as (3.11) are often called *normalized residuals* to distinguish them from their studentized counterparts.

The REML method is a popular alternative to the ML method for fitting mixed-effects models. However, as explained in Section 1.12.2, we do not use REML in this book because it does not provide a joint covariance matrix of the parameter estimates, which is needed for analysis of method comparison data.

3.2.4 Model Diagnostics

The mixed-effects model (3.1) involves a number of assumptions. After fitting a model, it is a good idea to verify that the assumptions are adequate before proceeding with the inference. Of particular importance is the assumption about the within-subject errors $\mathbf{e}_i$ that they follow independent $\mathcal{N}_{M_i}(\mathbf{0}, \mathbf{R}_i)$ distributions. This assumption is equivalent to assuming that the elements of the standardized errors $\mathbf{R}_i^{-1/2}\mathbf{e}_i$ are distributed as independent draws from a standard normal distribution. Essentially, there are four assumptions here for the standardized errors: (a) they have mean zero, (b) they are homoscedastic, (c) they are normally distributed, and (d) they are independent. These assumptions are assessed using standardized residuals, defined in (3.11). The model also assumes that the random effects $\mathbf{u}_i$ follow independent $\mathcal{N}_q(\mathbf{0}, \mathbf{G})$ distributions. It is assessed using estimated BLUPs of the random effects, given by (3.10). The errors and residuals do not have identical distributions, and the same holds for the random effects and their predicted values. Notwithstanding this fact, as far as model checking is concerned, the residuals and the predicted random effects serve as adequate proxies for the errors and the random effects, respectively. We will rely on diagnostic plots to examine compliance with the model assumptions.

Consider first the assumptions of zero mean and homoscedasticity for the standardized errors. The residual plot—the plot of standardized residuals against the fitted values—is the key diagnostic for checking these assumptions. If the assumptions hold, the points in the plot would be scattered around zero in a random manner. In particular, the presence in the plot of a trend or a nonconstant vertical scatter casts doubt on the respective assumptions of zero mean and homoscedasticity. In the specific context of method comparison studies, these violations are critical as they affect validity of the overall conclusions. Sometimes the violations can be corrected by a log transformation of the data. But if this transformation fails, then instead of looking for other more sophisticated transformations, we prefer explicit modeling of the heteroscedasticity or the trend. These topics are covered in Chapters 6 and 8, respectively.

It is often helpful to examine some variations of the basic residual plot. For example, the plot of absolute values of residuals against the fitted values makes it easier to check for heteroscedasticity because now one has to look for a trend rather than a nonconstant vertical scatter. In addition, this plot would suggest a model for the trend, essentially providing a model for the heteroscedasticity. Also, separate residual plots for different levels of important categorical covariates, for example, measurement method or gender of the subject, may reveal hidden patterns of dependence that may be missed in the basic plot. Moreover, if the error variances are suspected to depend on a continuous covariate such as age, then the residuals or their absolute values should also be plotted against that covariate.

Next, we take up the normality assumption. For errors, this can be checked by examining the normal quantile-quantile (Q-Q) plot of the standardized residuals. If the assumption holds, the points in the plot should fall on a straight line. In the same manner, the normality of each random effect can be examined using the Q-Q plot of its predicted values. However, this assessment of normality of marginals may not be enough if the random effects are jointly multivariate normal. In this case, we can examine a Q-Q plot of $\hat{\mathbf{u}}_i^T \hat{\mathbf{G}}^{-1} \hat{\mathbf{u}}_i$ using a χ^2 distribution with q degrees of freedom as the reference distribution. This diagnostic is based on the fact if $\mathbf{u}_i \sim \mathcal{N}_q(\mathbf{0}, \mathbf{G})$ then $\mathbf{u}_i^T \mathbf{G}^{-1} \mathbf{u}_i$ has a χ^2 distribution with q degrees of freedom. Using the proxy $\hat{\mathbf{u}}_i^T \hat{\mathbf{G}}^{-1} \hat{\mathbf{u}}_i$ in place of $\mathbf{u}_i^T \mathbf{G}^{-1} \mathbf{u}_i$ is an approximation that is adequate for the assessment of normality. The evaluation of joint normality is typically not needed for errors. It may be noted that mild to moderate departures from normality of either residuals or random effects are not of much concern in method comparison studies because generally they do not result in seriously incorrect estimates of parameters of interest and their standard errors.

The residual plot and the Q-Q plots may also reveal outliers. If these are seen and they cannot be attributed to data coding errors, a sensitivity analysis should be performed. At the minimum, this involves comparing the conclusions of interest with and without the outliers. If outliers exert substantial effect on the conclusions, then alternative modeling strategies, for example, using a nonparametric approach or an approach that replaces the normality of errors by a heavy-tailed distribution may be employed. A nonparametric approach is presented in Chapter 10. References are provided in the Bibliographic Note (Section 3.6) for mixed-effects models for skewed and heavy-tailed data.

Finally, there is the assumption of independence of standardized errors from the same subject. This may be an issue when a subject's measurements are collected over a period of time, for example, as in longitudinal data. The independence can be checked by examining the plot of autocorrelation of standardized residuals. We consider such plots in Chapter 9.

3.3 A LARGE-SAMPLE APPROACH TO INFERENCE

We now describe the standard *asymptotic* or *large-sample* methodology for statistical inference that is used throughout the book. This methodology assumes that the number of subjects n is large. It applies to any parametric model fit by the ML method, including the mixed-effects model (3.1) and the bivariate normal model of Chapter 4. We assume that the model is parameterized in terms of a $K \times 1$ unknown parameter vector θ. Its ML estimator is $\hat{\theta}$.

3.3.1 Approximate Distributions

When n is large, under some regularity conditions, the sampling distribution of $\hat{\boldsymbol{\theta}}$ can be approximated as

$$\hat{\boldsymbol{\theta}} \overset{\text{approx}}{\sim} \mathcal{N}_K\left(\boldsymbol{\theta}, \hat{\mathbf{H}}^{-1}\right), \tag{3.12}$$

where

$$\hat{\mathbf{H}} = -\left.\frac{\partial^2 \log\{L(\boldsymbol{\theta})\}}{\partial \boldsymbol{\theta} \partial \boldsymbol{\theta}^T}\right|_{\boldsymbol{\theta}=\hat{\boldsymbol{\theta}}} \tag{3.13}$$

is the $K \times K$ *Hessian matrix* of second-order partial derivatives of the negative log-likelihood function evaluated at the ML estimate. It is also known as the *observed information matrix*. While this matrix may be available in closed-form for some simple models, it is often computed using numerical differentiation techniques. Its inverse serves as the approximate covariance matrix of $\hat{\boldsymbol{\theta}}$. The regularity conditions needed for the normal approximation to hold are usually satisfied in practice. It follows from (3.12) that $\hat{\theta}_k$—the kth element of $\hat{\boldsymbol{\theta}}$—is approximately normal with mean θ_k, and its approximate standard error is

$$\text{SE}(\hat{\theta}_k) = \left(k\text{th diagonal element of } \hat{\mathbf{H}}^{-1}\right)^{1/2}, \quad k = 1, \dots, K. \tag{3.14}$$

We are often interested in inference on one or more functions of $\boldsymbol{\theta}$. Let there be $Q\, (\geq 1)$ such functions denoted as $\phi_1 = \phi_1(\boldsymbol{\theta}), \dots, \phi_Q = \phi_Q(\boldsymbol{\theta})$. Their ML estimators are obtained by simply replacing $\boldsymbol{\theta}$ by $\hat{\boldsymbol{\theta}}$ to get $\hat{\phi}_1 = \phi_1(\hat{\boldsymbol{\theta}}), \dots, \hat{\phi}_Q = \phi_Q(\hat{\boldsymbol{\theta}})$. Let us collectively denote the vectors of these functions and their ML estimators by the $Q \times 1$ vectors $\boldsymbol{\phi}$ and $\hat{\boldsymbol{\phi}}$, respectively. These are defined as

$$\boldsymbol{\phi} = \boldsymbol{\phi}(\boldsymbol{\theta}) = \left(\phi_1(\boldsymbol{\theta}), \dots, \phi_Q(\boldsymbol{\theta})\right)^T, \quad \hat{\boldsymbol{\phi}} = \boldsymbol{\phi}(\hat{\boldsymbol{\theta}}) = \left(\phi_1(\hat{\boldsymbol{\theta}}), \dots, \phi_Q(\hat{\boldsymbol{\theta}})\right)^T.$$

Assuming that $\boldsymbol{\phi}$ is a differentiable function of $\boldsymbol{\theta}$, the sampling distribution of $\hat{\boldsymbol{\phi}}$ can be approximated by the *multivariate delta method* as

$$\hat{\boldsymbol{\phi}} \overset{\text{approx}}{\sim} \mathcal{N}_Q\left(\boldsymbol{\phi}, \hat{\mathbf{D}}^T \hat{\mathbf{H}}^{-1} \hat{\mathbf{D}}\right), \tag{3.15}$$

where $\hat{\mathbf{H}}$ is the $K \times K$ observed information matrix defined in (3.13) and

$$\hat{\mathbf{D}} = \left.\frac{\partial \boldsymbol{\phi}(\boldsymbol{\theta})}{\partial \boldsymbol{\theta}}\right|_{\boldsymbol{\theta}=\hat{\boldsymbol{\theta}}} = \left.\begin{pmatrix} \frac{\partial \phi_1(\boldsymbol{\theta})}{\partial \theta_1} & \cdots & \frac{\partial \phi_Q(\boldsymbol{\theta})}{\partial \theta_1} \\ \vdots & \vdots & \vdots \\ \frac{\partial \phi_1(\boldsymbol{\theta})}{\partial \theta_K} & \cdots & \frac{\partial \phi_Q(\boldsymbol{\theta})}{\partial \theta_K} \end{pmatrix}\right|_{\boldsymbol{\theta}=\hat{\boldsymbol{\theta}}} \tag{3.16}$$

is the $K \times Q$ *Jacobian matrix* of derivatives of $\boldsymbol{\phi}$ with respect to $\boldsymbol{\theta}$, evaluated at its ML estimate. The derivatives involved in this matrix are sometimes available in a closed-form but they are usually computed numerically. The $Q \times Q$ matrix $\hat{\mathbf{D}}^T \hat{\mathbf{H}}^{-1} \hat{\mathbf{D}}$ serves as the approximate covariance matrix for $\hat{\boldsymbol{\phi}}$. As before, it follows from (3.15) that $\hat{\phi}_q$—the qth element of $\hat{\boldsymbol{\phi}}$—is approximately normal with mean ϕ_q, and its standard error can be approximated as

$$\text{SE}(\hat{\phi}_q) = \left(q\text{th diagonal element of } \hat{\mathbf{D}}^T \hat{\mathbf{H}}^{-1} \hat{\mathbf{D}}\right)^{1/2}, \quad q = 1, \dots, Q. \tag{3.17}$$

3.3.2 Confidence Intervals

To construct a confidence interval, we need a *pivot*—a function of both estimator and parameter whose distribution is completely known. Pivots determine the form of the interval and their percentiles are used as critical points in the interval. For θ_k, the approximate normality of $\hat{\theta}_k$ calls for using

$$(\hat{\theta}_k - \theta_k)/\text{SE}(\hat{\theta}_k) \overset{\text{approx}}{\sim} \mathcal{N}_1(0, 1)$$

as a pivot. Recalling that z_α is the 100αth percentile of a $\mathcal{N}_1(0, 1)$ distribution and also that it is a symmetric distribution, we have

$$P\big(|\hat{\theta}_k - \theta_k|/\text{SE}(\hat{\theta}_k) \leq z_{1-\alpha/2}\big) \approx 1 - \alpha.$$

Here we presume that $1 - \alpha$ is large enough so that $z_{1-\alpha/2}$ is positive. Rearranging terms in the event on the left, we can write

$$P\big(\hat{\theta}_k - z_{1-\alpha/2}\,\text{SE}(\hat{\theta}_k) \leq \theta_k \leq \hat{\theta}_k + z_{1-\alpha/2}\,\text{SE}(\hat{\theta}_k)\big) \approx 1 - \alpha,$$

from which we can deduce that

$$\big(\hat{\theta}_k - z_{1-\alpha/2}\,\text{SE}(\hat{\theta}_k),\ \hat{\theta}_k + z_{1-\alpha/2}\,\text{SE}(\hat{\theta}_k)\big)$$

is an approximate two-sided $100(1-\alpha)\%$ confidence interval for θ_k. The actual confidence level approaches the nominal level $1 - \alpha$ as $n \to \infty$.

We also need two-sided confidence intervals as well as one-sided confidence bounds for the parametric functions ϕ_q. For the confidence intervals, we proceed as in the case of θ_k to see that

$$Z_q = (\hat{\phi}_q - \phi_q)/\text{SE}(\hat{\phi}_q) \overset{\text{approx}}{\sim} \mathcal{N}_1(0, 1) \tag{3.18}$$

is an obvious pivot for ϕ_q. As before, this allows us to write

$$P\big(|\hat{\phi}_q - \phi_q|/\text{SE}(\hat{\phi}_q) \leq z_{1-\alpha/2}\big) \approx 1 - \alpha,$$

implying that

$$P\big(\hat{\phi}_q - z_{1-\alpha/2}\,\text{SE}(\hat{\phi}_q) \leq \phi_q \leq \hat{\phi}_q + z_{1-\alpha/2}\,\text{SE}(\hat{\phi}_q)\big) \approx 1 - \alpha.$$

This readily gives

$$\big(\hat{\phi}_q - z_{1-\alpha/2}\,\text{SE}(\hat{\phi}_q),\ \hat{\phi}_q + z_{1-\alpha/2}\,\text{SE}(\hat{\phi}_q)\big) \tag{3.19}$$

as an approximate two-sided $100(1-\alpha)\%$ confidence interval for ϕ_q. To get the one-sided bounds, we can analogously write

$$P\big(z_\alpha \leq (\hat{\phi}_q - \phi_q)/\text{SE}(\hat{\phi}_q)\big) = P\big(\phi_q \leq \hat{\phi}_q - z_\alpha\,\text{SE}(\hat{\phi}_q)\big) \approx 1 - \alpha,$$

obtaining

$$\hat{\phi}_q - z_\alpha\,\text{SE}(\hat{\phi}_q) = \hat{\phi}_q + z_{1-\alpha}\,\text{SE}(\hat{\phi}_q) \tag{3.20}$$

as an approximate $100(1-\alpha)\%$ upper confidence bound for ϕ_q. We can also write

$$P\big((\hat{\phi}_q - \phi_q)/\text{SE}(\hat{\phi}_q) \leq z_{1-\alpha}\big) = P\big(\hat{\phi}_q - z_{1-\alpha}\,\text{SE}(\hat{\phi}_q) \leq \phi_q\big) \approx 1 - \alpha,$$

leading to

$$\hat{\phi}_q - z_{1-\alpha} \, \mathrm{SE}(\hat{\phi}_q) \tag{3.21}$$

as an approximate $100(1 - \alpha)\%$ lower confidence bound for ϕ_q.

The confidence intervals given thus far are *individual* ones in that each interval *separately* covers a single parameter with probability approximately equal to $1 - \alpha$. Sometimes we are also interested in *simultaneous* confidence intervals for multiple parameters, say, $\phi_1, \ldots, \phi_Q$. To get the pivots for them, consider the Z_q defined in (3.18). We know that, marginally, each Z_q has an approximately $\mathcal{N}_1(0, 1)$ distribution. Their joint distribution is approximately multivariate normal with mean vector $\mathbf{0}$, and the covariance matrix is obtained from a pre- and post-multiplication of $\hat{\mathbf{D}}^T \hat{\mathbf{H}}^{-1} \hat{\mathbf{D}}$, given in (3.15), by a diagonal matrix whose elements are reciprocals of the standard errors $\mathrm{SE}(\hat{\phi}_1), \ldots, \mathrm{SE}(\hat{\phi}_Q)$ (see Exercise 3.11). Now, define

$$Z_{\min} = \min_{q=1,\ldots,Q} Z_q, \;\; Z_{\max} = \max_{q=1,\ldots,Q} Z_q, \;\; |Z|_{\max} = \max_{q=1,\ldots,Q} |Z_q|. \tag{3.22}$$

These three functions serve as the pivots for the simultaneous confidence intervals—$Z_{\min}$ for the upper bounds, $Z_{\max}$ for the lower bounds, and $|Z|_{\max}$ for the two-sided intervals. They have known, albeit complicated skewed distributions.

Next, define the percentiles of these pivots as

$$a_{1-\alpha} = 100(1 - \alpha)\text{th percentile of } |Z|_{\max},$$
$$b_{\alpha} = 100\alpha\text{th percentile of } Z_{\min},$$
$$c_{1-\alpha} = 100(1 - \alpha)\text{th percentile of } Z_{\max}.$$

Since

$$\min_{q=1,\ldots,Q} Z_q = - \max_{q=1,\ldots,Q} (-Z_q)$$

and the associated multivariate normal pdf is symmetric around its mean vector $\mathbf{0}$, we get $b_{\alpha} = -c_{1-\alpha}$. The percentiles are computed numerically assuming that the normal approximation for $(Z_1, \ldots, Z_Q)$ is exact. They also depend on the number of functions Q and the covariance matrix of $(Z_1, \ldots, Z_Q)$, but this dependence is suppressed from their notation for convenience. Thus,

$$P(|Z|_{\max} \le a_{1-\alpha}) \approx 1 - \alpha, \;\; P(b_{\alpha} \le Z_{\min}) = P(Z_{\max} \le c_{1-\alpha}) \approx 1 - \alpha, \tag{3.23}$$

from which we can, respectively, deduce that (Exercise 3.12)

$$P\big(\hat{\phi}_q - a_{1-\alpha} \, \mathrm{SE}(\hat{\phi}_q) \le \phi_q \le \hat{\phi}_q + a_{1-\alpha} \, \mathrm{SE}(\hat{\phi}_q) \text{ for all } q = 1, \ldots, Q\big) \approx 1 - \alpha,$$
$$P\big(\phi_q \le \hat{\phi}_q - b_{\alpha} \, \mathrm{SE}(\hat{\phi}_q) \text{ for all } q = 1, \ldots, Q\big) \approx 1 - \alpha,$$
$$P\big(\hat{\phi}_q - c_{1-\alpha} \, \mathrm{SE}(\hat{\phi}_q) \le \phi_q \text{ for all } q = 1, \ldots, Q\big) \approx 1 - \alpha. \tag{3.24}$$

These probability statements imply that for $\phi_1, \ldots, \phi_Q$ we can take

$$\big(\hat{\phi}_q - a_{1-\alpha} \, \mathrm{SE}(\hat{\phi}_q), \; \hat{\phi}_q + a_{1-\alpha} \, \mathrm{SE}(\hat{\phi}_q)\big), \;\; q = 1, \ldots, Q, \tag{3.25}$$

as simultaneous approximate $100(1 - \alpha)\%$ two-sided intervals;

$$\hat{\phi}_q - b_{\alpha} \, \mathrm{SE}(\hat{\phi}_q) = \hat{\phi}_q + c_{1-\alpha} \, \mathrm{SE}(\hat{\phi}_q), \;\; q = 1, \ldots, Q, \tag{3.26}$$

as simultaneous approximate $100(1 - \alpha)\%$ upper confidence bounds; and

$$\hat{\phi}_q - c_{1-\alpha} \, \mathrm{SE}(\hat{\phi}_q), \quad q = 1, \ldots, Q, \tag{3.27}$$

as simultaneous approximate $100(1 - \alpha)\%$ lower confidence bounds. When $Q = 1$, the critical points used in the simultaneous intervals and bounds in (3.25), (3.26), and (3.27), respectively, reduce to the standard normal percentiles used in their individual counterparts in (3.19), (3.20), and (3.21).

For convenience, we often collectively refer to the confidence intervals and bounds considered in this section as having the form

estimate $\pm$ critical point $\times$ SE(estimate),

with the understanding that the appropriate confidence limit and the critical point, including its sign, will be clear from the context.

3.3.3   Parameter Transformation

The accuracy of the estimated standard errors and the corresponding confidence intervals considered so far crucially depend on the accuracy of the normal approximation of the ML estimators. If, however, a parameter (or a parametric function ϕ) is such that the range of its possible values does not constitute $(-\infty, \infty)$, the range of a normal random variable, the normal approximation to the distribution of its ML estimator may be poor. Take, for example, a variance whose range is $(0, \infty)$ and a correlation whose range is $(-1, 1)$. Transforming such parameters by applying a *normalizing transformation* often improves the normal approximation for the estimators. These transformations are one-to-one functions that make the real line as the range on the transformed scale. The inference on the transformed parameters proceeds exactly as described in preceding sections. Once the confidence limits are available on the transformed scale, the inverse transformation is applied to them to get the limits on the original scale (Exercise 3.10). The normalizing transformations are not unique and sometimes they are not helpful.

We now consider three specific situations where a parameter transformation is commonly employed. The first is a ϕ with range $(0, \infty)$, for example, a variance component or the TDI, defined by (2.29). In this case, a log transformation is applied as $\log(\phi)$ has range $(-\infty, \infty)$. If l is a confidence limit for $\log(\phi)$, then $\exp(l)$ is the corresponding confidence limit on the original scale.

The second is when ϕ represents a correlation-type parameter with range $(-1, 1)$, for example, Pearson correlation or the CCC, defined by (2.6). In this case, the Fisher's z-transformation $z(\phi) \equiv \tanh^{-1}(\phi)$, defined in (1.32), is applied as its range is $(-\infty, \infty)$. If l is a confidence limit on the transformed scale, then

$$\tanh(l) = \frac{\exp(2l) - 1}{\exp(2l) + 1}$$

is the corresponding limit on the original scale.

The last is a ϕ with range $(0, 1)$, for example, a probability. In this case, a logit transformation, defined as

$$\mathrm{logit}(\phi) = \log\left(\frac{\phi}{1 - \phi}\right), \tag{3.28}$$

with range $(-\infty, \infty)$, is applied. If l is a confidence limit on the transformed scale, then

$$\frac{\exp(l)}{1 + \exp(l)}$$

is the corresponding limit on the original scale.

Although by definition the correlation-type measures such as CCC may be negative, their expressions based on a mixed-effects model are often constrained to be positive, see, for example, (4.11). The Fisher's z-transformation is used in this case as well, even though the range of the transformed scale is not $(-\infty, \infty)$ (see Bibliographic Note for references).

3.3.4 Bootstrap Confidence Intervals

In the preceding section, we described the standard large-sample approach for constructing confidence intervals. This methodology requires the number of subjects n to be large to justify the normal approximation (3.12) for the sampling distribution of $\hat{\theta}$. If n is not large enough, the accuracy of this approximation and hence that of the confidence intervals based upon it are in doubt. Possible reasons for the inaccuracy include a bias in the estimator, underestimation of its standard error, and lack of symmetry in its sampling distribution. Although we do not know exactly how large n should be for this methodology to produce reasonably accurate conclusions, we believe that for n of less than 30, the accuracy may be short of being acceptable.

Therefore, we seek an alternative that works when n is not large enough for the application of the standard large-sample approach. This is where the resampling-based methodology of *bootstrap* is helpful. We may think of bootstrap as a generally more accurate alternative to the standard approach for small to moderate n. Of course, it can be used for a large n as well, but in this case bootstrap loses its accuracy advantage as its results tend to be similar to the standard approach while its computational costs increase.

In essence, the bootstrap methodology consists of employing a resampling strategy to obtain a large number of draws from the *bootstrap distribution* of the estimator. This distribution commonly provides a better approximation to the sampling distribution of the estimator than the usual normal approximation. The bootstrap draws are then used to approximate features of the sampling distribution such as percentiles. There are a variety of techniques that fall under the umbrella of bootstrap. Here we restrict attention to the technique of *parametric studentized bootstrap* as we have found it to work well in method comparison applications. The interval produced by this method has the same form as the ordinary large-sample interval, but the critical points are percentiles of the bootstrap distribution of the pivot employed.

To describe the studentized bootstrap methodology, we focus on the confidence intervals, both individual and simultaneous, for the components of the vector ϕ of Q functions of the model parameter vector θ. The confidence intervals for θ become a special case. The ordinary large-sample intervals of ϕ were constructed in Section 3.3.2. The underlying setup there can be summarized as follows: we have independent observations $\mathbf{Y}_1, \ldots, \mathbf{Y}_n$ following a model that depends on an unknown parameter vector θ. Fitting this model by the ML method yields the ML estimator $\hat{\theta}$. From (3.12), its approximate covariance matrix is $\mathrm{var}(\hat{\theta}) = \hat{\mathbf{H}}^{-1}$. The ML estimator of the parametric function vector ϕ is $\hat{\phi}$. From (3.15), its approximate covariance matrix is $\mathrm{var}(\hat{\phi}) = \hat{\mathbf{D}}^T \hat{\mathbf{H}}^{-1} \hat{\mathbf{D}}$. The estimates of elements of ϕ and their standard errors are used to compute the pivots $Z_1, \ldots, Z_Q$ defined in (3.18), for the individual intervals; and also the pivots $Z_{\min}$, $Z_{\max}$, and $|Z|_{\max}$ defined in (3.22), for the simultaneous intervals.

We now provide the steps needed for computing the percentiles of these pivots. The percentiles will be used as critical points in studentized bootstrap intervals. In what follows, a quantity associated with resampled data is marked by an asterisk (*) to distinguish it from its counterpart based on the original data.

Step 1. Simulate n observations $\mathbf{Y}_1^*, \ldots, \mathbf{Y}_n^*$ independently from the assumed model by taking $\theta = \hat{\theta}$. These simulated data constitute a parametric resample of the original data.

Step 2. Fit the assumed model to the resampled data by the ML method. Let $\hat{\theta}^*$ be the resulting ML estimator of θ. Compute the bootstrap counterparts of

$$\text{var}(\hat{\theta}), \ \hat{\phi}, \ \text{var}(\hat{\phi}), \ Z_1, \ldots, Z_Q, \ Z_{\min}, \ Z_{\max}, \ |Z|_{\max}$$

by replacing $(\mathbf{Y}_1, \ldots, \mathbf{Y}_n)$ with $(\mathbf{Y}_1^*, \ldots, \mathbf{Y}_n^*)$ and $\hat{\theta}$ with $\hat{\theta}^*$, obtaining

$$\text{var}^*(\hat{\theta}^*), \ \hat{\phi}^*, \ \text{var}^*(\hat{\phi}^*), \ Z_1^*, \ldots, Z_Q^*, \ Z_{\min}^*, \ Z_{\max}^*, \ |Z|_{\max}^*.$$

Step 3. Repeat Steps 1 and 2 a large number of times, say B. Only the draws of the pivots need to be saved. Denote the draws of the pivots in the bth repetition as

$$Z_{b,1}^*, \ldots, Z_{b,Q}^*, Z_{b,\min}^*, Z_{b,\max}^*, |Z|_{b,\max}^*, \ \ b = 1, \ldots, B.$$

Order the B draws of each pivot from smallest to largest. Denote the ordered draws of the pivot Z_q^*, whose actual draws are $Z_{1,q}^*, \ldots, Z_{B,q}^*$, as $Z_{(1),q}^*, \ldots, Z_{(B),q}^*$. Use a similar notation to denote the ordered draws of the other pivots.

Step 4. Compute appropriate sample percentiles of the bootstrap draws obtained in Step 3 for each pivot. Assuming that B is chosen so that $(B+1)\alpha$ is a positive integer, the $(B+1)\alpha$th ordered draw of a pivot can be taken as its 100αth sample percentile. Thus, the 100αth percentiles of the pivots Z_q^*, $q = 1, \ldots, Q$, $|Z|_{\max}^*$, $Z_{\min}^*$, and $Z_{\max}^*$ can be, respectively, approximated as:

$$z_{\alpha,q}^* = Z_{((B+1)\alpha),q}^*, \ \ q = 1, \ldots, Q,$$
$$a_\alpha^* = |Z|_{((B+1)\alpha),\max}^*, \ b_\alpha^* = Z_{((B+1)\alpha),\min}^*, \ c_\alpha^* = Z_{((B+1)\alpha),\max}^*. \tag{3.29}$$

Replacing the normality-based percentiles in the intervals for $\phi_1, \ldots, \phi_Q$ in Section 3.3.2 by their counterparts from (3.29) gives the corresponding studentized bootstrap $100(1-\alpha)\%$ intervals. Upon doing so in (3.19), (3.20) and (3.21) we, respectively, get the individual two-sided intervals and one-sided upper and lower bounds for ϕ_q as

$$\left(\hat{\phi}_q - z_{1-\alpha/2,q}^* \, \text{SE}(\hat{\phi}_q), \ \hat{\phi}_q - z_{\alpha/2,q}^* \, \text{SE}(\hat{\phi}_q)\right),$$
$$\hat{\phi}_q - z_{\alpha,q}^* \, \text{SE}(\hat{\phi}_q), \ \ \hat{\phi}_q - z_{1-\alpha,q}^* \, \text{SE}(\hat{\phi}_q), \ \ q = 1, \ldots, Q. \tag{3.30}$$

However, unlike normal distributions, the bootstrap distributions are discrete and nonsymmetric. Consequently, $z_{\alpha,q}^* \neq -z_{1-\alpha,q}^*$, implying that one has to compute upper and lower percentiles from separate calculations. Proceeding in a similar manner, we, respectively, get simultaneous two-sided intervals and one-sided upper and lower bounds for $\phi_1, \ldots, \phi_Q$ from (3.25), (3.26), and (3.27) as

$$\left(\hat{\phi}_q - a_{1-\alpha}^* \, \text{SE}(\hat{\phi}_q), \; \hat{\phi}_q + a_{1-\alpha}^* \, \text{SE}(\hat{\phi}_q) \right),$$

$$\hat{\phi}_q - b_\alpha^* \, \text{SE}(\hat{\phi}_q), \; \hat{\phi}_q - c_{1-\alpha}^* \, \text{SE}(\hat{\phi}_q), \; q = 1, \ldots, Q. \tag{3.31}$$

The bootstrap process can get computationally intensive, especially if the model is complex, because almost all the computations involved in model fitting and estimating standard errors must be repeated B times. The B should be a relatively large number for accurate estimation of the percentiles. Moreover, just like the ordinary large-sample intervals, the studentized bootstrap intervals also benefit from parameter transformation (Section 3.3.3). Finally, we must emphasize that bootstrap is a not a panacea for data with small n. It may not work satisfactorily if n is too small, say, less than 15 or so.

3.3.5 Confidence Bands

Sometimes we are interested in inference on a scalar parametric function ϕ that also depends on a covariate $x \in \mathcal{X}$. The covariate may be categorical or continuous. If it is categorical, let it have Q levels $x_1, \ldots, x_Q$. If it is continuous, we discretize its domain $\mathcal{X}$ into a moderately large grid of Q points $x_1, \ldots, x_Q$. Often, 20 to 30 points on the grid are good enough in practice. The points may be equally spaced in the domain, or they may be the observed values of the covariate or the percentiles thereof. In any case, define

$$\phi_q = \phi(x_q), \; q = 1, \ldots, Q.$$

Now, the methodology for constructing one- and two-sided confidence intervals developed in Section 3.3.2 or 3.3.4 can be applied to get individual and simultaneous intervals for $\phi_1, \ldots, \phi_Q$. If x is continuous, the individual intervals form a *pointwise band* and the simultaneous intervals form a band with approximate simultaneous coverage probability $1 - \alpha$. The latter, an approximate *simultaneous band*, is usually more useful in practice because it allows inference for the function $\phi(x)$ simultaneously over its *entire* domain $\mathcal{X}$.

3.3.6 Test of Homogeneity

Let $\phi_1, \ldots, \phi_Q$ denote values of a scalar parametric function ϕ under Q different settings. Sometimes we want to test the hypotheses

$$H_0 : \phi_1 = \ldots = \phi_Q \; \text{versus} \; H_1 : \text{At least one of the } \phi_q \text{ differs from the rest.}$$

The test of this null hypothesis of equality is often called a *test of homogeneity*. Using the matrix notation, the hypotheses can be reformulated as

$$H_0 : \mathbf{C}\phi = \mathbf{0} \; \text{versus} \; H_1 : \mathbf{C}\phi \neq \mathbf{0},$$

where $\mathbf{C}$ is the $(Q-1) \times Q$ matrix

$$\mathbf{C} = \begin{pmatrix} 1 & -1 & 0 & \ldots & 0 \\ 1 & 0 & -1 & \ldots & \\ \vdots & \vdots & \vdots & \vdots & \vdots \\ 1 & 0 & 0 & \ldots & -1 \end{pmatrix}.$$

These hypotheses can be tested using a *Wald test*. Its test statistic is

$$(\mathbf{C}\hat{\phi})^T \mathbf{C}\hat{\mathbf{D}}^T \hat{\mathbf{H}}^{-1} \hat{\mathbf{D}} \mathbf{C}^T (\mathbf{C}\hat{\phi}) = \hat{\phi}^T \mathbf{C}^T \mathbf{C}\hat{\mathbf{D}}^T \hat{\mathbf{H}}^{-1} \hat{\mathbf{D}} \mathbf{C}^T \mathbf{C}\hat{\phi},$$

with the matrix $\hat{\mathbf{D}}^T \hat{\mathbf{H}}^{-1} \hat{\mathbf{D}}$ given by (3.15). When n is large, under certain regularity conditions, the null distribution of the statistic can be approximated by a χ^2 distribution with $Q - 1$ degrees of freedom. Therefore, the p-value for the test can be approximated by the probability under this distribution to the right of the observed value of the statistic. This p-value can be used to decide whether to accept or reject the null hypothesis at a given significance level.

3.3.7 Model Comparison

Often we are interested in comparing fits of two models to the same data where one model is a special case of the other. Such models are called *nested*. Suppose the larger model has K_2 and the smaller model has K_1 $(K_1 < K_2)$ unknown parameters. Because of nesting, we can assume without loss of generality that the smaller model is obtained by fixing $K_2 - K_1$ parameters in the larger model at known values, usually zeros. This means the problem of comparing two nested models can be formulated as the problem of testing a null hypothesis that assigns known values to these $K_2 - K_1$ parameters, against the alternative hypothesis that represents the complement of the null. If the null hypothesis is accepted, the smaller is adequate. But if it is rejected, the larger model is taken to provide a better fit than the smaller model.

These hypotheses can be tested using the *likelihood ratio test*. Suppose L_2 is the maximum likelihood for the larger model, that is, its likelihood function evaluated at the ML estimate, and L_1 is the maximum likelihood for the smaller model. The test statistic for the likelihood ratio test is

$$2\log(L_2/L_1) = 2\{\log(L_2) - \log(L_1)\}. \tag{3.32}$$

This statistic is non-negative because by construction we have $L_2 \geq L_1$, implying $\log(L_2) \geq \log(L_1)$. Under certain regularity conditions, when n is large, the null distribution of the test statistic can be approximated by a χ^2 distribution with $K_2 - K_1$ degrees of freedom. Thus, the p-value for the test can be approximated by the probability under this distribution to the right of the observed value of the statistic. The p-value can be used to decide whether to accept the null hypothesis and select the smaller model, or reject the null hypothesis and select the larger model.

In the context of mixed-effects models, the smaller model is often obtained by setting the variance of a random effect in the larger model equal to zero. This results in violation of one of the regularity conditions for the likelihood ratio test, which requires the parameters under the null hypothesis to be in the interior of the parameter space. Although the test can still be used to compare the two models, it becomes conservative in that its p-value is greater than what it should be (see Bibliographic Note).

An alternative to comparing models using likelihood ratio tests is to use information theoretic criteria such as *Akaike information criterion* (AIC) and *Bayesian information criterion* (BIC). For a given model with $\boldsymbol{\theta}$ as the $K \times 1$ vector of unknown parameters that is fit by the ML method to a dataset consisting of N observations, these are defined as

$$\text{AIC} = -2\log\{L(\hat{\boldsymbol{\theta}})\} + 2K,$$
$$\text{BIC} = -2\log\{L(\hat{\boldsymbol{\theta}})\} + K\log(N), \tag{3.33}$$

where $\hat{\boldsymbol{\theta}}$ is the ML estimator of $\boldsymbol{\theta}$. One can think of these criteria as representing a compromise between the goodness-of-fit of the model, as measured by the first term in the sum on the right, and the complexity of the model, as measured by the second term. We would like the model to provide a good fit without being overly complex. The principle of "smaller is better" is used for comparing two or more models using these criteria. In other words, the model with the smallest value of a criterion is preferred on the basis of that criterion. As is obvious from (3.33), the two criteria differ in the penalty for model complexity—$2K$ in the case of AIC versus $K\log(N)$ in the case of BIC. If $N > 8$, we have $\log(N) > 2$, implying that BIC > AIC for the same data. The converse is true for $N \leq 7$. Unlike the likelihood ratio test, these model comparison criteria do not require the models to be nested and provide a less formal approach for model selection.

3.4 MODELING AND ANALYSIS OF METHOD COMPARISON DATA

In a method comparison study, we have measurements from two or more methods on each subject in the study. The data on the same subject are dependent while those from different subjects are independent. This particular feature of the data makes it particularly attractive for modeling by a mixed-effects model of the form (3.1). Our task now is to develop a general framework for mixed-effects modeling and analysis of method comparison data.

To fix ideas, consider a method comparison study involving $J\,(\geq 2)$ methods and n subjects. The subjects are indexed as $i = 1, \ldots, n$, and the methods as $j = 1, \ldots, J$. Let there be m_{ij} measurements from method j on subject i. The $m_{ij} \times 1$ vector of these measurements is $\mathbf{Y}_{ij}$. Let $M_i = \sum_{j=1}^{J} m_{ij}$ and $N = \sum_{i=1}^{n} M_i$ denote the total number of measurements on subject i and in the study, respectively.

We would like the modeling framework to be flexible enough to allow for more than two methods, multiple measurements from each method on every subject, balanced or unbalanced designs, covariates, and heteroscedasticity. Besides these basic requirements, some additional considerations regarding multilevel fixed effects, random effects, and within-subject errors arise while developing a general framework. These include the following:

- There may be two types of fixed effects. One at the level of subjects that do not depend on the methods, for example, the effects of gender or age of the subject, and the other at the level of methods that may or may not depend on the subjects. For example, the main effect of the methods themselves and the method × gender interaction effects are both method-level fixed effects, but the main effect of the methods does not depend on the subjects, whereas the interaction does.

- There may be two types of random effects as well. One at the level of subjects that do not depend on the method, for example, the effects of the subjects themselves, and the other at the level of methods that are nested within the subjects, for example, subject × method interactions.

- The within-subject errors necessarily depend on the methods, but the parameters of their distributions may also be of two types. One that changes with the method, for example, the error variances, and the other that is common across all the methods, for example, an autocorrelation parameter.

Further, the nature of the method comparison problem itself suggests that the data from each method should be modeled in a similar way so as to allow differences in marginal characteristics of the methods to be reflected in the measures of similarity. In particular, this means that the models for data from different methods should be identical except for possible differences in values of the model parameters and aspects of models that are tied to the study design, for example, the number of measurements on a subject.

These considerations suggest a mixed-effects model of the following form for the data vectors $\mathbf{Y}_{ij}, j = 1, \ldots, J, i = 1, \ldots, n$:

$$\mathbf{Y}_{ij} = \mathbf{X}_{ij}^{(0)}\boldsymbol{\beta}_0 + \mathbf{X}_{ij}^{(1)}\boldsymbol{\beta}_j + \mathbf{Z}_{ij}^{(0)}\mathbf{u}_{i0} + \mathbf{Z}_{ij}^{(1)}\mathbf{u}_{ij} + \mathbf{e}_{ij}, \tag{3.34}$$

where

- $\boldsymbol{\beta}_0$ is the vector of fixed effects common to all methods,

- $\boldsymbol{\beta}_j$ is the vector of fixed effects of method j,

- $\mathbf{u}_{i0}$ is the vector of random effects of subject i common to all methods,

- $\mathbf{u}_{ij}$ is the vector of random effects of subject i specific to method j,

- $\mathbf{X}_{ij}^{(0)}, \mathbf{X}_{ij}^{(1)}, \mathbf{Z}_{ij}^{(0)}$, and $\mathbf{Z}_{ij}^{(1)}$ are full rank design matrices associated with $\boldsymbol{\beta}_0, \boldsymbol{\beta}_j, \mathbf{u}_{i0}$, and $\mathbf{u}_{ij}$, respectively, and

- $\mathbf{e}_{ij}$ is the vector of within-subject random errors of method j.

It is also assumed that, with appropriate dimensions,

- $\mathbf{u}_{i0}$ follow independent $\mathcal{N}(\mathbf{0}, \mathbf{G}_0)$ distributions,

- $\mathbf{u}_{ij}$ follow independent $\mathcal{N}(\mathbf{0}, \mathbf{G}_j)$ distributions,

- $\mathbf{e}_{ij}$ follow independent $\mathcal{N}(\mathbf{0}, \mathbf{R}_{ij})$ distributions, and

- $\mathbf{u}_{i0}, \mathbf{u}_{ij}$, and $\mathbf{e}_{ij}$ are mutually independent.

The covariance matrices are positive definite. They are generally represented in terms of a relatively small number of parameters. We have deliberately avoided specifying dimensions of the vectors and matrices involved in this model to avoid introducing much new notation. They should be clear from the context.

The marginal models for the J methods are of the same form in that their mean vectors and covariance matrices of random effects as well as errors are parameterized identically. The models may differ in values of the parameters but the parameters hold the same interpretation across the J models. This, in particular, implies that the columns of the design matrices correspond to identical effects. This way the differences

$$\boldsymbol{\beta}_j - \boldsymbol{\beta}_l, \ \mathbf{u}_{ij} - \mathbf{u}_{il},$$

for $j \neq l$ are well defined even though $\mathbf{Y}_{ij}$ and $\mathbf{Y}_{il}$ may have different dimensions. The model (3.34) can be written in the form of the general mixed-effects model (3.1) by defining the various vectors and matrices as (Exercise 3.14)

$$
\mathbf{Y}_i = \begin{pmatrix} \mathbf{Y}_{i1} \\ \mathbf{Y}_{i2} \\ \vdots \\ Y_{iJ} \end{pmatrix}, \; \mathbf{X}_i = \begin{pmatrix} \mathbf{X}_{i1}^{(0)} & \mathbf{X}_{i1}^{(1)} & \mathbf{0} & \cdots & \mathbf{0} \\ \mathbf{X}_{i2}^{(0)} & \mathbf{0} & \mathbf{X}_{i2}^{(1)} & \cdots & \mathbf{0} \\ \vdots & \vdots & \vdots & \vdots & \vdots \\ \mathbf{X}_{iJ}^{(0)} & \mathbf{0} & \mathbf{0} & \cdots & \mathbf{X}_{iJ}^{(1)} \end{pmatrix}, \; \boldsymbol{\beta} = \begin{pmatrix} \boldsymbol{\beta}_0 \\ \boldsymbol{\beta}_1 \\ \vdots \\ \boldsymbol{\beta}_J \end{pmatrix},
$$

$$
\mathbf{Z}_i = \begin{pmatrix} \mathbf{Z}_{i1}^{(0)} & \mathbf{Z}_{i1}^{(1)} & \mathbf{0} & \cdots & \mathbf{0} \\ \mathbf{Z}_{i2}^{(0)} & \mathbf{0} & \mathbf{Z}_{i2}^{(1)} & \cdots & \mathbf{0} \\ \vdots & \vdots & \vdots & \vdots & \vdots \\ \mathbf{Z}_{iJ}^{(0)} & \mathbf{0} & \mathbf{0} & \cdots & \mathbf{Z}_{iJ}^{(1)} \end{pmatrix}, \; \mathbf{u}_i = \begin{pmatrix} \mathbf{u}_{i0} \\ \mathbf{u}_{i1} \\ \vdots \\ \mathbf{u}_{iJ} \end{pmatrix}, \; \mathbf{e}_i = \begin{pmatrix} \mathbf{e}_{i1} \\ \mathbf{e}_{i2} \\ \vdots \\ \mathbf{e}_{iJ} \end{pmatrix},
$$

$$
\mathbf{G} = \operatorname{diag}\{\mathbf{G}_0, \ldots, \mathbf{G}_J\}, \; \mathbf{R}_i = \operatorname{diag}\{\mathbf{R}_{i1}, \ldots, \mathbf{R}_{iJ}\}. \tag{3.35}
$$

It follows from the assumptions for the model (3.34) that $(\mathbf{Y}_{i1}, \ldots, \mathbf{Y}_{iJ})$—the vector of all observations on subject i—jointly follows independent multivariate normal distributions for $i = 1, \ldots, n$ with (Exercise 3.13)

$$
E(\mathbf{Y}_{ij}) = \mathbf{X}_{ij}^{(0)} \boldsymbol{\beta}_0 + \mathbf{X}_{ij}^{(1)} \boldsymbol{\beta}_j,
$$

$$
\operatorname{var}(\mathbf{Y}_{ij}) = \mathbf{Z}_{ij}^{(0)} \mathbf{G}_0 \mathbf{Z}_{ij}^{(0)T} + \mathbf{Z}_{ij}^{(1)} \mathbf{G}_j \mathbf{Z}_{ij}^{(1)T} + \mathbf{R}_{ij},
$$

$$
\operatorname{cov}(\mathbf{Y}_{ij}, \mathbf{Y}_{il}) = \mathbf{Z}_{ij}^{(0)} \mathbf{G}_0 \mathbf{Z}_{il}^{(0)T}, \; j \neq l = 1, \ldots, J. \tag{3.36}
$$

The mixed-effects model (3.34) offers a general framework for handling method comparison. It allows modeling of the mean functions through both common and method-specific fixed effects. It also allows for dependence in a subject's multiple measurements from the same method through both common and method-specific random effects of the subject. Dependence in a subject's measurements from different methods is modeled through common random effects. It lets the covariance matrices of the within-subject errors vary with subject and method, allowing one to account for correlation and certain forms of heteroscedasticity in the errors as well. Special cases of (3.34) are used throughout the book to model various types of continuous data. The model assumes that the method-specific random effects of a subject are independent and so are the within-subject errors of the methods. These assumptions are informed by what we have seen in practice. They may need to be relaxed in some applications.

While employing this model in practice, one has to ensure that the model is *identifiable*. A model is called identifiable if no two different combinations of its parameter values lead to the same data distribution. It becomes non-identifiable if it is overparameterized and in this case there is not enough information in the data to estimate all the model parameters (see Section 1.6.1 for an example). To make matters worse, a model fitting software generally does not check for identifiability and may happily provide estimates without any warning. However, at least some of the estimates will be meaningless. The remedy for this includes simplifying the model by reducing the number of parameters, changing the model, or collecting more data, though not by simply increasing the number of subjects.

Even if the model is identifiable, it may happen that estimates of some of its parameters are not reliable in that they have unrealistically large standard errors. This often happens when the data do not have enough information to *reliably* estimate all parameters of the model. A prime example of this is the mixed-effects model (1.19) for paired measurements data (see Chapter 4). This model is identifiable, but the estimate of at least one within-subject variance is frequently unreliable. The remedies for this problem are the same as those for a non-identifiable model.

The principle of model parsimony calls for not having more parameters in the model than what is really necessary. However, a key goal in the analysis of method comparison data is evaluation of similarity and agreement of the methods. On one extreme, if all method-specific parameters are equal across the methods, then the methods are as similar as they possibly can be and they may seem to agree well. But this is just an artifact of the model assumptions. On the other extreme, if all method-specific parameters are assumed unequal, then this may result in a non-identifiable model. In practice, we need to be somewhere between these extremes. Therefore, the guiding principle for us is to let the method-specific parameters that are crucial for evaluating similarity and agreement differ across the methods without worrying about model parsimony. At the minimum, we let the methods have their own fixed intercepts and error variances and include a random subject-specific intercept in the model, provided that the model remains identifiable and the parameters are estimated reliably.

After building an adequate model, the attention shifts to the evaluation of similarity and agreement of the measurement methods. This requires two-sided confidence intervals for measures of similarity and one-sided confidence bounds for measures of agreement. To construct these intervals and bounds, usually we first define $\mathbf{Y} = (Y_1, \ldots, Y_J)^T$ as the vector of a single measurement from each of the methods on a randomly selected subject from population. One may think of this $\mathbf{Y}$ as representing typical measurements from the methods. Next, we determine the joint distribution of $\mathbf{Y}$ that is induced by the assumed model. The mechanics of how this is done is illustrated in later chapters. The distribution of $\mathbf{Y}$ depends on the vector θ of model parameters. Then we use this distribution to derive expressions for measures of similarity and agreement as functions ϕ of θ. In the next step, we use the methodology outlined in Section 3.3 to estimate these measures and construct appropriate confidence bounds and intervals for them (see Chapters 4, 5, and 7). If the distribution of $\mathbf{Y}$ depends on a covariate, this computation is repeated over the range of values of the covariate that may be of interest (see Chapters 6, 8, and 9).

3.5   CHAPTER SUMMARY

1. A mixed-effects model offers a flexible framework for modeling data where the observations on the same subject are dependent and those on different subjects are independent.

2. The method comparison data are naturally modeled by a mixed-effects model.

3. Standard large-sample inference based on a mixed-effects model assumes that the number of subjects is large and uses normal sampling distributions.

4. If the number of subjects is not large, bootstrap confidence intervals tend to be more accurate and are recommended.

3.6 BIBLIOGRAPHIC NOTE

Pinheiro and Bates (2000) provide a good introduction to linear mixed-effects models. These authors provide a succinct but lucid account of estimation theory as well as computational details. They use a large number of examples to illustrate how their `nlme` package for fitting mixed-effects model can be used to analyze real data. These examples deal with the whole gamut of issues involved in data analysis—from plots and exploratory analysis to model diagnostics and inference. They also discuss testing for zero variance of a random effect. Searle et al. (1992) and McCulloch et al. (2008) discuss prediction in mixed-effects models in detail.

For data with outliers and skewness, a number of authors propose replacing the normality assumption for random effects or errors with generalizations of the normal distribution. In particular, Verbeke and Lesaffre (1996) consider a finite mixture of normals as the distribution of the random effects. Zhang and Davidian (2001) use a semi-nonparametric representation of random effects. Pinheiro et al. (2001) use a joint t distribution for random effects and errors. Independent multivariate skew-normal distributions for random effects and errors are assumed in Arellano-Valle et al. (2005). Ho and Lin (2010) assume a joint skew-t distribution for random effects and errors. Choudhary et al. (2014) and Sengupta et al. (2015) use a skew-t distribution for random effects and an independent t distribution for errors.

Lehmann (1998) gives an excellent introduction to large-sample theory of inference, including that of the ML estimators. The regularity conditions needed for the asymptotic normality of ML estimators to hold can also be found in Chapter 7 of this book. Efron and Tibshirani (1993) and Davison and Hinkley (1997) provide clear comprehensive accounts of bootstrap, including its applications.

To compute simultaneous confidence intervals and bounds, one needs percentiles of appropriate functions of multivariate normally distributed pivots (Section 3.3.2). These can be computed, for example, using the `multcomp` package of Hothorn et al. (2008) in R. It uses an algorithm of Genz (1992) for efficient computation of multivariate normal probabilities.

Specific mixed-effects models for method comparison data have been considered by a number of authors, including Carrasco and Jover (2003), Quiroz (2005), Lai and Shiao (2005), Carstensen et al. (2008), and Choudhary (2008). These authors also consider likelihood-based inference on specific agreement measures. For example, Carstensen et al. (2008) and Lai and Shiao (2007) focus on limits of agreement; Choudhary (2008) considers TDI; and Carrasco and Jover (2003) and Quiroz (2005) focus on CCC. Lin et al. (2007) also consider a mixed-effects model and discuss inference on several agreement measures, including TDI and CCC. But they use a generalized estimating equations approach (GEE; Hardin and Hilbe, 2012) to fit the model instead of the ML approach. Carrasco and Jover (2003) and Lin et al. (2007) use Fisher's z-transformation for inference on CCC even though the range on the transformed scale does not constitute the real line.

EXERCISES

3.1 Verify that the marginal distribution of $\mathbf{Y}_1, \ldots, \mathbf{Y}_n$ following the mixed-effects model (3.1) is given by (3.2).

3.2 Consider the mixed-effects model (3.1).

    (a) Verify that the joint distribution of $(\mathbf{u}_i, \mathbf{Y}_i)$ is given by (3.3).

    (b) Deduce that the conditional distribution of $\mathbf{u}_i|\mathbf{Y}_i$ is given by (3.4).

3.3 Suppose Y and u are continuous univariate random variables. We want to predict u using a function $\tilde{u}$ of Y. The predictor's error is measured using its *mean absolute prediction error*, $E(|\tilde{u} - u|)$.

    (a) Show that the constant c that minimizes $E(|u - c|)$ is the median of u.

    (b) Deduce that the predictor $\tilde{u}$ that minimizes $E\{(|\tilde{u} - u|)|Y\}$ is the conditional median of u given Y.

    (c) Show that the conditional median in (b) is also the best predictor in the sense of minimizing the mean absolute prediction error.

    (d) Assume now that Y and u are independent and the median u_0 of u is known. Deduce that u_0 is the best predictor $\tilde{u}$.

3.4 (Brockwell and Davis, 2001) Suppose Y and u are random variables with $\mu = E(u)$ and $\sigma^2 = \text{var}(u)$. We want to predict u using a function $\tilde{u}$ of Y. The predictor's error is measured using its mean squared prediction error, $E(\tilde{u} - u)^2$.

    (a) Show that the constant c that minimizes $E(u - c)^2$ is $c = \mu$. What is the minimum value?

    (b) Deduce that the predictor $\tilde{u}$ that minimizes $E\{(\tilde{u} - u)^2|Y\}$ is $\tilde{u} = E(u|Y)$.

    (c) Show that $\tilde{u} = E(u|Y)$ is also the best predictor in the sense of minimizing the mean squared prediction error.

    (d) Assume now that Y and u are independent and μ is known. Deduce that the best predictor is $\tilde{u} = \mu$.

3.5 (A generalization of Exercise 3.4; Brockwell and Davis, 2001) Suppose $Y_1, \ldots, Y_n$ and u are random variables with $\mu = E(u)$ and $\sigma^2 = \text{var}(u)$. We would like to predict u using a function $\tilde{u}$ of $Y_1, \ldots, Y_n$, with error measured by the predictor's mean squared prediction error.

    (a) Show that the predictor $\tilde{u}$ that minimizes $E\{(\tilde{u} - u)^2|Y_1, \ldots, Y_n\}$ is $\tilde{u} = E(u|Y_1, \ldots, Y_n)$.

    (b) Deduce that $\tilde{u} = E(u|Y_1, \ldots, Y_n)$ is also the best predictor.

    (c) Assume now that $Y_1, \ldots, Y_n$ and u are i.i.d. and μ is known. Deduce that the best predictor is $\tilde{u} = \mu$.

    (d) Assume that the conditions of part (c) hold except that μ is now unknown. Consider *estimating* μ in terms of $Y_1, \ldots, Y_n$ using a linear unbiased estimator. Show that the sample mean $\overline{Y} = (Y_1 + \ldots + Y_n)/n$ is the best linear unbiased estimator of μ in that it minimizes the variance of the estimator.

    (e) Assume that the conditions of part (d) hold. Returning to prediction of u using $Y_1, \ldots, Y_n$, deduce that $\overline{Y}$ is the best linear unbiased predictor of u.

3.6 (Another generalization of Exercise 3.4) Suppose we want to predict a $q \times 1$ random vector $\mathbf{u}$ using an $m \times 1$ random vector $\mathbf{Y}$. The two vectors have a joint distribution. Suppose the error of a predictor $\tilde{\mathbf{u}}$—a $q \times 1$ function of $\mathbf{Y}$—is measured using

$$C = E\{(\tilde{\mathbf{u}} - \mathbf{u})^T \mathbf{B}(\tilde{\mathbf{u}} - \mathbf{u})\},$$

where $\mathbf{B}$ is a $q \times q$ positive definite symmetric matrix. The mean squared prediction error defined in (3.6) is obtained by taking $\mathbf{B}$ to be an identity matrix.

(a) Show that the best predictor that minimizes the above criterion is $\tilde{\mathbf{u}} = E(\mathbf{u}|\mathbf{Y})$.

(b) For the best predictor $\tilde{\mathbf{u}}$, establish the following claims:

 i. It is unbiased for $\mathbf{u}$.
 ii. The covariance matrix of its prediction error is $\mathrm{var}(\tilde{\mathbf{u}} - \mathbf{u}) = E\{\mathrm{var}(\mathbf{u}|\mathbf{Y})\}$.
 iii. $\mathrm{cov}(\tilde{\mathbf{u}}, \mathbf{u}) = \mathrm{var}(\tilde{\mathbf{u}})$.
 iv. $\mathrm{cov}(\tilde{\mathbf{u}}, \mathbf{Y}) = \mathrm{cov}(\mathbf{u}, \mathbf{Y})$.

3.7 Consider the same setup as in Exercise 3.6 but restricted to predictors $\tilde{\mathbf{u}}$ that are linear in $\mathbf{Y}$, that is, are of the form

$$\tilde{\mathbf{u}} = \mathbf{AY} + \mathbf{b},$$

where $\mathbf{A}$ is a $q \times m$ matrix and $\mathbf{b}$ is a $q \times 1$ vector. This exercise follows McCulloch et al. (2008, Chapter 13) to find the best linear predictor $\tilde{\mathbf{u}}$ by minimizing the generalized mean squared prediction error C given in Exercise 3.6 with respect to $\mathbf{A}$ and $\mathbf{b}$. (For an excellent introduction to vector calculus, see Graybill (2001).)

(a) Show that the criterion to be minimized can be written as

$$C = \mathbf{b}^T \mathbf{Bb} + E\{(\mathbf{AY} - \mathbf{u})^T \mathbf{B}(\mathbf{AY} - \mathbf{u})\} + 2\mathbf{b}^T \mathbf{B} E(\mathbf{AY} - \mathbf{u}).$$

(b) Solve $\partial C / \partial \mathbf{b} = \mathbf{0}$ for $\mathbf{b}$ and verify that the solution is

$$\mathbf{b} = -E(\mathbf{AY} - \mathbf{u}).$$

(c) Show that with $\mathbf{b}$ found in part (b) the criterion C can be expressed as

$$\mathrm{tr}\{\mathbf{B}\, \mathrm{var}(\mathbf{AY} - \mathbf{u})\}.$$

Deduce that minimizing this expression with respect to $\mathbf{A}$ is equivalent to minimizing $\mathrm{tr}(\mathbf{BE})$, where $\mathbf{E}$ is a $q \times q$ matrix given by

$$\mathbf{E} = \mathbf{A}\mathrm{var}(\mathbf{Y})\mathbf{A}^T - \mathbf{A}\mathrm{cov}(\mathbf{Y}, \mathbf{u}) - \mathrm{cov}(\mathbf{u}, \mathbf{Y})\mathbf{A}^T.$$

Denoting the ith row of $\mathbf{A}$ as $\mathbf{a}_i^T$ and the jth column of $\mathrm{cov}(\mathbf{Y}, \mathbf{u})$ as $\mathbf{c}_j$, the (i, j)th element of $\mathbf{E}$ can be written as

$$\mathbf{a}_i^T \mathrm{var}(\mathbf{Y})\mathbf{a}_j - \mathbf{a}_i^T \mathbf{c}_j - \mathbf{c}_i^T \mathbf{a_j}, \quad i, j = 1, \ldots, q.$$

(d) Solve $\partial \mathrm{tr}(\mathbf{BE}) / \partial \mathbf{a}_i = \mathbf{0}$ for $\mathbf{a}_i$ and verify that the solution is

$$\mathbf{a}_i = \mathrm{var}(\mathbf{Y})^{-1} \mathbf{c}_i, \quad i = 1, \ldots, q.$$

The solutions can be written in the matrix form as

$$\mathbf{A} = \operatorname{cov}(\mathbf{u}, \mathbf{Y})\operatorname{var}(\mathbf{Y})^{-1}.$$

(e) Deduce from parts (b) and (d) that the desired best linear predictor is

$$\tilde{\mathbf{u}} = E(\mathbf{u}) + \operatorname{cov}(\mathbf{u}, \mathbf{Y})\operatorname{var}(\mathbf{Y})^{-1}\{\mathbf{Y} - E(\mathbf{Y})\}.$$

(f) Argue that solving $\partial C/\partial \mathbf{b} = \mathbf{0}$ in part (b) to get $\mathbf{b}$ and solving $\partial \operatorname{tr}(\mathbf{BE})/\partial \mathbf{a}_i = 0$, $i = 1, \ldots, q$ in (d) to get $\mathbf{A}$ defined there are equivalent to solving

(i) $E(\text{prediction error}) = \mathbf{0}$,   (ii) $\operatorname{cov}(\text{prediction error}, \mathbf{Y}) = \mathbf{0}$.

The equations (i) and (ii) above, respectively, imply that the best linear predictor is unbiased and its error is uncorrelated with $\mathbf{Y}$.

(g) Show that covariance matrix of the prediction error $\tilde{\mathbf{u}} - \mathbf{u}$ of the best linear predictor is

$$\operatorname{var}(\tilde{\mathbf{u}} - \mathbf{u}) = \operatorname{var}(\mathbf{u}) - \operatorname{cov}(\mathbf{u}, \mathbf{Y})\operatorname{var}(\mathbf{Y})^{-1}\operatorname{cov}(\mathbf{Y}, \mathbf{u}).$$

3.8 Suppose that $\mathbf{Y}$ follows the mixed-effects model

$$\mathbf{Y} = \mathbf{X}\boldsymbol{\beta} + \mathbf{Z}\mathbf{u} + \mathbf{e},$$

where

$$E\begin{pmatrix}\mathbf{u}\\\mathbf{e}\end{pmatrix} = \begin{pmatrix}\mathbf{0}\\\mathbf{0}\end{pmatrix}, \quad \operatorname{cov}\begin{pmatrix}\mathbf{u}\\\mathbf{e}\end{pmatrix} = \begin{pmatrix}\mathbf{G} & \mathbf{0}\\\mathbf{0} & \mathbf{R}\end{pmatrix}.$$

The dimensions of these vectors and matrices can be taken from (3.3) applied to a single subject i. Also, as before, $\mathbf{V} = \mathbf{Z}\mathbf{G}\mathbf{Z}^T + \mathbf{R}$ is $\operatorname{var}(\mathbf{Y})$ and $\operatorname{cov}(\mathbf{u}, \mathbf{Y}) = \mathbf{G}\mathbf{Z}^T$. Assume that $\boldsymbol{\beta}$ is unknown but $\mathbf{G}$ and $\mathbf{R}$ are known. We would like to jointly estimate $\boldsymbol{\beta}$ and $\mathbf{u}$. This exercise follows McCulloch et al. (2008, Chapter 13) to find the BLUP of the scalar quantity

$$\mathbf{s}^T\mathbf{X}\boldsymbol{\beta} + \mathbf{t}^T\mathbf{u},$$

where $\mathbf{s}$ and $\mathbf{t}$ are arbitrary known vectors. This involves finding a predictor of the form $\mathbf{a}^T\mathbf{Y}$ that minimizes the mean squared prediction error

$$E\{(\mathbf{a}^T\mathbf{Y} - \mathbf{s}^T\mathbf{X}\boldsymbol{\beta} - \mathbf{t}^T\mathbf{u})^2\}$$

with respect to the vector $\mathbf{a}$, subject to the unbiasedness condition

$$E(\mathbf{a}^T\mathbf{Y}) = E(\mathbf{s}^T\mathbf{X}\boldsymbol{\beta} + \mathbf{t}^T\mathbf{u}).$$

(a) Show that the unbiasedness condition is equivalent to $\mathbf{X}^T\mathbf{a} = \mathbf{X}^T\mathbf{s}$. Deduce that, under this condition, the mean squared prediction error is the variance of the prediction error, given as

$$\operatorname{var}(\mathbf{a}^T\mathbf{Y} - \mathbf{s}^T\mathbf{X}\boldsymbol{\beta} - \mathbf{t}^T\mathbf{u}) = \mathbf{a}^T\mathbf{V}\mathbf{a} + \mathbf{t}^T\mathbf{G}\mathbf{t} - 2\mathbf{a}^T\mathbf{Z}\mathbf{G}\mathbf{t}.$$

(b) Let $2\boldsymbol{\lambda}$ be a vector of *Lagrange multipliers*. Then, the expression to be minimized with respect to $\mathbf{a}$ and $\boldsymbol{\lambda}$ is

$$\operatorname{var}(\mathbf{a}^T\mathbf{Y} - \mathbf{s}^T\mathbf{X}\boldsymbol{\beta} - \mathbf{t}^T\mathbf{u}) + 2\boldsymbol{\lambda}^T(\mathbf{X}^T\mathbf{a} - \mathbf{X}^T\mathbf{s}).$$

Show that **a** and λ that minimize this expression are solutions of

$$\begin{pmatrix} \mathbf{V} & \mathbf{X} \\ \mathbf{X}^T & \mathbf{0} \end{pmatrix} \begin{pmatrix} \mathbf{a} \\ \lambda \end{pmatrix} = \begin{pmatrix} \mathbf{ZGt} \\ \mathbf{X}^T \mathbf{s} \end{pmatrix}.$$

(c) Show that solving for **a** leads to the desired BLUP of $\mathbf{s}^T \mathbf{X} \beta + \mathbf{t}^T \mathbf{u}$ as

$$\mathbf{a}^T \mathbf{Y} = \mathbf{s}^T \mathbf{X} \tilde{\beta} + \mathbf{t}^T \mathbf{G} \mathbf{Z}^T \mathbf{V}^{-1} (\mathbf{Y} - \mathbf{X}\tilde{\beta}),$$

where

$$\tilde{\beta} = \left(\mathbf{X}^T \mathbf{V}^{-1} \mathbf{X} \right)^{-1} \mathbf{X}^T \mathbf{V}^{-1} \mathbf{Y}$$

is the BLUE of β. It is also the generalized least squares estimator of β.

(d) Deduce that $\mathbf{G} \mathbf{Z}^T \mathbf{V}^{-1} (\mathbf{Y} - \mathbf{X}\tilde{\beta})$ is the BLUP of **u**.

(e) Compare the BLUP with the best linear predictor found in Exercise 3.7, part (e).

3.9 Consider the setup of Exercises 3.6 and 3.7. Assume in addition that $(\mathbf{u}, \mathbf{Y})$ jointly follow a multivariate normal distribution. Show that the best predictor and the best linear predictor of **u** are identical.

3.10 Suppose the interval (L, U) is a $100(1-\alpha)\%$ confidence interval for a monotonically increasing function g of parameter θ. Let g^{-1} be the inverse function of g.

(a) Show that $\left(g^{-1}(L), g^{-1}(U)\right)$ is a $100(1-\alpha)\%$ confidence interval for θ.

(b) Suppose $0 < \theta < 1$ and $g(\theta) = \log\{\theta/(1-\theta)\}$. Determine g^{-1}.

(c) What will be the confidence interval for θ if g is a monotonically decreasing function of θ?

3.11 Consider the pivots $Z_1, \ldots, Z_Q$ defined in (3.18). Use (3.15) to show that the joint distribution of the Z_q can be approximated by a Q-variate normal distribution with mean vector $\mathbf{0}$ and covariance matrix obtained by pre- and post-multiplying $\hat{\mathbf{D}}^T \hat{\mathbf{H}}^{-1} \hat{\mathbf{D}}$ by a diagonal matrix whose elements are reciprocals of the standard errors $\mathrm{SE}(\hat{\phi}_1), \ldots, \mathrm{SE}(\hat{\phi}_Q)$, given by (3.17).

3.12 Show that the probability statements in (3.24) follow from (3.23).

3.13 Show that the joint distribution of $(\mathbf{Y}_{i1}, \ldots, \mathbf{Y}_{iJ})$ under the mixed-effects model (3.34) is multivariate normal with parameters given by (3.36).

3.14 Verify that the model (3.34) can be written in the form (3.1) by using the vectors and matrices defined in (3.35).

CHAPTER 4

PAIRED MEASUREMENTS DATA

4.1 PREVIEW

Even though the paired measurements design is not a good choice for method comparison studies, it remains by far the most commonly used design in practice. This chapter coalesces ideas from previous chapters to present a methodology for analysis of paired measurements data. The methodology follows the steps outlined in Section 1.16. Modeling of data via either a mixed-effects model or a bivariate normal model is considered. Evaluation of similarity and agreement under the assumed model is taken up next. Three case studies are used to illustrate the methodology.

4.2 MODELING OF DATA

4.2.1 Mixed-Effects Model

The data consist of paired measurements (Y_{i1}, Y_{i2}), $i = 1, \ldots, n$, by two measurement methods on n randomly selected subjects from a population. In principle, there are two choices for modeling these data (Section 1.12). The preferred one is the mixed-effects model (1.19), which is written as

$$Y_{i1} = b_i + e_{i1}, \ \ Y_{i2} = \beta_0 + b_i + e_{i2}, \ \ i = 1, \ldots, n, \tag{4.1}$$

where

Measuring Agreement: Models, Methods, and Applications. By P. K. Choudhary and H. N. Nagaraja
Copyright © 2017 John Wiley & Sons, Inc.

- the true values b_i follow independent $\mathcal{N}_1(\mu_b, \sigma_b^2)$ distributions,

- the random errors e_{ij} follow independent $\mathcal{N}_1(0, \sigma_{ej}^2)$ distributions, $j = 1, 2$, and

- the true values and the random errors are mutually independent.

This model implicitly assumes that the methods have the same scale (Section 1.12.2). The paired measurements are i.i.d. as (Y_1, Y_2), and their differences $D_i = Y_{i2} - Y_{i1}$ are i.i.d. as D. From (1.20), (1.21), and (1.24), we have

$$\begin{pmatrix} Y_1 \\ Y_2 \end{pmatrix} \sim \mathcal{N}_2 \left(\begin{pmatrix} \mu_b \\ \beta_0 + \mu_b \end{pmatrix}, \begin{pmatrix} \sigma_b^2 + \sigma_{e1}^2 & \sigma_b^2 \\ \sigma_b^2 & \sigma_b^2 + \sigma_{e2}^2 \end{pmatrix} \right), \quad D \sim \mathcal{N}_1 \left(\beta_0, \sigma_{e1}^2 + \sigma_{e2}^2 \right).$$
(4.2)

The ML estimates—$(\hat{\beta}_0, \hat{\mu}_b, \hat{\sigma}_b^2, \hat{\sigma}_{e1}^2, \hat{\sigma}_{e2}^2)$—of model parameters can be obtained by using a statistical software for fitting mixed-effects models. In fact,

$$\hat{\beta}_0 = \overline{Y}_{\cdot 2} - \overline{Y}_{\cdot 1}, \quad \hat{\mu}_b = \overline{Y}_{\cdot 1},$$
(4.3)

and often the other estimates can be obtained explicitly as well (Exercise 4.2). It is a good idea to examine especially the estimates of error variances and their standard errors to ensure that they are estimated reliably (Section 1.12.2). The predicted random effects $\hat{b}_i$ are

$$\hat{b}_i = \hat{\mu}_b + \frac{\hat{\sigma}_b^2 \{ \hat{\sigma}_{e2}^2 (Y_{i1} - \overline{Y}_{\cdot 1}) + \hat{\sigma}_{e1}^2 (Y_{i2} - \overline{Y}_{\cdot 2}) \}}{(\hat{\sigma}_b^2 + \hat{\sigma}_{e1}^2)(\hat{\sigma}_b^2 + \hat{\sigma}_{e2}^2) - \hat{\sigma}_b^4},$$
(4.4)

and the fitted values $\hat{Y}_{ij}$ and the residuals $\hat{e}_{ij}$ are (Exercise 4.3)

$$\hat{Y}_{i1} = \hat{b}_i, \quad \hat{Y}_{i2} = \hat{\beta}_0 + \hat{b}_i, \quad \hat{e}_{ij} = Y_{ij} - \hat{Y}_{ij}, \quad j = 1, 2.$$
(4.5)

The model adequacy is checked by performing model diagnostics (Section 3.2.4). Mild departures from normality of either residuals or random effects are not of much concern because generally they do not lead to seriously incorrect estimates of parameters of interest and their standard errors. However, presence of a trend or nonconstant scatter in the residual plot casts doubt on the respective assumptions of independence of true values and errors and homoscedasticity of error distributions. Moreover, a trend in the Bland-Altman plot (Section 1.13) may indicate violation of the equal scales assumption. These violations may not be benign because, in this case, the extent of agreement between the methods depends on the magnitude of measurement, contradicting what is implied by the model. Often, these assumptions hold after a log transformation of the data. These plots may also reveal outliers. If they are present and cannot be attributed to coding errors, their influence should be examined as well. At the minimum, this involves analyzing data with and without the outliers and comparing the key conclusions. During model evaluation we are not interested in checking whether a submodel with $\beta_0 = 0$ or $\sigma_{e1}^2 = \sigma_{e2}^2$ provides an equally good but a more parsimonious fit to the data. We let each of the two methods have its own accuracy and precision-related parameters under our model, and use inference on measures of similarity (Section 1.7) to examine their closeness. The differences in these marginal characteristics of the methods are also reflected in the measures of agreement.

4.2.2 Bivariate Normal Model

Quite often, the error variances in the mixed-effects model (4.1) are not estimated reliably (Section 1.12.2). This is evident when at least one of the estimates has a rather large standard error, or when one of the estimates is nearly zero and the other is substantially larger. Generally this happens because the paired measurements do not have enough information to reliably estimate the error variances. In this case, we fit the bivariate normal model (Section 1.12.3), which simply postulates that the paired measurements are i.i.d. as (Y_1, Y_2), where

$$\begin{pmatrix} Y_1 \\ Y_2 \end{pmatrix} \sim \mathcal{N}_2 \left(\begin{pmatrix} \mu_1 \\ \mu_2 \end{pmatrix}, \begin{pmatrix} \sigma_1^2 & \sigma_{12} \\ \sigma_{12} & \sigma_2^2 \end{pmatrix} \right), \tag{4.6}$$

with $\sigma_{12} = \rho\sigma_1\sigma_2$ and ρ denoting the correlation. It follows that the differences D_i are i.i.d. as D, where

$$D \sim \mathcal{N}_1 \left(\xi = \mu_2 - \mu_1, \tau^2 = \sigma_1^2 + \sigma_2^2 - 2\sigma_{12} \right). \tag{4.7}$$

Unlike (4.1), this model does not make any assumptions about the relationship between the observed measurements, their underlying true values, and the random errors. Neither does it require the assumption of a common scale for the methods. Further, the methods have a positive correlation under (4.1), whereas there is no such constraint here. However, the methods in practice do tend to have a positive correlation.

The use of a bivariate normal model has consequences for evaluation of similarity of methods (Section 1.12.3), but reliable estimation of its parameters is generally not an issue. The ML estimators of these parameters and of their functions appearing in (4.7) are given by their sample counterparts (Exercise 4.1),

$$\hat{\mu}_j = \overline{Y}_{\cdot j}, \ \hat{\sigma}_j^2 = \frac{n-1}{n} S_j^2, \ j = 1, 2, \ \hat{\sigma}_{12} = \frac{n-1}{n} S_{12}, \ \hat{\rho} = R,$$

$$\hat{\xi} = \overline{D}, \ \hat{\tau}^2 = \frac{n-1}{n} S_D^2, \tag{4.8}$$

where the sample moments are from (1.16) and (1.17).

Checking the adequacy of the fitted bivariate normal model involves examining the assumptions of normality and homoscedasticity of data. Bivariate normality can be assessed by using normal Q-Q plots to examine marginal normality of paired measurements as well as their linear combinations such as means and differences. The marginal Q-Q plots can be supplemented by a χ^2 Q-Q plot for direct assessment of bivariate normality (Section 3.2.4). The homoscedasticity assumption can be verified by examining the Bland-Altman plot (Section 1.13.3) and a trellis plot of the data. Absence of a trend in the Bland-Altman plot is suggestive of common scales for the methods. In this case, the mean difference $\mu_2 - \mu_1$ can be interpreted as the fixed bias difference β_0 (Section 1.7). These plots may also reveal outliers. As usual, if outliers are present, their influence needs to be investigated by analyzing data with and without them and comparing the conclusions of interest.

Here we have presented the bivariate normal model (4.6) as a fallback to the mixed-effects model (4.1) for the situation when the estimation of error variances is problematic. However, if $\rho > 0$, one may think of (4.6) as (4.1) with model parameters reparameterized as first- and second-order population moments of (Y_1, Y_2),

$$\begin{pmatrix} \mu_1 \\ \mu_2 \end{pmatrix} = \begin{pmatrix} \mu_b \\ \beta_0 + \mu_b \end{pmatrix}, \begin{pmatrix} \sigma_1^2 & \sigma_{12} \\ \sigma_{12} & \sigma_2^2 \end{pmatrix} = \begin{pmatrix} \sigma_b^2 + \sigma_{e1}^2 & \sigma_b^2 \\ \sigma_b^2 & \sigma_b^2 + \sigma_{e2}^2 \end{pmatrix}. \tag{4.9}$$

Under certain conditions (given in Exercise 4.2), the ML estimators of these moments are identical under the two models.

4.3 EVALUATION OF SIMILARITY AND AGREEMENT

Under the mixed-effects model, the methods have the same scale and hence their sensitivity ratio is identical to the precision ratio (Section 1.7). Therefore, the methods differ only in two marginal characteristics—fixed biases and precisions. Thus, similarity can be evaluated by examining estimates and two-sided confidence intervals for the intercept β_0 and the precision ratio $\lambda = \sigma_{e1}^2/\sigma_{e2}^2$. If λ is not estimated reliably, possibly because the estimated error variances have large standard errors, the confidence interval of λ will be unreliable. In this case, we have to forgo comparing precisions of the methods. This point is moot if we switch to the bivariate normal model.

The bivariate normal model does not allow inference on any measure of similarity (Section 1.12.3). Nevertheless, one can compare the means and variances of the methods by examining estimates and two-sided confidence intervals for the mean difference $\mu_2 - \mu_1$ and the variance ratio σ_2^2/σ_1^2. Of course, $\mu_2 - \mu_1$ equals β_0 under the equal scales assumption, but in general the two may differ because the differences in fixed biases and scales of the methods get confounded in $\mu_2 - \mu_1$, see (1.10). Even then, if the mean difference is close to zero we can often conclude that the methods have similar fixed biases and scales. The inference on variance ratio, however, may not be that informative. From (1.8), the differences in scales and error variances get confounded in σ_2^2/σ_1^2. Since the between-subject variation typically dominates the within-subject variation, the variance ratio may be close to 1 regardless of whether or not the precision ratio is close to 1.

To evaluate agreement between the methods, we can take any scalar agreement measure that is a function of parameters of the bivariate distribution of (Y_1, Y_2), replace the population quantities in its definition by their counterparts under the assumed model, and examine its estimate and appropriate one-sided confidence bound. For example, recall the CCC and TDI defined by (2.6) and (2.29), respectively. They are

$$\text{CCC} = \frac{2\sigma_{12}}{(\mu_1 - \mu_2)^2 + \sigma_1^2 + \sigma_2^2}, \quad \text{TDI}(p) = \left\{\tau^2 \chi_{1,p}^2 \left(\xi^2/\tau^2\right)\right\}^{1/2}. \tag{4.10}$$

These measures can be used directly under the bivariate normal model. Under the mixed-effects model, these can be expressed by replacing the population moments of (Y_1, Y_2) and D by their model-based counterparts in (4.2) to obtain

$$\text{CCC} = \frac{2\sigma_b^2}{\beta_0^2 + 2\sigma_b^2 + \sigma_{e1}^2 + \sigma_{e2}^2},$$

$$\text{TDI}(p) = \left\{(\sigma_{e1}^2 + \sigma_{e2}^2) \chi_{1,p}^2 \left(\beta_0^2/\{\sigma_{e1}^2 + \sigma_{e2}^2\}\right)\right\}^{1/2}. \tag{4.11}$$

For both the mixed-effects and bivariate models, the ML estimators of measures of similarity and agreement are obtained by replacing the model parameters in their definitions with their ML estimators. Then, the large-sample theory of ML estimators is used to compute standard errors and confidence bounds and intervals (Section 3.3). Further, the 95% limits of agreement are given as

$$\hat{\xi} \pm 1.96\,\hat{\tau}, \tag{4.12}$$

where $\hat{\xi}$ and $\hat{\tau}$ are given in (4.8).

For the mixed-effects model, if the difference β_0 in fixed biases is appreciable, it may be reasonable to reevaluate agreement by transforming method 2 measurements as $Y_{i2}^* = Y_{i2} - \beta_0$ and $Y_2^* = Y_2 - \beta_0$. For this, one can simply repeat the analysis by subtracting $\hat{\beta}_0$ from method 2 measurements. We can achieve a similar end for the bivariate normal model by using the mean difference $\mu_2 - \mu_1$ in place of β_0, provided the equal scales assumption holds.

4.4 CASE STUDIES

We now revisit the three datasets introduced in Section 1.13 and analyze them using the methodology described in this chapter. The analysis follows the five key steps outlined in Section 1.16, namely, visualization, modeling, evaluation of similarity, evaluation of agreement, and review of causes of disagreement. The last step is aimed at a recalibration strategy to increase agreement between the methods. Here and elsewhere in the book the unit of measurement is generally mentioned with the data description and is omitted thereafter for brevity.

4.4.1 Oxygen Saturation Data

This dataset, introduced in Section 1.13.1, consists of measurements of percent saturation of hemoglobin with oxygen in 72 adults, obtained using an oxygen saturation monitor (OSM, method 1) and a pulse oximetry screener (POS, method 2). The scatterplot and the Bland-Altman plot of these data shown in Figure 1.3 indicate that the methods are highly correlated and have similar scales. The trellis plot of these data displayed in Figure 4.1 shows some overlap in the readings produced by the methods, but it is also apparent that POS measurements tend to be smaller than OSM, especially in the middle of the measurement range. The data appear homoscedastic.

We first fit the mixed-effects model (4.1). But $\hat{\sigma}_{e1}^2$ has a large standard error (Exercise 4.4), leading us to question the reliability of the estimate. Therefore, we prefer the bivariate normal model (4.6). The resulting ML estimates and standard errors are presented in Table 4.1. None of the estimates has an unusually large standard error. The adequacy of bivariate normality is checked in Exercise 4.4. Substituting these estimates in (4.6) gives the *fitted distributions* of (Y_1, Y_2) and D as follows:

$$\begin{pmatrix} Y_1 \\ Y_2 \end{pmatrix} \sim \mathcal{N}_2 \left(\begin{pmatrix} 89.50 \\ 89.09 \end{pmatrix}, \begin{pmatrix} 74.57 & 74.42 \\ 74.42 & 75.72 \end{pmatrix} \right), \quad D \sim \mathcal{N}_1 \left(-0.41, 1.45 \right).$$

Clearly, POS measurements are on average a bit smaller than OSM, and both methods have similar variabilities. The correlation between the methods is 0.99. The differences in measurements have a standard deviation of 1.2. Further, the 95% limits of agreement from (4.12) are $(-2.77, 1.94)$.

For similarity evaluation under the bivariate normal model, we must be content with inference on the mean difference $\mu_2 - \mu_1$ and the variance ratio σ_2^2/σ_1^2. The estimate of $\mu_2 - \mu_1$ is -0.41 and its 95% confidence interval is $(-0.69, -0.13)$. Thus, there is evidence that the mean for POS is slightly smaller than OSM. But this difference may be considered negligibly small because the measurements range between 70 and 100, with

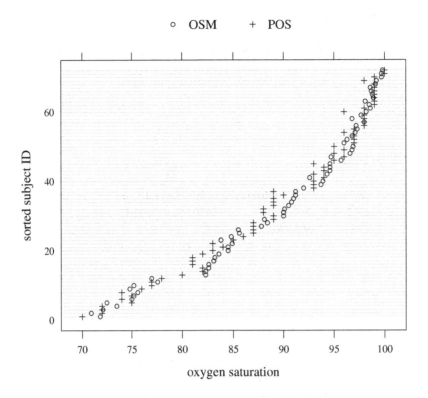

Figure 4.1 Trellis plot of oxygen saturation data.

the average around 89. Note that this $\mu_2 - \mu_1$ can be interpreted as β_0 as the equal scales assumption appears reasonable for these data. The estimate of σ_2^2/σ_1^2 is 1.02 and its 95% confidence interval is $(0.95, 1.08)$, confirming similar variances for the methods.

The next step is evaluation of agreement. Table 4.1 also provides estimates and 95% one-sided confidence bounds for agreement measures CCC and TDI(0.90). A lower bound is provided for CCC, whereas an upper bound is provided for TDI. For greater accuracy in estimation, the confidence bounds are computed by first applying the Fisher's z-transformation to CCC and the log transformation to TDI, and then transforming the results back to the original scale (Section 3.3.3). The estimate 0.989 and the lower bound 0.984 for CCC indicate a high degree of agreement between the methods. Nonetheless, a high CCC is almost guaranteed here because the between-subject variation in the data is much greater than the within-subject variation (see Figure 4.1). More informative are the estimate 2.09 and upper bound 2.40 for TDI(0.90). From the tolerance interval interpretation of TDI's upper bound (Section 2.8), it follows that 90% of differences in OSM and POS measurements lie within ± 2.40 with 95% confidence. Given that the measurements range between 70 and 100, a difference of 2.4 may be considered too small to be clinically important.

As the methods differ in means (or fixed biases under the equal scales assumption), it is of interest to recalibrate POS by subtracting $\hat{\mu}_2 - \hat{\mu}_1 = -0.41$ from its measurements, and reevaluate its agreement with OSM. Of course, the estimated means are identical after

Parameter	Estimate	SE
μ_1	89.50	1.02
μ_2	89.08	1.03
$\log(\sigma_1^2)$	4.31	0.17
$\log(\sigma_2^2)$	4.33	0.17
$z(\rho)$	2.67	0.12
$z(\text{CCC})$	2.61	0.12
$\log\{\text{TDI}(0.90)\}$	0.74	0.08

Similarity Evaluation		
Measure	Estimate	95% Interval
$\mu_2 - \mu_1$	-0.41	$(-0.69, -0.13)$
σ_2^2/σ_1^2	1.02	$(0.95, 1.08)$

Agreement Evaluation		
Measure	Estimate	95% Bound
CCC	0.989	0.984
TDI(0.90)	2.091	2.397

Table 4.1 Summary of estimates of bivariate normal model parameters and measures of similarity and agreement for oxygen saturation data. Lower bound for CCC and upper bound for TDI are presented. Methods 1 and 2 refer to OSM and pulse, respectively.

recalibration, but there is only a slight improvement in the extent of agreement. The estimate of CCC and its lower bound, respectively, increase to 0.990 and 0.986, and the estimate of TDI(0.90) and its upper bound, respectively, decrease to 1.98 and 2.27. The conclusion here is that if a difference in OSM and POS of 2.4 is considered clinically unimportant, then these methods agree sufficiently well to be used interchangeably. This conclusion holds regardless of whether POS is recalibrated or not.

4.4.2 Plasma Volume Data

This dataset, introduced in Section 1.13.2, consists of measurements of plasma volume in 99 subjects using the Hurley method (method 1) and the Nadler method (method 2). Unlike the oxygen saturation data, these data show a difference in proportional biases of the methods. But it vanishes after a log transformation and the assumption of equal scales is satisfied for log-scale measurements. The trellis plot in Figure 1.10 shows that, with only a few exceptions, the Nadler measurements are higher than Hurley's by nearly a constant amount. Of course, this indicates unequal fixed biases of the methods. The data seem homoscedastic.

First we fit the mixed-effects model (4.1) and Table 4.2 summarizes the results. None of the standard errors is especially large, and $\hat{\beta}_0$ has a small standard error. This is not surprising given the near constancy of differences seen in the trellis plot. Figure 4.2 presents the residual plot from the fitted model. Lack of any discernible pattern in this plot supports the model. Evaluation of normality assumption is taken up in Exercise 4.5. For comparison, Table 4.2 also presents estimates resulting from fitting the bivariate normal model to the

Mixed-Effects Model			Bivariate Normal Model		
Parameter	Estimate	SE	Parameter	Estimate	SE
β_0	0.10	0.002	μ_1	4.48	0.02
μ_b	4.48	0.02	μ_2	4.58	0.02
$\log(\sigma_b^2)$	−3.69	0.14	$\log(\sigma_1^2)$	−3.67	0.14
$\log(\sigma_{e1}^2)$	−8.07	1.11	$\log(\sigma_2^2)$	−3.68	0.14
$\log(\sigma_{e2}^2)$	−8.78	2.25	$z(\rho)$	2.69	0.10

Both Models		
Parameter	Estimate	SE
$z(\text{CCC})$	1.19	0.07
$\log\{\text{TDI}(0.90)\}$	−2.07	0.02

Similarity Evaluation		
Measure	Estimate	95% Interval
β_0 (or $\mu_2 - \mu_1$)	0.099	$(0.095, 0.103)$
σ_2^2/σ_1^2	0.994	$(0.942, 1.048)$

Agreement Evaluation		
Measure	Estimate	95% Bound
CCC	0.830	0.792
TDI(0.90)	0.127	0.132

Table 4.2   Summary of estimates of model parameters and measures of similarity and agreement for log-scale plasma volume data. Lower bound for CCC and upper bound for TDI are presented. Methods 1 and 2 refer to Hurley and Nadler methods, respectively.

data. As expected, both models lead to the same fitted distributions of (Y_1, Y_2) and D;

$$\begin{pmatrix} Y_1 \\ Y_2 \end{pmatrix} \sim \mathcal{N}_2 \left(\begin{pmatrix} 4.48 \\ 4.58 \end{pmatrix}, \begin{pmatrix} 2.54 & 2.50 \\ 2.50 & 2.52 \end{pmatrix} \times 10^{-2} \right), \quad D \sim \mathcal{N}_1 \left(0.10, 4.7 \times 10^{-4} \right).$$

We see that log-scale measurements of Nadler exceed those of Hurley by 0.10 on average, the measurements have similar variabilities, and their correlation is 0.99. From (1.4), both methods have reliabilities around 0.99. The differences have a small standard deviation. The 95% limits of agreement are $(−0.04, 0.23)$.

To evaluate similarity, Table 4.2 provides an estimate of 0.10 and a 95% confidence interval of $(0.095, 0.103)$ for β_0. The interval is tight around 0.10, confirming unequal fixed biases of the methods. As in the previous case study, we have to forgo inference on the precision ratio λ because its estimate has a large standard error (Exercise 4.5). Nevertheless, the estimated variance ratio σ_2^2/σ_1^2 is practically 1 with 95% confidence interval $(0.94, 1.05)$.

To evaluate agreement, Table 4.2 provides estimates and 95% one-sided confidence bounds for CCC and TDI(0.90). These are 0.83 and 0.79, respectively, for CCC; and 0.127 and 0.132, respectively, for TDI. The TDI bound shows that 90% of differences in

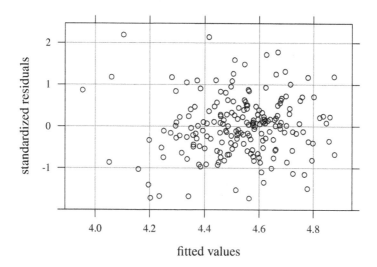

Figure 4.2 Residual plot for log-scale plasma volume data.

log-scale measurements fall within ± 0.132 with 95% confidence. This means that, with 95% confidence, 90% of Nadler over Hurley ratios fall between $\exp(-0.132) = 0.88$ and $\exp(0.132) = 1.14$. At best, this indicates a modest agreement between the methods.

It is apparent that the lack of agreement is mainly due to a difference in the fixed biases of the methods. Since the Nadler's measurements are consistently smaller than Hurley's, it is imperative that we recalibrate Nadler's log-scale measurements by subtracting $\hat{\beta}_0 = 0.10$ from them and reevaluating its agreement with Hurley method. After the recalibration, $\hat{\beta}_0 = 0$, and the estimate of CCC and its lower bound both increase to 0.99. In addition, the estimate of TDI and its upper bound decrease to 0.035 and 0.040, respectively. This allows us to conclude that the two methods agree quite well on log-scale after the recalibration. On the original untransformed scale, the bound of 0.04 implies that 90% of Nadler over Hurley ratios fall between $\exp(-0.04) = 0.96$ and $\exp(0.04) = 1.04$, a spread of ± 0.04. Thus, the agreement on the original scale is also quite good after the recalibration, which amounts to multiplying a Nadler's original measurement by $\exp(0.10) = 1.11$.

4.4.3 Vitamin D Data

This dataset, introduced in Section 1.13.3, consists of concentrations of vitamin D in 34 samples measured using two assays. There are two noteworthy features of these data. First, they exhibit heteroscedasticity and a log transformation of the data removes it, making them suitable for analysis using the models of this chapter. Second, there are four outliers in the data—three horizontal and one vertical (see panel (d) of Figure 1.5 on page 28). The horizontal outliers allow us to compare the assays over the measurement range of 0–250 instead of 0–50. The vertical outlier becomes apparent only after the log transformation. The assumption of equal scales also appears reasonable for the log-scale data. Figure 4.3

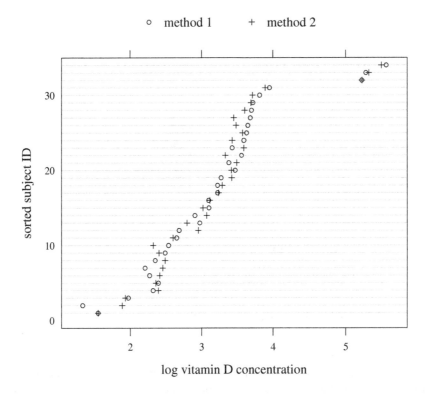

Figure 4.3   Trellis plot of log-scale vitamin D data.

shows their trellis plot. Although the measurements are close and the methods appear to have similar means, there is not a lot of overlap between the measurements.

Our next task is to find a suitable model for these data. Fitting the mixed-effects model produces a virtually zero value for $\hat{\sigma}_{e2}^2$ with a large standard error (Exercise 4.6). Therefore, we favor the bivariate normal model. Table 4.3 summarizes the results. The assumption of normality is checked in Exercise 4.6. From (4.6) and (4.7), the fitted distributions of (Y_1, Y_2) and D are

$$\begin{pmatrix} Y_1 \\ Y_2 \end{pmatrix} \sim \mathcal{N}_2 \left(\begin{pmatrix} 3.18 \\ 3.19 \end{pmatrix}, \begin{pmatrix} 0.88 & 0.82 \\ 0.82 & 0.79 \end{pmatrix} \right), \quad D \sim \mathcal{N}_1 \left(0.01, 0.026 \right).$$

On log-scale, method 1's mean exceeds that of method 2 only by a negligibly small amount, but its variance is about 10% smaller than that of method 2. The correlation of the methods is about 0.99. The differences in measurements have a somewhat large standard deviation ($\sqrt{0.026} = 0.161$). The 95% limits of agreement are $(-0.31, 0.32)$.

Table 4.3 provides estimates and confidence intervals for $\mu_2 - \mu_1$ and σ_2^2/σ_1^2. We can safely conclude that the methods have similar means and similar fixed biases because the equal scales assumption seems to hold here. But there is some evidence that the variability of method 2 is less than that of method 1. From Figure 4.3, we see that this may be partly due to an outlying method 1 observation in the bottom left corner. This is the same observation that showed up as a vertical outlier in the Bland-Altman plot in Figure 1.5.

Parameter	Estimate	SE
μ_1	3.18	0.16
μ_2	3.19	0.15
$\log(\sigma_1^2)$	-0.13	0.24
$\log(\sigma_2^2)$	-0.24	0.24
$z(\rho)$	2.48	0.17
$z(\text{CCC})$	2.43	0.16
$\log\{\text{TDI}(0.90)\}$	-1.33	0.12

Similarity Evaluation		
Measure	Estimate	95% Interval
$\mu_2 - \mu_1$	0.01	$(-0.05, 0.06)$
σ_2^2/σ_1^2	0.90	$(0.80, 1.00)$

Agreement Evaluation		
Measure	Estimate	95% Bound
CCC	0.985	0.974
$\text{TDI}(0.90)$	0.263	0.322

Table 4.3 Summary of estimates of bivariate normal model parameters and measures of similarity and agreement for vitamin D data. Lower bound for CCC and upper bound for TDI are presented.

To evaluate agreement, Table 4.3 provides estimates and confidence bounds for CCC and TDI(0.90). The lower bound of 0.97 for CCC suggests a high degree of agreement. But CCC is misleading here as these data have high between-subject variation compared to within-subject variation (see Figure 4.3). More informative is TDI's upper bound of 0.32, allowing us to claim with 95% confidence that 90% of differences in log-scale measurements fall within ± 0.32. At best, this suggests a rather modest level of agreement between the methods on log-scale. On the original scale, the ratios of measurements may fall within $\exp(-0.32) = 0.73$ and $\exp(0.32) = 1.38$. Because this interval is rather large around one, we cannot conclude good agreement for practical use.

In contrast with the plasma volume data, we cannot find a simple recalibration here that would bring the methods closer. The situation improves somewhat when the vertical outlier is removed. The 95% confidence intervals for $\mu_2 - \mu_1$ and σ_2^2/σ_1^2, respectively, become $(-0.05, 0.03)$ and $(0.95, 1.05)$. Further, TDI's upper bound reduces to 0.26, but this does not alter our final conclusion regarding agreement. We also saw three horizontal outliers in Figure 1.5. Removing them in addition to the vertical outlier leads to confidence intervals for $\mu_2 - \mu_1$ and σ_2^2/σ_1^2 as $(-0.06, 0.04)$ and $(0.76, 1.04)$, respectively; and confidence bounds for CCC and TDI become 0.95 and 0.28, respectively. Since these lead to conclusions that are qualitatively similar to the ones based on the complete data, there is no reason to exclude the outliers. This is especially true for the horizontal outliers because they allow the conclusions to hold over a wider measurement range. It is interesting to note that the removal of all four outliers leads to a slight decrease in CCC. This happens because the between-subject variation decreases while the within-subject variation remains virtually unchanged.

4.5 CHAPTER SUMMARY

1. The methodology of this chapter assumes homoscedastic data.

2. The ML method is used to estimate model parameters.

3. The assumption of equal scales is necessary for the mixed-effects model. Making this assumption simplifies the interpretation of mean difference $\mu_2 - \mu_1$ as the fixed bias difference β_0.

4. A log transformation of data may remove a difference in scales of the methods. It may also make the data homoscedastic.

5. The paired measurements data generally do not have enough information to reliably estimate error variances in the mixed-effects model.

6. If these error variances cannot be reliably estimated, the analysis is based on the bivariate normal model.

7. When both the estimated error variances are away from zero, the two models generally lead to similar results.

8. The bivariate normal model does not allow inference on measures of similarity such as the fixed bias difference β_0 and precision ratio λ. It, however, allows inference on the mean difference $\mu_2 - \mu_1$, which equals β_0 under the equal scales assumption, and the variance ratio σ_2^2 / σ_1^2.

9. If the between-subject variation in the data is high relative to the within-subject variation, the variance ratio σ_2^2 / σ_1^2 may be nearly 1 despite a considerable difference in precisions of the methods.

10. If the estimate of either β_0 or $\mu_2 - \mu_1$ is non-negligible, one of the methods can be recalibrated to improve agreement between the two methods.

11. The methodology requires a large number of subjects for the estimation of standard errors and construction of confidence bounds and intervals.

4.6 TECHNICAL DETAILS

4.6.1 Mixed-Effects Model

To represent the mixed-effects model (4.1) in the notation of Chapter 3 wherein the random effect has mean zero, define

$$\beta_1 = \mu_b, \ \beta_2 = \beta_0 + \mu_b, \ u_i = b_i - \mu_b.$$

Then, (4.1) can be written as

$$Y_{ij} = \beta_j + u_i + e_{ij}, \ j = 1, 2, \ i = 1, \ldots, n. \tag{4.13}$$

Taking

$$\mathbf{Y}_i = \begin{pmatrix} Y_{i1} \\ Y_{i2} \end{pmatrix}, \ \mathbf{e}_i = \begin{pmatrix} e_{i1} \\ e_{i2} \end{pmatrix}, \ \mathbf{X} = \mathbf{I}_2, \ \boldsymbol{\beta} = \begin{pmatrix} \beta_1 \\ \beta_2 \end{pmatrix}, \ \mathbf{Z} = \mathbf{1}_2, \tag{4.14}$$

we can write this model in the matrix notation of Chapter 3 as

$$\mathbf{Y}_i = \mathbf{X}\boldsymbol{\beta} + \mathbf{Z}u_i + \mathbf{e}_i, \ i = 1, \ldots, n, \tag{4.15}$$

where

$$u_i \sim \mathcal{N}_1(0, G = \sigma_b^2), \ \mathbf{e}_i \sim \mathcal{N}_2\left(\mathbf{0}, \mathbf{R} = \text{diag}\{\sigma_{e1}^2, \sigma_{e2}^2\}\right).$$

It follows that

$$\mathbf{Y}_i \sim \mathcal{N}_2\left(\mathbf{X}\boldsymbol{\beta}, \mathbf{V} = \mathbf{Z}G\mathbf{Z}^T + \mathbf{R}\right),$$

where the mean vector $\mathbf{X}\boldsymbol{\beta}$ and the covariance matrix $\mathbf{V}$ simplify to the expressions in (4.2). The matrices $\mathbf{X}, \mathbf{Z}, \mathbf{R}$, and $\mathbf{V}$ do not depend on i. Letting

$$\boldsymbol{\theta} = \left(\beta_0, \mu_b, \log(\sigma_b^2), \log(\sigma_{e1}^2), \log(\sigma_{e2}^2)\right)^T$$

denote the vector of transformed model parameters, the log-likelihood function is

$$\log\{L(\boldsymbol{\theta})\} = -n\log(2\pi) - \frac{n}{2}\log(|\mathbf{V}|) - \frac{1}{2}\sum_{i=1}^{n}(\mathbf{y}_i - \mathbf{X}\boldsymbol{\beta})^T\mathbf{V}^{-1}(\mathbf{y}_i - \mathbf{X}\boldsymbol{\beta}).$$

Its maximization gives the ML estimator $\hat{\boldsymbol{\theta}}$. Quite often, $\hat{\boldsymbol{\theta}}$ can be obtained explicitly (Exercise 4.2). It can also be computed using a software that fits mixed-effects models. From (3.9), the predicted random effects $\hat{u}_i$—the estimated BLUP of u_i, the fitted values $\hat{\mathbf{Y}}_i$, and the residuals $\hat{\mathbf{e}}_i$ are, respectively,

$$\hat{u}_i = \hat{G}\mathbf{Z}^T\hat{\mathbf{V}}^{-1}(\mathbf{Y}_i - \mathbf{X}\hat{\boldsymbol{\beta}}), \ \hat{\mathbf{Y}}_i = \mathbf{X}\hat{\boldsymbol{\beta}} + \mathbf{Z}\hat{u}_i, \ \hat{\mathbf{e}}_i = \mathbf{Y}_i - \hat{\mathbf{Y}}_i, \tag{4.16}$$

where $\hat{\boldsymbol{\beta}}, \hat{G}$, and $\hat{\mathbf{V}}$ are ML estimators of their population counterparts. These expressions reduce to the ones given in (4.4) and (4.5).

4.6.2 Bivariate Normal Model

For the bivariate normal model (4.6), the (transformed) model parameter vector is

$$\boldsymbol{\theta} = \left(\mu_1, \mu_2, \log(\sigma_1^2), \log(\sigma_2^2), z(\rho)\right)^T,$$

where $z(\rho)$ represents the Fisher's z-transformation of ρ, see (1.32). Letting

$$\boldsymbol{\mu} = \begin{pmatrix} \mu_1 \\ \mu_2 \end{pmatrix}, \ \mathbf{V} = \begin{pmatrix} \sigma_1^2 & \sigma_{12} \\ \sigma_{12} & \sigma_2^2 \end{pmatrix}, \tag{4.17}$$

the likelihood function is

$$L(\boldsymbol{\theta}) = \frac{1}{(2\pi)^n |\mathbf{V}|^{n/2}} \exp\left\{-\frac{1}{2}\sum_{i=1}^{n}(\mathbf{y}_i - \boldsymbol{\mu})^T\mathbf{V}^{-1}(\mathbf{y}_i - \boldsymbol{\mu})\right\}. \tag{4.18}$$

This likelihood can be explicitly maximized with respect to μ and $\mathbf{V}$ to get their ML estimators as (Exercise 4.1)

$$\hat{\mu} = \begin{pmatrix} \hat{\mu}_1 \\ \hat{\mu}_2 \end{pmatrix}, \ \hat{\mathbf{V}} = \begin{pmatrix} \hat{\sigma}_1^2 & \hat{\sigma}_{12} \\ \hat{\sigma}_{12} & \hat{\sigma}_2^2 \end{pmatrix},$$

where the various elements are defined by (4.8). Therefore,

$$\hat{\boldsymbol{\theta}} = \left(\hat{\mu}_1, \hat{\mu}_2, \log(\hat{\sigma}_1^2), \log(\hat{\sigma}_2^2), z(\hat{\rho}) \right)^T$$

is the ML estimator of $\boldsymbol{\theta}$.

Under either model, a scalar measure $\phi(\boldsymbol{\theta})$ of similarity or agreement is estimated as $\phi(\hat{\boldsymbol{\theta}})$. The standard error of this estimator and an appropriate confidence bound or interval for the measure can be computed using the large-sample approach described in Section 3.3.

4.7 BIBLIOGRAPHIC NOTE

Lin (1989) considers inference on CCC under a bivariate normal model. Carrasco and Jover (2003) estimate CCC under a mixed-effects model, somewhat different from (4.1). Inference on TDI for normally distributed differences is considered in Lin (2000), Lin et al. (2002), and Choudhary and Nagaraja (2007). Escaramis et al. (2010) compare existing procedures for estimating TDI assuming a mixed-effects model. Choudhary and Nagaraja (2007) also discuss bootstrap for inference on TDI for moderately large samples. A similar approach can be used for other measures of similarity and agreement. See Davison and Hinkley (1997) for an introduction to bootstrap. Johnson and Wichern (2002, pages 177-189) discuss assessment of bivariate normality through normal and χ^2 Q-Q plots.

EXERCISES

4.1 Assume that the paired measurements data follow the bivariate normal model (4.6). The goal of this exercise is to show that $\hat{\mu}_1$, $\hat{\mu}_2$, $\hat{\sigma}_1^2$, $\hat{\sigma}_2^2$, and $\hat{\sigma}_{12}$ given by (4.8) are ML estimators of their respective parameters. For convenience we will use the matrix notation from Section 4.6.2. By definition, the covariance matrix $\mathbf{V}$ and its sample counterpart $\hat{\mathbf{V}}$ are arbitrary *positive definite* matrices.

(a) Show that the likelihood L given by (4.18) can be written as a function of μ and $\mathbf{V}$ as

$$L(\boldsymbol{\mu}, \mathbf{V}) = \frac{1}{(2\pi)^n |\mathbf{V}|^{n/2}}$$
$$\times \exp \left[-\frac{1}{2} \left\{ n \operatorname{tr}(\mathbf{V}^{-1} \hat{\mathbf{V}}) + n(\hat{\boldsymbol{\mu}} - \boldsymbol{\mu})^T \mathbf{V}^{-1} (\hat{\boldsymbol{\mu}} - \boldsymbol{\mu}) \right\} \right].$$

(b) Deduce that for a given $\mathbf{V}$, $L(\boldsymbol{\mu}, \mathbf{V})$ is maximized with respect to μ at $\mu = \hat{\mu}$.

(c) Show that $L(\hat{\boldsymbol{\mu}}, \mathbf{V})$ is maximized with respect to $\mathbf{V}$ at $\mathbf{V} = \hat{\mathbf{V}}$ to obtain the desired result.

[*Hint:* Use the following matrix inequality result from Johnson and Wichern (2002, page 170). Given a $p \times p$ symmetric positive definite matrix $\mathbf{B}$ and a scalar $b > 0$,

$$\frac{1}{|\mathbf{V}|^b} \exp\left\{-\frac{1}{2}\text{tr}(\mathbf{V}^{-1}\mathbf{B})\right\} \leq \frac{1}{|\mathbf{B}|^b}(2b)^{pb}\exp(-bp)$$

for all positive definite $\mathbf{V}$, with equality holding only for $\mathbf{V} = (1/2b)\mathbf{B}$.]

4.2 Consider the mixed-effects model (4.1).

(a) Show that ML estimators of β_0 and μ_b are given by (4.3).

(b) Show that if $(\hat{\sigma}_1^2, \hat{\sigma}_2^2, \hat{\sigma}_{12})$ defined in (4.8) are such that $\hat{\sigma}_{12} > 0$ and $\hat{\sigma}_1^2 - \hat{\sigma}_{12}$, $\hat{\sigma}_2^2 - \hat{\sigma}_{12} \geq 0$, then ML estimators of $(\sigma_b^2, \sigma_{e1}^2, \sigma_{e2}^2)$ are

$$\hat{\sigma}_b^2 = \hat{\sigma}_{12}, \quad \hat{\sigma}_{e1}^2 = \hat{\sigma}_1^2 - \hat{\sigma}_{12}, \quad \hat{\sigma}_{e2}^2 = \hat{\sigma}_2^2 - \hat{\sigma}_{12}.$$

(c) Can these $(\hat{\sigma}_b^2, \hat{\sigma}_{e1}^2, \hat{\sigma}_{e2}^2)$ still be ML estimators if the non-negativity restriction does not hold? If not, how can they be obtained?

[*Hint:* Use Exercise 4.1 along with the reparameterization (4.9) of model parameters.]

4.3 Use (4.16) to verify the expressions for predicted random effects $\hat{b}_i$ given in (4.4) and fitted values $\hat{Y}_{ij}$ given in (4.5).

4.4 Consider the oxygen saturation data (Sections 1.13.1 and 4.4.1).

(a) Fit model (4.1). Find standard error of $\hat{\sigma}_{e1}^2$. Is σ_{e1}^2 estimated reliably?

(b) Fit model (4.6) and verify the results in Table 4.1.

(c) Perform diagnostics for model (4.6), including an assessment of bivariate normality. Does this model fit reasonably well? Explain.

4.5 Consider the log-scale plasma volume data (Sections 1.13.2 and 4.4.2).

(a) Fit both models (4.1) and (4.6), and verify the results in Table 4.2.

(b) Find the standard error of estimated precision ratio $\hat{\lambda}$. Do you think λ is estimated well? Explain.

(c) Check adequacy of both models. Be sure to evaluate the normality assumption.

4.6 Consider the log-scale vitamin D data (Sections 1.13.3 and 4.4.3).

(a) Fit model (4.1). Find standard error of $\hat{\sigma}_{e2}^2$ and comment on whether σ_{e2}^2 is estimated reliably.

(b) Fit model (4.6), and verify the results in Table 4.3.

(c) Evaluate goodness-of-fit of model (4.6). Does the bivariate normality assumption seem appropriate?

4.7 (Continuation of Exercise 1.8)

(a) Use the five steps outlined in Section 1.16 to analyze the IPI angle data.

(b) Justify the choice of your model and check its adequacy.

(c) Is there a need to transform the data for better adherence to model assumptions?

(d) Do the methods agree well enough to be used interchangeably, possibly after a recalibration?

4.8 Table 4.4 provides measurements of cardiac output (l/min) in 23 ventilated patients, made noninvasively by two observers using Doppler echocardiography.

(a) Repeat Exercise 4.7 for these data.

(b) Redo the analysis using bootstrap confidence intervals and bounds (Section 3.3.4) and note any differences in conclusions.

Patient	Observer A	Observer B	Patient	Observer A	Observer B
1	4.80	5.80	13	7.70	8.50
2	5.60	5.10	14	7.70	9.50
3	6.00	7.70	15	8.20	9.10
4	6.40	7.80	16	8.20	10.00
5	6.50	7.60	17	8.30	9.10
6	6.60	8.10	18	8.50	10.80
7	6.80	8.00	19	9.30	11.50
8	7.00	8.10	20	10.20	11.50
9	7.00	6.60	21	10.40	11.20
10	7.20	8.10	22	10.60	11.50
11	7.40	9.50	23	11.40	12.00
12	7.60	9.60			

Reprinted from Müller and Büttner (1994), ©1994 Wiley, with permission from Wiley.

Table 4.4   Cardiac output (l/min) data for Exercise 4.8.

4.9 Consider Dataset A of the oxygen consumption data introduced in Table 2.1 on page 67.

(a) Perform an exploratory data analysis using appropriate plots.

(b) Given that the data come from a test-retest experiment where the true values during the test and the corresponding retest may not be the same, does it seem appropriate to model them using (4.1)? How about using the model (4.6)? Justify your answers.

(c) Analyze these data by fitting model (4.6). Does this model provide an adequate fit? Do the test-retest measurements agree well? Explain.

(d) Repeat the above steps using Dataset B in Table 2.1. Compare your conclusions for the two datasets.

CHAPTER 5

REPEATED MEASUREMENTS DATA

5.1 PREVIEW

This chapter presents a methodology for the analysis of studies comparing two methods wherein both take multiple measurements on each subject. It focuses on two types of repeated measurements data—*unlinked* and *linked*. The usual steps in analysis consist of displaying data, modeling of data via a mixed-effects model, and associated evaluation of similarity and agreement. With repeated measurements, one can also evaluate *repeatability* of each method, which amounts to self-agreement. The methodology is illustrated with two case studies.

5.2 INTRODUCTION

Let Y_{ijk} denote the kth repeated measurement of the jth method on the ith subject. The data consist of Y_{ijk}, $k = 1, \ldots, m_{ij}$, $j = 1, 2$, $i = 1, \ldots, n$. Here n is the number of subjects in the study and m_{ij} is the number of measurements of method j on subject i. It is assumed that $m_{ij} \geq 2$. Let $M_i = m_{i1} + m_{i2}$ and $N = \sum_{i=1}^{n} M_i$, respectively, denote the total number of measurements on the ith subject and in the entire dataset. When $m_{i1} = m_{i2}$, we will use m_i to denote the common value. Moreover, when the m_i are equal, the common value will be denoted by m. The design is *balanced* if each method has the same number m of measurements on every subject, otherwise it is *unbalanced*. Measurements on the same subject are dependent, whereas those from different subjects

Measuring Agreement: Models, Methods, and Applications. By P. K. Choudhary and H. N. Nagaraja
Copyright © 2017 John Wiley & Sons, Inc.

are assumed to be independent. It is necessary to appropriately model the dependence among the repeated measurements on the same subject to get accurate estimates.

5.2.1   Types of Data

Often "repeated measurements data" is used as a catch-all term to refer to any type of data wherein multiple measurements are available on each subject. Here we distinguish between three types of repeated measurements, viz., *unlinked*, *linked*, and *longitudinal*. This distinction is important as it affects how the data are modeled. These data types are described next.

The repeated measurements on a subject are *unlinked* (or *unpaired*) if the measurements from the two methods are obtained separately, and a method's multiple measurements on a subject are independent replications of the same underlying measurement. By *replication*, we mean repeating a measurement under identical conditions, ensuring that the true value of the subject remains unchanged during the measurement period. The methods need not have the same number of measurements on a subject. Essentially a method's unlinked repeated measurements are identically distributed. They may arise, for example, when the multiple measurements are taken in quick succession or when a subject's homogeneous specimen is subsampled to get the multiple measurements. The assumption of independence holds if the multiple measurements are taken without influencing each other. The kiwi data to be introduced in Section 5.2.3 is an example of unlinked repeated measurements data.

The repeated measurements on a subject are *linked* (or *paired*) when the measurements from the two methods are made together in pairs as (Y_{i1k}, Y_{i2k}), $k = 1, \ldots, m_i$. The measurements in each pair are linked by a common condition k, which we call "time." Often this time factor is an actual measurement occasion. Obviously, the contribution of each subject to the data consists of two paired trajectories over time, one for each method. Unlike the unlinked case, the methods necessarily have an equal number of measurements on a subject. This means $m_{i1} = m_{i2} = m_i$ in our notation, but m_i may vary from subject to subject. In addition, the true value need not remain constant over time, and usually it does not. For this reason, we refrain from calling the repeated pairs as replications. Naturally, the order in which the linked measurements are made matters. However, it is assumed that there is no systematic effect of time on the paired trajectories beyond the dependence induced in them by the common measurement time. Linked repeated measurements may arise when the quantity being measured itself keeps changing, for example, blood pressure or heart rate, and it is the instantaneous measurement that is of interest. The oximetry data in Section 5.2.3 is an example of such data.

The repeated measurements on a subject are *longitudinal* when the measurements from both methods are made over a period of time, and unlike the linked case, there is a systematic fixed effect of time or a time-dependent covariate on the measurements. Thus, the contribution of each subject consists of two trajectories over time, but these may or may not be paired over the measurement times. The true value of the subject necessarily changes, making the time of measurement important. The time may be a discrete quantity with a small number of values (e.g., before and after an intervention or a visit number), or it may be a continuous quantity (e.g., age of subject at the time of measurement). Unlike linked and unlinked data, longitudinal data necessitates modeling the measurement trajectories as functions of time, warranting a special treatment of its own. Therefore, this chapter only considers unlinked and linked data; longitudinal data is the subject of Chapter 9.

5.2.2   Individual versus Average Measurement

The analysis of repeated measurements data involves a decision as to whether a subject's individual measurements or their average value should be the object of analysis. This issue is generally relevant only for the unlinked data because they consist of replications of the same underlying measurements. Linked and longitudinal data are usually not structured like this; but when they do consist of such replications, this issue would be relevant there as well.

The decision about the object of analysis is informed by how the methods are used in common practice. If it is customary to replicate measurements but use their average value, obviously the individual measurements should be averaged, and the methodology of Chapter 4 should be applied to the paired averages. If, however, we want to use the multiple measurements individually, which is usually the case in practice, the methodology of this chapter is appropriate. The measurements in this case should not be averaged prior to analysis because doing so will make the methods seem more precise, and hence the methods will exhibit more agreement than observed in practice. Even though a single measurement may be the standard procedure, it is a good idea to replicate the measurements anyway because this allows reliable estimation of precisions of the methods.

5.2.3   Example Datasets

We now introduce two datasets that will be used as illustrative examples in this chapter.

5.2.3.1   *Kiwi Eggshell Data*   These data were collected in a study of thickness of avian eggshell, a quantity of particular interest to ecologists because it has a direct bearing on the strength of the eggshell. The thickness of the shell of an egg is not uniform; the shell is thinnest and most uniform at the equator, and thickest at the two poles. The study compared two methods for measuring eggshell thickness. One is the usual caliper type micrometer (method 1) and the other is a scanning electron microscope (method 2). A micrometer is portable, cost-effective, and can be easily used anywhere. However, its use may be unsuitable if the fragility of eggshells is of concern. This may happen, for instance, if the eggshells come from museum collections. The microscope offers a less invasive alternative than the micrometer, but it has disadvantages of its own. They include its cost, time, and electricity requirement, restricting its usage, for example, in remote locations.

In the study, the thickness of eggshell fragments from the equatorial region of eggs of 16 North Island brown kiwis (*Apteryx mantelli*), which are small flightless birds native to New Zealand, was measured (in μm) at three randomly selected locations using both methods. The three locations for each method were different. Each eggshell fragment came from a different egg and the same individual took all the measurements. The design of this study is balanced. Repeated measurements here are unlinked because the two methods measure at different locations and the true value at these locations are considered same due to uniformity of thickness in the equatorial region.

5.2.3.2   *Oximetry Data*   The oximetry data come from a study conducted in infants at Royal Children's Hospital in Melbourne, Australia. It compared two methods for measuring percent oxygen saturation in blood, namely, pulse oximetry (method 1) and CO-oximetry (method 2). The former is a noninvasive method that indirectly measures oxygen saturation using a sensor placed on a thin body part, for example, fingertip. The latter uses a blood

specimen to directly measure oxygen saturation. The study involved 61 infants. Among them, 56 were measured on three occasions, four were measured on two occasions, and one was measured on only one occasion. Thus, the study design was unbalanced. The repeated measurements here are linked because they are paired over the measurement times.

5.3 DISPLAYING DATA

5.3.1 Basic Plots

Basic graphical tools for displaying paired data wherein each subject contributes a pair of measurements are the trellis plot, the scatterplot, and the Bland-Altman plot. These plots need to be adapted to display repeated measurements data. A key consideration is that, in addition to displaying the usual data features, they should also allow us the ability to effectively examine the within- and between-subject variations—a key motivation for collecting repeated measurements in the first place.

5.3.1.1 Trellis Plot By design, the vertical axis of this plot is divided into rows and each row displays all data on a subject using method-specific symbols. Thus, for unlinked as well as linked data, each row will now have multiple measurements per method instead of a single measurement it had for the paired data. Figures 5.1 and 5.2 show trellis plots of kiwi and oximetry data, respectively. The first data are unlinked, whereas the second data are linked. A trellis plot, in addition to allowing examination of the overlap of the data produced by the two methods and comparison of their biases, makes it easy to see a number of data features of interest. It shows how the within-subject variations of the two methods compare, whether they change with magnitude of measurement or not, and how they relate to the between-subject variation. It also shows whether there is any subject × method interaction. It, however, does not preserve information about the pairing that is inherent in the linked data. Detailed interpretation of the plots is postponed until Section 5.7, where the case studies are presented.

5.3.1.2 Scatterplot and Bland-Altman Plot Ordinarily, these plots display one measurement pair per subject and the data from different subjects are independent, justifying using the same plotting symbol for each subject. With linked repeated measurements, each subject contributes multiple *dependent* measurement pairs. This dependence structure can be shown in the plot by using a subject-specific plotting symbol. Otherwise that information will be lost and the plots will often give a wrong impression of the dependence structure. A numerical subject ID is a natural choice for the subject-specific plotting symbol. In practice, however, it may be hard to distinguish between the subjects if a large number of them cluster together. This happens in the top panel of Figure 5.3, where scatterplot and Bland-Altman plot are shown for the oximetry data. Another possibility is to use the same symbol for all data but connect the points coming from the same subject by a line. This version is presented in the bottom panel of Figure 5.3. Both versions essentially convey the same information, and they do not show the within-subject variation as clearly as the trellis plot.

The unlinked data do not have natural pairings of a subject's multiple measurements from the two methods. However, to display them in a scatterplot or a Bland-Altman plot, we need to identify one pair per subject. There are two ways to form such pairs. One

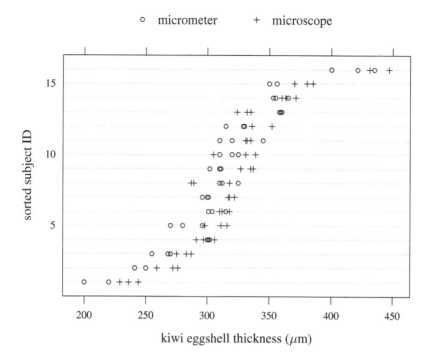

Figure 5.1 Trellis plot of kiwi data.

is to randomly select one measurement per method from the available measurements of a subject. The justification for this is that the unlinked repeated measurements data are assumed to exhibit a distributional symmetry. Randomly choosing only one measurement per method to display in the plot preserves the essential information and is supported by this symmetry. The other alternative is to compute method-specific averages for each subject. But the averaging will make the methods appear more precise and show better agreement than shown by individual pairs, especially if the within-subject variation is large. In either case, the resulting plots may look sparse if n is small. In addition, their construction masks the within-subject variation. Figure 5.4 displays both versions of the scatterplot and the Bland-Altman plot for the kiwi data. The effect of averaging is more visible in the Bland-Altman plot in the form of reduced range for the difference on the vertical axis.

For linked data we have not considered plots based on either single measurements or averages. This is because the true values therein may change over the measurement period. Taking only a single measurement or an average will result in substantial loss of information, making this an inadequate choice. We also see that none of the modified versions of the scatterplot shows the within-subject variation as clearly as a trellis plot. Nonetheless, the scatterplots as well as the Bland-Altman plots are useful because they provide complementary information, just like in the case of paired data.

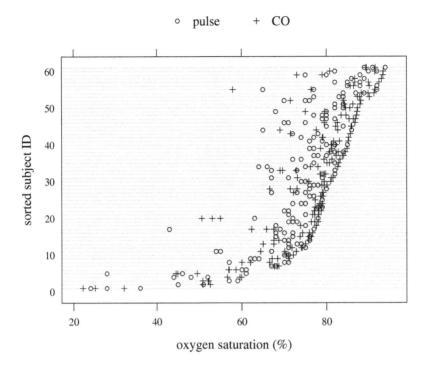

Figure 5.2   Trellis plot of oximetry data.

5.3.2 Interaction Plots

Repeated measurements data also allow us to incorporate certain interactions in the analysis that may be present in the data (see Section 5.4). The two interactions of particular interest are subject × method interaction, relevant for both unlinked and linked data, and subject × time interaction, relevant only for the latter. While it may be possible to see evidence of their presence in the aforementioned plots, it is formally explored through *interaction plots*. To describe them, let

$$\overline{Y}_{ij\cdot} = \frac{1}{m_{ij}} \sum_{k=1}^{m_{ij}} Y_{ijk}, \ \ j = 1, 2, \ i = 1, \ldots, n,$$

be the average over the repeated measurements for method j, and

$$\overline{Y}_{i \cdot k} = \frac{Y_{i1k} + Y_{i2k}}{2}, \ \ k = 1, \ldots, m_i,$$

be the average over the methods at time k. The latter is relevant only for linked data, in which case $m_{ij} = m_i$.

For subject × method interaction, we can plot average $\overline{Y}_{ij\cdot}$ against method j $(j = 1, 2)$, separately for each subject i, with points for each subject connected by a line. Similarly, for subject × time interaction, we can plot average $\overline{Y}_{i \cdot k}$ against time k $(k = 1, \ldots, m_i)$, separately for each subject i, with points for each subject connected by lines. Both these

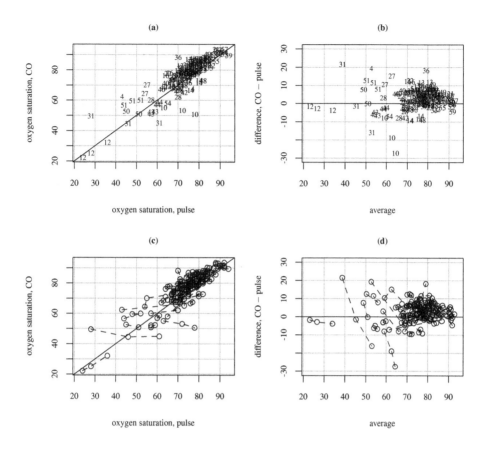

Figure 5.3 Plots for oximetry data. Top panel (left to right): Scatterplot with line of equality and Bland-Altman plot with zero line, with subject ID (1 to 61) as plotting symbol. Bottom panel (left to right): Same as top panel but with a common plotting symbol and points from the same subject joined by a broken line.

interaction plots consist of n connected lines, one for each subject. In either case, there is evidence of interaction if the lines are not parallel.

Figure 5.5 displays a subject × method interaction plot for kiwi data. Figure 5.6 displays two interaction plots for oximetry data—one for subject × method interaction and the other for subject × time interaction. All show clear evidence of interaction.

5.4 MODELING OF DATA

Models for repeated measurements data depend on whether they are unlinked or linked. We consider these scenarios in turn.

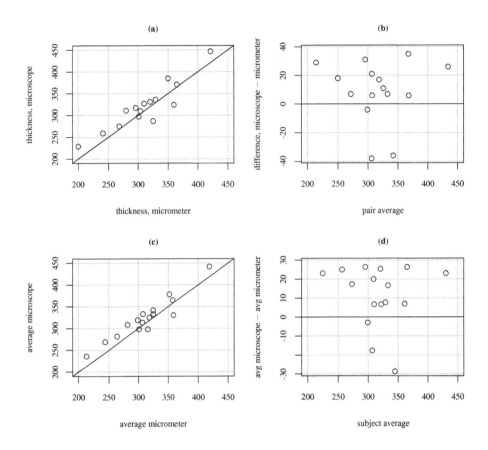

Figure 5.4 Plots for kiwi eggshell thickness data. Top panel (left to right): Scatterplot with line of equality and Bland-Altman plot with zero line based on 16 randomly formed measurement pairs. Bottom panel (left to right): Same as top panel but based on 16 average measurements.

5.4.1 Unlinked Data

Here the data consist of Y_{ijk}, $k = 1, \ldots, m_{ij}$, $j = 1, 2$, $i = 1, \ldots, n$, where a method's multiple measurements on a subject are replications of the same underlying measurement. The two methods are replicated separately, implying that their measurements on a subject are dependent but not paired. The measurements from different subjects are assumed to be independent, as always. To model these data, we consider the basic mixed-effects model (4.1) for paired measurements data and add to it a random subject × method inter-action term b_{ij}. Thus, the model can be written as

$$Y_{i1k} = b_i + b_{i1} + e_{i1k}, \quad Y_{i2k} = \beta_0 + b_i + b_{i2} + e_{i2k}, \tag{5.1}$$

$k = 1, \ldots, m_{ij}$, $j = 1, 2$, $i = 1, \ldots, n$. As in (4.1), the methods are assumed to have the same scale. Moreover, b_i remains the true unobservable measurement of the ith subject, β_0 remains the difference in the fixed biases of the methods, and e_{ijk} are random errors.

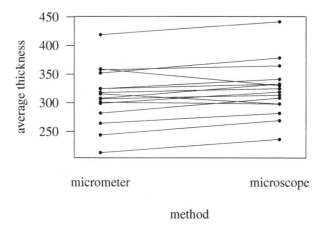

Figure 5.5   Interaction plot for kiwi data depicting subject × method interaction. Lines join points from the same subject.

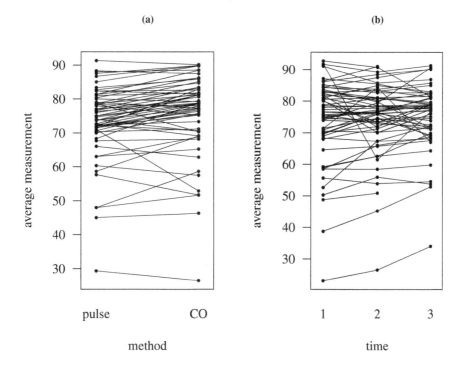

Figure 5.6   Interaction plots for oximetry data depicting subject × method interaction (left panel) and subject × time interaction (right panel). Lines join points from the same subject.

We now consider interpreting the interaction term b_{ij}. One way is to think of it as the effect of method j on subject i. In other words, these interactions are subject-specific biases of the methods. For another interpretation, recall that b_i and $\beta_0 + b_i$ are, respectively, the true values of methods 1 and 2 for subject i (Section 1.6). However, their error-free values under (5.1) are $b_i + b_{i1}$ and $\beta_0 + b_i + b_{i2}$, respectively. The true values and the error-free values differ by b_{ij} in the case of method j. This suggests that b_{ij} can be interpreted as an *error in equation* of method j. The equation error b_{ij} is different from the random error e_{ijk}. The former is a characteristic of the method-subject combination that remains stable during the measurement period. The latter fluctuates from measurement to measurement within a subject. While we call b_{ij} as an interaction in keeping with the terminology in mixed-effects modeling, it is indeed called an equation error in measurement error modeling. It is also known as a *matrix effect* in analytical chemistry. A matrix refers to a substance that dissolves a chemical of interest. It plays the role of a subject in our terminology.

To complete the specification of the model (5.1), we make the usual normality and independence assumptions for the random quantities:

- b_i follow independent $\mathcal{N}_1(\mu_b, \sigma_b^2)$ distributions,

- b_{ij} follow independent $\mathcal{N}_1(0, \psi^2)$ distributions,

- e_{ijk} follow independent $\mathcal{N}_1(0, \sigma_{ej}^2)$ distributions, and

- b_i, b_{ij}, and e_{ijk} are mutually independent.

The random errors have method-specific variances, but the interaction effects have a common variance for the two methods. It is also possible to let the variance of the interaction term depend on the method. Although the resulting model is identifiable, reliable estimation of both the variances becomes an issue. A similar situation arose in Chapter 4 for estimation of two error variances with paired data. Therefore, we assume a common variance for the interactions for the time being. This assumption is relaxed in Chapter 7, where more than two methods are compared.

In model (5.1), the effect of a subject manifests on the measurements through three independent quantities, namely, b_i, b_{i1}, and b_{i2}. Upon averaging out the subject effects we see that the vectors of $M_i = m_{i1} + m_{i2}$ measurements on subject $i = 1, \ldots, n$ follow independent M_i-variate normal distributions with means (Exercise 5.1)

$$E(Y_{i1k}) = \mu_b, \quad E(Y_{i2k}) = \beta_0 + \mu_b \tag{5.2}$$

and variances

$$\mathrm{var}(Y_{ijk}) = \sigma_b^2 + \psi^2 + \sigma_{ej}^2. \tag{5.3}$$

Further,

$$\mathrm{cov}(Y_{ijk}, Y_{ijl}) = \sigma_b^2 + \psi^2, \quad k \neq l \tag{5.4}$$

is the common covariance between two replications of the same method, and

$$\mathrm{cov}(Y_{i1k}, Y_{i2l}) = \sigma_b^2 \tag{5.5}$$

is the common covariance between any two measurements from different methods on the same subject. The first covariance involves two variance components because a method's replications on a subject i shares two random effects—the true measurement b_i and the interaction effect b_{ij}. The second covariance involves only one variance component because the measurements from different methods share only the b_i. The model (5.1) has a total of six unknown parameters, namely, $(\beta_0, \mu_b, \sigma_b^2, \psi^2, \sigma_{e1}^2, \sigma_{e2}^2)$.

Even though we have replicated measurements, our ultimate interest is in evaluating how close a measurement from one method on a subject is to a measurement from the other method on the same subject. This evaluation requires examination of measures of similarity and agreement derived from the distribution of (Y_1, Y_2), a pair of measurements by the two methods on a randomly selected subject from the population (Section 1.7). The assumed model (5.1) induces a distribution for (Y_1, Y_2). Drop the subscripts i and k in (5.1) to obtain the companion model for (Y_1, Y_2) as

$$Y_1 = b + b_1 + e_1, \quad Y_2 = \beta_0 + b + b_2 + e_2, \tag{5.6}$$

where b, b_j, and e_j are identically distributed as b_i, b_{ij}, and e_{ijk}, respectively. Proceeding as before gives (Exercise 5.2)

$$\begin{pmatrix} Y_1 \\ Y_2 \end{pmatrix} \sim \mathcal{N}_2 \left(\begin{pmatrix} \mu_b \\ \beta_0 + \mu_b \end{pmatrix}, \begin{pmatrix} \sigma_b^2 + \psi^2 + \sigma_{e1}^2 & \sigma_b^2 \\ \sigma_b^2 & \sigma_b^2 + \psi^2 + \sigma_{e2}^2 \end{pmatrix} \right). \tag{5.7}$$

It follows that
$$D = Y_2 - Y_1 \sim \mathcal{N}_1 \left(\beta_0, 2\psi^2 + \sigma_{e1}^2 + \sigma_{e2}^2 \right). \tag{5.8}$$

Notice that taking the difference eliminates the effect of true value b_i but the effect of interaction b_{ij} remains. The measures of similarity and agreement based on these distributions are derived in Section 5.5.

5.4.2 Linked Data

The data in the linked case consist of paired measurements (Y_{i1k}, Y_{i2k}) over time $k = 1, \ldots, m_i$. These data are also modeled as (5.1) except that we add a term b_{ik}^* representing the random effect of the common time k on the measurements. This random effect links the measurements at the time k. The model becomes

$$Y_{i1k} = b_i + b_{i1} + b_{ik}^* + e_{i1k}, \quad Y_{i2k} = \beta_0 + b_i + b_{i2} + b_{ik}^* + e_{i2k}. \tag{5.9}$$

The b_{ik}^* follow independent $\mathcal{N}_1(0, \sigma_{b*}^2)$ distributions and they are mutually independent of b_i, b_{ij}, and e_{ijk}, which continue to follow the assumptions made for model (5.1). The distribution of b_{ik}^* does not depend on either method or time.

The effect b_{ik}^* can also be interpreted as a subject $\times$ time interaction. In other words, b_{ik}^* is a subject-specific bias that gets introduced in the measurements at time k. It is instructive to contrast the interactions b_{ij} and b_{ik}^*. The former is a characteristic that depends on method but remains stable over time. The latter is a characteristic that does not depend on method and captures the change in the true value of the ith subject over time. Both effects, however, vary from subject to subject and these variations are modeled via normal distributions.

The effect of a subject on the measurements now manifests through independent random variables b_i, b_{ij}, and b_{ik}^*. The distributions of vectors of M_i $(= 2m_i)$ measurements on subject $i = 1, \ldots, n$ are independent M_i-variate normals with means (Exercise 5.3)

$$E(Y_{i1k}) = \mu_b, \quad E(Y_{i2k}) = \beta_0 + \mu_b \tag{5.10}$$

and variances

$$\text{var}(Y_{ijk}) = \sigma_b^2 + \psi^2 + \sigma_{b^*}^2 + \sigma_{ej}^2. \tag{5.11}$$

In addition, there are three distinct covariances. The first is the covariance between two measurements of the same method,

$$\text{cov}(Y_{ijk}, Y_{ijl}) = \sigma_b^2 + \psi^2, \ \ k \neq l. \tag{5.12}$$

This covariance is attributed to two random effects—b_i and b_{ij}—that the measurements have in common. The second is the covariance between measurements from different methods taken at the same time,

$$\text{cov}(Y_{i1k}, Y_{i2k}) = \sigma_b^2 + \sigma_{b^*}^2. \tag{5.13}$$

This covariance is also attributed to two random effects—b_i and b_{ik}^*—that the measurements share. Notice how the random effect of time k induces covariance in the two measurements taken at the particular time point. The last is the common covariance between measurements from different methods taken at different times,

$$\text{cov}(Y_{i1k}, Y_{i2l}) = \sigma_b^2, \ \ k \neq l. \tag{5.14}$$

This covariance is attributed to the only random effect b_i that the measurements share. The model (5.9) has seven unknown parameters, namely, $(\beta_0, \mu_b, \sigma_b^2, \psi^2, \sigma_{b^*}^2, \sigma_{e1}^2, \sigma_{e2}^2)$.

Recall from Section 5.2.1 that even though we have linked measurements over a period of time, we are interested in comparing methods with respect to their measurements on a subject at any particular instant. This means we again need to find the distribution of a single measurement pair (Y_1, Y_2) induced by the assumed model (5.9). We now proceed as in the unlinked case to obtain this distribution. Dropping the subscripts i and k in (5.9), the companion model for (Y_1, Y_2) can be written as

$$Y_1 = b + b_1 + b^* + e_1, \ \ Y_2 = \beta_0 + b + b_2 + b^* + e_2, \tag{5.15}$$

where b, b_j, b^*, and e_j are identically distributed as b_i, b_{ij}, b_{ik}^*, and e_{ijk}, respectively. It follows that (Exercise 5.4)

$$\begin{pmatrix} Y_1 \\ Y_2 \end{pmatrix} \sim \mathcal{N}_2 \left(\begin{pmatrix} \mu_b \\ \beta_0 + \mu_b \end{pmatrix}, \begin{pmatrix} \sigma_b^2 + \psi^2 + \sigma_{b^*}^2 + \sigma_{e1}^2 & \sigma_b^2 + \sigma_{b^*}^2 \\ \sigma_b^2 + \sigma_{b^*}^2 & \sigma_b^2 + \psi^2 + \sigma_{b^*}^2 + \sigma_{e2}^2 \end{pmatrix} \right). \tag{5.16}$$

This implies

$$D \sim \mathcal{N}_1 \left(\beta_0, 2\psi^2 + \sigma_{e1}^2 + \sigma_{e2}^2 \right). \tag{5.17}$$

There are two noteworthy features of this distribution. First, it does not involve any effect of time. Second, it is identical to the one obtained in (5.8) for the unlinked case even though the two data models are different. This happens because the effect of the true value at a given time is eliminated upon differencing, and only the effects of random errors and subject × method interactions remain in the difference. We return to these distributions in Section 5.5 to obtain measures of similarity and agreement.

5.4.3 Model Fitting and Evaluation

The models for both unlinked and linked data can be fit by the ML method using a statistical software that fits mixed-effects models (see Section 5.9 for some technical details). For (5.1), we will have the ML estimates $(\hat{\beta}_0, \hat{\mu}_b, \hat{\sigma}_b^2, \hat{\psi}^2, \hat{\sigma}_{e1}^2, \hat{\sigma}_{e2}^2)$ of the model parameters, predicted values $(\hat{b}_i, \hat{b}_{i1}, \hat{b}_{i2})$ of the random effects, and the fitted values

$$\hat{Y}_{i1k} = \hat{b}_i + \hat{b}_{i1}, \quad \hat{Y}_{i2k} = \hat{\beta}_0 + \hat{b}_i + \hat{b}_{i2}.$$

Analogously, for (5.9), we will have the ML estimates $(\hat{\beta}_0, \hat{\mu}_b, \hat{\sigma}_b^2, \hat{\psi}^2, \hat{\sigma}_{b^*}^2, \hat{\sigma}_{e1}^2, \hat{\sigma}_{e2}^2)$ of the model parameters, predicted values $(\hat{b}_i, \hat{b}_{i1}, \hat{b}_{i2}, \hat{b}_{i1}^*, \ldots, \hat{b}_{im_i}^*)$ of the random effects, and the fitted values

$$\hat{Y}_{i1k} = \hat{b}_i + \hat{b}_{i1} + \hat{b}_{ik}^*, \quad \hat{Y}_{i2k} = \hat{\beta}_0 + \hat{b}_i + \hat{b}_{i2} + \hat{b}_{ik}^*.$$

In both cases, the residuals are $\hat{e}_{ijk} = Y_{ijk} - \hat{Y}_{ijk}$, and $\hat{e}_{ijk}/\hat{\sigma}_{ej}$ are their standardized counterparts.

Both models involve a number of assumptions. These can be verified by the usual model diagnostics. In particular, one can examine the Bland-Altman plot for the equal scales assumption, the plot of standardized residuals against fitted values for the homoscedasticity and the zero mean assumptions for random errors, and Q-Q plots of standardized residuals and predicted random effects for the normality assumptions. It is often a good idea to examine residual and Q-Q plots for the two methods separately to reveal any method-specific structures that may be present.

Moreover, as in Chapter 4, we do not normally look for submodels of the original models (5.1) and (5.9) with the intent of obtaining a more parsimonious description of data. The original models are basic to begin with, and we prefer to use measures of similarity and agreement based on these models to quantify any differences in the method-specific parameters.

It often happens that not all variance components in model (5.1) or (5.9) are estimated reliably with the data available. This is evident when at least one of the estimated variance components is near zero or has an unusually large standard error. In this case, we may proceed by either dropping the interaction term b_{ij} from the model, or adopting a model where the b_i term is dropped and (b_{i1}, b_{i2}) are assumed to be i.i.d. draws from a bivariate normal distribution with mean vector (β_1, β_2) and an unstructured covariance matrix (see also Exercise 7.12). The methodology of the next two sections can be easily modified to accommodate these changes to the model.

5.5 EVALUATION OF SIMILARITY AND AGREEMENT

Evaluation of similarity calls for examining differences in marginal distributions of Y_1 and Y_2 through estimates and two-sided confidence intervals (Section 1.7). The distributions of Y_1 and Y_2 are given in (5.7) for unlinked and in (5.16) for linked data. The similarity measures of interest include the intercept β_0, representing the difference in the fixed biases of the methods, and the precision ratio $\lambda = \sigma_{e1}^2/\sigma_{e2}^2$. This λ compares only the random errors of the two methods; it ignores their equation errors, that is, the subject $\times$ method interactions. They can also be included in the comparison by replacing σ_{ej}^2 with $\psi^2 + \sigma_{ej}^2$

to get the following modification of λ:

$$\lambda_1 = \frac{\psi^2 + \sigma_{e1}^2}{\psi^2 + \sigma_{e2}^2}. \tag{5.18}$$

Often, however, both λ and λ_1 lead to the same conclusion regarding similarity.

To evaluate agreement, one has to examine estimates and one-sided confidence bounds for measures of agreement based upon the joint distribution of (Y_1, Y_2). The two agreement measures of specific interest are CCC and TDI. From its definition in (2.6), CCC for unlinked data can be written as

$$\text{CCC} = \frac{2\sigma_b^2}{\beta_0^2 + 2(\sigma_b^2 + \psi^2) + \sigma_{e1}^2 + \sigma_{e2}^2}, \tag{5.19}$$

and CCC for linked data is

$$\text{CCC} = \frac{2(\sigma_b^2 + \sigma_{b*}^2)}{\beta_0^2 + 2(\sigma_b^2 + \psi^2 + \sigma_{b*}^2) + \sigma_{e1}^2 + \sigma_{e2}^2}. \tag{5.20}$$

The TDI measure is based on the difference D. We saw from (5.8) and (5.17) that D has the same distribution for unlinked as well as linked data. Therefore, TDI has the same expression in both cases. From its definition in (2.29),

$$\text{TDI}(p) = \left\{ (2\psi^2 + \sigma_{e1}^2 + \sigma_{e2}^2) \, \chi_{1,p}^2 \big(\beta_0^2 / \{2\psi^2 + \sigma_{e1}^2 + \sigma_{e2}^2\} \big) \right\}^{1/2}. \tag{5.21}$$

As before, the ML estimators of measures of similarity and agreement are obtained by replacing the unknown parameters in their expressions by their respective ML estimators. Furthermore, the large-sample theory is used to compute standard errors and confidence bounds and intervals (Section 5.9). One can also use the distribution of D to compute the 95% limits of agreement in both unlinked and linked cases as

$$\hat{\beta}_0 \pm 1.96 \times \sqrt{2\hat{\psi}^2 + \hat{\sigma}_{e1}^2 + \hat{\sigma}_{e2}^2}. \tag{5.22}$$

5.6 EVALUATION OF REPEATABILITY

Repeatability of a method refers to its agreement with itself. It is important to evaluate this intra-method agreement because, if a method does not agree well with itself, it cannot be expected to agree well with another method. The evaluation of a method's repeatability is essentially an evaluation of its error variation. The repeated measurements data make this evaluation possible.

Repeatability measures are distinct from the measures of agreement that quantify how much the two methods agree, and the measures of similarity that quantify differences in marginal distributions of the methods. The extent of intra-method agreement that a repeatability measure quantifies serves as a benchmark for the extent of inter-method agreement quantified by an agreement measure.

From the viewpoint of benchmarking, an attractive way to measure intra-method agreement is to adapt the measures of agreement that have been developed for measuring inter-method agreement. The inference on them proceeds exactly in the same manner as the agreement measures. Such repeatability measures are derived next.

5.6.1 Unlinked Data

Here the repeated measurements are replications of the same underlying measurement. We have been using (Y_1, Y_2) to denote measurements by the two methods on a randomly selected subject from the population. Now let Y_1^* be a replication of Y_1 and Y_2^* be a replication of Y_2 on the same subject. By definition, Y_j and Y_j^* have the same marginal distribution. To find their joint distribution, recall that the assumed data model (5.1) induces a companion model (5.6) for (Y_1, Y_2). Similarly, it also induces a companion model for (Y_1^*, Y_2^*) as:

$$Y_1^* = b + b_1 + e_1^*, \quad Y_2^* = \beta_0 + b + b_2 + e_2^*, \tag{5.23}$$

where e_1^* and e_2^* are independent copies of e_1 and e_2, respectively, both of which are defined in (5.6). It follows from the two companion models (5.6) and (5.23) that (Exercise 5.2)

$$\begin{pmatrix} Y_1 \\ Y_1^* \end{pmatrix} \sim \mathcal{N}_2 \left(\begin{pmatrix} \mu_b \\ \mu_b \end{pmatrix}, \begin{pmatrix} \sigma_b^2 + \psi^2 + \sigma_{e1}^2 & \sigma_b^2 + \psi^2 \\ \sigma_b^2 + \psi^2 & \sigma_b^2 + \psi^2 + \sigma_{e1}^2 \end{pmatrix} \right), \tag{5.24}$$

and

$$\begin{pmatrix} Y_2 \\ Y_2^* \end{pmatrix} \sim \mathcal{N}_2 \left(\begin{pmatrix} \beta_0 + \mu_b \\ \beta_0 + \mu_b \end{pmatrix}, \begin{pmatrix} \sigma_b^2 + \psi^2 + \sigma_{e2}^2 & \sigma_b^2 + \psi^2 \\ \sigma_b^2 + \psi^2 & \sigma_b^2 + \psi^2 + \sigma_{e2}^2 \end{pmatrix} \right). \tag{5.25}$$

Define $D_j = Y_j - Y_j^*$ as the difference in two replications of method j. From (5.24) and (5.25), we have

$$D_j \sim \mathcal{N}_1(0, 2\sigma_{ej}^2), \quad j = 1, 2. \tag{5.26}$$

We know that an agreement measure is a function of parameters of the bivariate distribution of (Y_1, Y_2). Taking the same function of parameters but of the bivariate distribution of (Y_j, Y_j^*) yields a measure of repeatability (or intra-method agreement) of method j. This approach would produce an analog of any agreement measure for measuring self-agreement. For example, the repeatability versions of CCC and TDI are (Exercise 5.2)

$$\mathrm{CCC}_j = \frac{\sigma_b^2 + \psi^2}{\sigma_b^2 + \psi^2 + \sigma_{ej}^2}, \quad \mathrm{TDI}_j(p) = \left\{ 2\sigma_{ej}^2 \, \chi_{1,p}^2(0) \right\}^{1/2}, \quad j = 1, 2. \tag{5.27}$$

Notice that CCC_j is simply the intraclass correlation between Y_j and Y_j^* as the two measurements have identical means and variances. A comparison with (1.4) shows that CCC_j is in fact the reliability of method j because it can be interpreted as the proportion of total variation not explained by the within-subject errors. Notice also that TDI_j is just a constant multiple of the error variation of method j. These expressions essentially reinforce that a repeatability measure is a measure of a method's error variation. The distribution of D_j in (5.26) can also be used to get the repeatability analog of the 95% limits of agreement for method j as

$$\pm 1.96 \times \sqrt{2} \, \hat{\sigma}_{ej}, \quad j = 1, 2. \tag{5.28}$$

5.6.2 Linked Data

Paralleling the above development, let (Y_1^*, Y_2^*) be another pair of measurements taken by the two methods on the same subject that gives (Y_1, Y_2) but at another time. We do not call (Y_1^*, Y_2^*) a replication of (Y_1, Y_2) as the underlying true value may not be the same.

The companion model for (Y_1, Y_2) induced by the data model (5.9) is given by (5.15). The corresponding companion model for (Y_1^*, Y_2^*) is

$$Y_1^* = b + b_1 + b^{**} + e_1^*, \quad Y_2^* = \beta_0 + b + b_2 + b^{**} + e_2^*, \tag{5.29}$$

where b^{**}, e_1^*, and e_2^* are independent copies of b^*, e_1, and e_2, respectively, all defined in (5.15). As before, it can be seen from (5.15) and (5.29) that (Exercise 5.4)

$$\begin{pmatrix} Y_1 \\ Y_1^* \end{pmatrix} \sim \mathcal{N}_2 \left(\begin{pmatrix} \mu_b \\ \mu_b \end{pmatrix}, \begin{pmatrix} \sigma_b^2 + \psi^2 + \sigma_{b^*}^2 + \sigma_{e1}^2 & \sigma_b^2 + \psi^2 \\ \sigma_b^2 + \psi^2 & \sigma_b^2 + \psi^2 + \sigma_{b^*}^2 + \sigma_{e1}^2 \end{pmatrix} \right), \tag{5.30}$$

and

$$\begin{pmatrix} Y_2 \\ Y_2^* \end{pmatrix} \sim \mathcal{N}_2 \left(\begin{pmatrix} \beta_0 + \mu_b \\ \beta_0 + \mu_b \end{pmatrix}, \begin{pmatrix} \sigma_b^2 + \psi^2 + \sigma_{b^*}^2 + \sigma_{e2}^2 & \sigma_b^2 + \psi^2 \\ \sigma_b^2 + \psi^2 & \sigma_b^2 + \psi^2 + \sigma_{b^*}^2 + \sigma_{e2}^2 \end{pmatrix} \right). \tag{5.31}$$

Moreover,

$$D_j \sim \mathcal{N}_1 \left(0, 2(\sigma_{b^*}^2 + \sigma_{ej}^2) \right), \quad j = 1, 2. \tag{5.32}$$

Notice the effect of time on D_j in the form of the variance component $\sigma_{b^*}^2$. To see where this comes from, use (5.15) and (5.29) to write

$$D_j = Y_j - Y_j^* = b^* - b^{**} + e_j - e_j^*,$$

making it explicit that D_j has two sources of variation—the difference in effects of times as well as errors. This contrasts with the unlinked case where the effect of time is absent.

As before, versions of CCC and TDI for measuring repeatability can be deduced from (5.30), (5.31), and (5.32) as (Exercise 5.4)

$$\mathrm{CCC}_j = \frac{\sigma_b^2 + \psi^2}{\sigma_b^2 + \psi^2 + \sigma_{b^*}^2 + \sigma_{ej}^2},$$

$$\mathrm{TDI}_j(p) = \left\{ 2(\sigma_{b^*}^2 + \sigma_{ej}^2) \chi_{1,p}^2(0) \right\}^{1/2}, \quad j = 1, 2. \tag{5.33}$$

Although this CCC_j is also the intraclass correlation between Y_j and Y_j^*, it is not a reliability measure in the strict sense of (1.4) because it does not represent the proportion of total variation not explained by the errors. This interpretation is possible if we think of the effect of time as a part of the error. It also allows TDI_j to be interpreted as a constant times the error variation of method j, just like the unlinked case. Moreover, the 95% limits of intra-method agreement for method j using (5.32) are:

$$\pm 1.96 \times \sqrt{2(\hat{\sigma}_{b^*}^2 + \hat{\sigma}_{ej}^2)}, \quad j = 1, 2. \tag{5.34}$$

It is instructive to ask: "Can a method agree more with another method than with itself?" Intuitively, we expect the answer to be no in general. This is indeed the case for unlinked data, but the linked data are a different matter altogether; see, for example, the analysis of the oximetry data in the next section and also Exercise 5.5.

5.7 CASE STUDIES

5.7.1 Kiwi Data

The kiwi data, introduced in Section 5.2.3, consist of measurements of thickness (in μm) of $n = 16$ kiwi eggshells from a micrometer (method 1) and a scanning electron microscope (method 2). The data are unlinked and we have a balanced design with $m = 3$ replications. We have already seen a number of plots of these data—a trellis plot in Figure 5.1, scatterplots and Bland-Altman plots of 16 randomly selected and of average over replications in Figure 5.4, and a subject × method interaction plot in Figure 5.5. The trellis plot clearly shows that microscope measurements are larger than micrometer for almost all subjects, indicating a difference in fixed biases of the methods. The difference between the methods does not seem to be constant over the subjects, implying a subject × method interaction, which is confirmed by the crossings of the lines in the interaction plot. The trellis plot also shows that the within-subject variation of both methods are comparable and are small in comparison with the between-subject variation. The data appear homoscedastic because the within-subject variation does not seem to vary much over the measurement range. The scatterplots of both individual and average measurements show high correlation between the methods. The microscope's tendency to produce higher readings is confirmed by both sets of scatterplots and Bland-Altman plots. The latter plots do not exhibit any trend, implying that the methods can be assumed to have equal scales. This assumption is needed for modeling of data using the mixed-effects model (5.1).

The next step is to fit this model. The resulting residual plot in Figure 5.7 is centered at zero and does not exhibit any pattern. The normality assumption for errors and random effects is checked in Exercise 5.6. On the whole, the model appears to fit reasonably well.

Table 5.1 presents ML estimates of model parameters and their standard errors. Both methods have considerable random error variation ($\hat{\sigma}_{e1} = 9.3$, $\hat{\sigma}_{e2} = 8.9$). Their magnitudes are comparable to that of the subject × method interaction ($\hat{\psi} = 9.8$). Substitution of the estimates in (5.7) and (5.8) gives the fitted distributions of (Y_1, Y_2) and $D = Y_2 - Y_1$ as

$$\begin{pmatrix} Y_1 \\ Y_2 \end{pmatrix} \sim \mathcal{N}_2 \left(\begin{pmatrix} 311.81 \\ 323.26 \end{pmatrix}, \begin{pmatrix} 2204.4 & 2022.4 \\ 2022.4 & 2198.7 \end{pmatrix} \right), \quad D \sim \mathcal{N}_1(11.35, 358.4). \quad (5.35)$$

On average, a measurement of thickness of a specimen from the microscope exceeds that from the micrometer by 11.35. The methods have comparable variances and their correlation is 0.92. The differences in measurements have a standard deviation of $\sqrt{358.4} = 18.9$. Both the errors and the interactions contribute about equally to the variation in D. From (5.22), the 95% limits of agreement between the methods are $11.35 \pm 1.96 * 18.9 = (-26, 48)$.

Substitution of the parameter estimates in (5.24) and (5.25) gives the fitted distributions of (Y_1, Y_1^*) and (Y_2, Y_2^*). The marginal distribution of Y_j^* is the same as that of Y_j and their correlation is 0.96 for both methods. From (5.26), the fitted distributions of the intra-method differences D_j are:

$$D_1 \sim \mathcal{N}_1(0, 171.6), \quad D_2 \sim \mathcal{N}_1(0, 160.1).$$

These have zero means by definition, and their standard deviations are about 13. Thus, from (5.28), the 95% limits of intra-method agreement are $\pm 1.96\sqrt{171.6} = \pm 26$ for micrometer, and $\pm 1.96\sqrt{160.1} = \pm 25$ for microscope.

Table 5.1 provides estimates and 95% confidence intervals for β_0 and λ for similarity evaluation. The interval for β_0 is $(4, 19)$. It confirms larger fixed bias of microscope compared to micrometer as the lower limit is above zero. The interval for λ is $(0.5, 2)$. Although the estimated λ of 1.1 shows slightly better precision for microscope, the confidence interval allows us to conclude that the methods have practically the same precision.

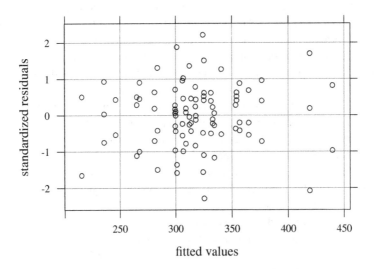

Figure 5.7   Residual plot for kiwi data.

An identical conclusion follows from the 95% confidence interval $(0.7, 1.4)$ for λ_1 (not presented in the table). This modification of λ, defined in (5.18), incorporates the variation of subject $\times$ method interactions in the comparison in addition to that of the errors.

Table 5.1 also provides estimates and one-sided 95% confidence bounds for intra-method versions of CCC and TDI (0.90) for evaluating repeatability. Clearly, the methods have similar repeatability on both measures. This finding, however, is not surprising since repeatability is essentially a measure of error variation and we just saw that the methods have similar precisions. More revealing are the actual values of the estimates and the bounds. The CCC estimates, which also represent the estimated reliabilities, are 0.96. This essentially shows that the error variations are a small portion of the total variation in the measurements. The TDI bounds of 26 imply that 90% of the time the difference between two replicate measurements from the same method on the same eggshell falls within ± 26. This bound of 26 is about 8% of $\hat{\mu}_b = 312$. The measurements themselves range between 200 and 450. This extent of repeatability was acceptable to the ecologists conducting the study.

Next, we proceed to the evaluation of agreement. From Table 5.1, the estimates and 95% confidence bounds are, respectively, 0.89 and 0.79 for CCC and 36 and 45 for TDI (0.90). These suggest a modest level of agreement between the methods. In particular, the TDI bound of 45 is about 14% of $\hat{\mu}_b$. It indicates that 90% of differences in measurements of the two methods range between ± 45. It is clear from the evaluations of similarity and repeatability that a difference in fixed biases of the methods and their somewhat large error variations are two key contributors to disagreement. Reducing the error variations may not be a simple task, but the estimated biases can be made equal by subtracting $\hat{\beta}_0 = 11.35$ from the microscope's measurements. Doing so increases the estimate and the lower bound of CCC to 0.92 and 0.84, respectively, and decreases the estimate and the upper bound of TDI to 31 and 38, respectively. The agreement now is slightly better than before. Nevertheless,

Parameter	Estimate	SE
β_0	11.35	3.94
μ_b	311.81	11.58
$\log(\sigma_b^2)$	7.61	0.36
$\log(\psi^2)$	4.57	0.46
$\log(\sigma_{e1}^2)$	4.45	0.25
$\log(\sigma_{e2}^2)$	4.38	0.25

Similarity Evaluation		
Measure	Estimate	95% Interval
β_0	11.35	$(3.64, 19.07)$
λ	1.07	$(0.54, 2.14)$

Repeatability Evaluation		
Measure	Estimate	95% Bound
CCC_1	0.96	0.92
CCC_2	0.96	0.93
$TDI_1(0.90)$	21.55	26.47
$TDI_2(0.90)$	20.81	25.55

Agreement Evaluation		
Measure	Estimate	95% Bound
CCC	0.89	0.79
TDI(0.90)	36.27	44.82

Table 5.1 Summary of estimates of model parameters and measures of similarity, repeatability, and agreement for kiwi data. Lower bounds for CCC and upper bounds for TDI are presented. Methods 1 and 2 refer to micrometer and microscope, respectively.

the ecologists deemed the two methods to have "reasonable" agreement even without the correction for bias differences.

The above confidence intervals were computed using the standard large-sample approach (Section 3.3.2). However, given that $n = 16$ here is not large, the bootstrap approach (Section 3.3.4) may yield more accurate intervals. The reader is asked to explore both approaches in Exercise 5.6.

5.7.2 Oximetry Data

This dataset, introduced in Section 5.2.3, contains measurements of percent oxygen saturation in blood of $n = 61$ infants obtained using pulse oximetry (method 1) and CO-oximetry (method 2). There are between one and three paired measurements over time by the two methods on each infant. The data are linked and have an unbalanced design. The measurements range from 20 to 100, with most values falling between 70 and 90. The normal range for oxygen saturation in infants is 95 to 100. But most infants in this study had below normal values because they were sick.

These data have also been already displayed in several plots. Their trellis plot in Figure 5.2 leads us to a number of observations. First, CO yields higher readings than pulse for most subjects. This is more easily seen from the scatterplots in Figure 5.3 where most points are above the line of equality. Second, the differences between the methods vary considerably from subject to subject, suggesting a strong subject × method interaction. This is confirmed by the interaction plot in left panel of Figure 5.6. Third, the within-subject variation for pulse is higher than for CO, and both are small compared to the between-subject variation. Fourth, there is some evidence of nonconstant within-subject variation over the measurement range. Finally, in Figure 5.3 there seem to be a few outlying observations, mostly coming from pulse, but they appear moderate except for those from subjects 10 and 31. The scatterplots show moderate correlation between the methods. The Bland-Altman plots in Figure 5.3 suggest that the methods may be assumed to have equal scales. The interaction plot in the right panel of Figure 5.6 shows a strong subject × time interaction.

These initial findings from the data justify modeling them using the mixed-effects model (5.9). Figure 5.8 presents separate plots of standardized residuals against fitted values for each method in its top panel. The residuals are centered at zero and exhibit no clear pattern. There are three residuals, all from pulse, that exceed three in absolute value. Two of these belong to subject 31 and one belongs to subject 4. We will comment on the impact of these three outliers on the analysis later. The bottom panel of Figure 5.8 displays absolute values of the residuals against the fitted values, superimposed with a nonparametric smooth. The smooth for each method may be taken as essentially a horizontal line, implying that the errors can be considered homoscedastic. Verifying the normality assumption for errors and random effects is left to Exercise 5.7. Here we proceed assuming that the fitted model is adequate.

The ML estimates of model parameters and their functions of interest are summarized in Table 5.2. Upon replacing the parameters in (5.16) and (5.17) with their estimates, we get the fitted distributions of (Y_1, Y_2) and D as

$$\begin{pmatrix} Y_1 \\ Y_2 \end{pmatrix} \sim \mathcal{N}_2 \left(\begin{pmatrix} 73.17 \\ 75.64 \end{pmatrix}, \begin{pmatrix} 150.1 & 125.9 \\ 125.9 & 139.6 \end{pmatrix} \right), \quad D \sim \mathcal{N}_1 \left(2.47, 37.9 \right). \tag{5.36}$$

As expected, CO has larger mean but smaller variance than pulse. Their correlation of 0.87 is moderately high. Their differences have mean 2.5 and standard deviation $\sqrt{37.9} = 6.1$. The 95% limits of inter-method agreement are $2.5 \pm 1.96\sqrt{37.9} = (-9.6, 14.6)$. From (5.30) and (5.31), the correlation between two repeated measurements is 0.82 for pulse and 0.88 for CO. Further, the fitted distributions of the intra-method differences D_j from (5.32) are as follows:

$$D_1 \sim \mathcal{N}_1(0, 54.4), \quad D_2 \sim \mathcal{N}_1(0, 33.4). \tag{5.37}$$

Based on these, the 95% limits of intra-method agreement are $\pm 1.96\sqrt{54.4} = \pm 14.5$ for pulse and $\pm 1.96\sqrt{33.4} = \pm 11.3$ for CO.

Consider next the evaluation of similarity using estimates and 95% confidence intervals for β_0 and λ provided in Table 5.2. The estimate 2.5 and interval $(1.2, 3.7)$ for β_0 confirms a larger mean for CO than pulse, although the difference is not substantial. The estimate 3.0 and interval $(1.3, 7.0)$ for λ clearly shows CO's higher precision than pulse.

For evaluation of repeatability, Table 5.2 provides estimates and one-sided 95% confidence bounds for intra-method versions of CCC and TDI (0.90). Obviously, CO's better

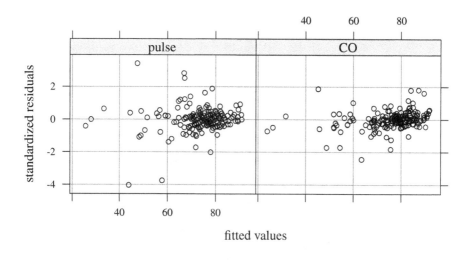

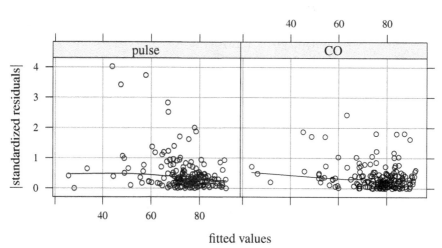

Figure 5.8 Plots of residuals (top panel) and their absolute values (bottom panel) against fitted values for each separate method in oximetry data. A nonparametric smooth is added to the bottom plots.

precision translates into higher repeatability over pulse. The estimates of CCC, represented by intraclass correlations, are 0.82 for pulse and 0.88 for CO, the same as reported previously. The TDI bounds for pulse and CO are 13.5 and 10.6, respectively. Thus, 90% of differences in two pulse measurements lie within ± 13.5. A similar interpretation holds in the case of CO. Given that the observations range from 20 to 100 with $\hat{\mu}_b = 73$ and these bounds are more than 15% of $\hat{\mu}_b$, it is safe to say that both methods exhibit poor repeatability.

For evaluation of agreement, the estimates and 95% confidence bounds reported in Table 5.2 are, respectively, 0.85 and 0.80 for CCC and 10.9 and 12.1 for TDI (0.90).

Parameter	Estimate	SE
β_0	2.47	0.63
μ_b	73.17	1.47
$\log(\sigma_b^2)$	4.74	0.20
$\log(\psi^2)$	2.15	0.26
$\log(\sigma_{b*}^2)$	2.45	0.19
$\log(\sigma_{e1}^2)$	2.75	0.17
$\log(\sigma_{e2}^2)$	1.64	0.35

Similarity Evaluation		
Measure	Estimate	95% Interval
β_0	2.47	$(1.23, 3.71)$
λ	3.04	$(1.32, 7.00)$

Repeatability Evaluation		
Measure	Estimate	95% Bound
CCC_1	0.82	0.76
CCC_2	0.88	0.83
$\text{TDI}_1(0.90)$	12.13	13.48
$\text{TDI}_2(0.90)$	9.51	10.60

Agreement Evaluation		
Measure	Estimate	95% Bound
CCC	0.85	0.80
TDI(0.90)	10.91	12.14

Table 5.2   Summary of estimates of model parameters and measures of similarity, repeatability, and agreement for the oximetry data. Lower bounds for CCC and upper bounds for TDI are presented. Methods 1 and 2 refer to pulse oximetry and CO-oximetry, respectively.

The TDI bound is about 17% of $\hat{\mu}_b$. It shows that 90% of the time the differences in measurements fall within ± 12. These numbers suggest a weak agreement between the methods. Upon comparing the intra- and inter-method estimates for both measures, we come to the curious conclusion that the pulse method agrees more with the CO method than with itself! To explain this, one needs to look no further than the fitted distributions of D (CO-pulse difference) and D_1 (pulse-pulse difference) given in (5.36) and (5.37), respectively. These distributions have comparable means but the variance of D_1 is higher than D. Alternatively, one may verify that the condition given in Exercise 5.5 for inter-method agreement to exceed intra-method agreement holds with parameters replaced by estimates.

It is also apparent that the weak agreement between the methods is mostly due to their relatively poor repeatability. Transforming pulse measurements by adding $\hat{\beta}_0$ to them makes the estimated fixed biases of the methods equal but does not help much with agreement. The CCC and TDI bounds improve slightly to 0.82 and 11.2, respectively. On the whole, we may prefer CO because of its higher precision than pulse, but CO's precision itself is not as high as one would hope.

We now assess the sensitivity of the results to the three observations of pulse identified earlier as outliers. For this we remove them and their paired counterparts to preserve the pairings, and repeat the analysis. This reduces pulse's error standard deviation from 3.95 to 2.50, whereas the CO's remains virtually unchanged (2.27 versus 2.25). It also reduces the estimate of λ, from 3.04 to 1.23, and its new confidence interval $(0.53, 2.88)$ implies that the methods may be considered to have the same precision. The new confidence bounds for intra-method agreement of pulse and CO are, respectively, 0.82 and 0.83 for CCC and 11.05 and 10.71 for TDI. The same bounds for inter-method agreement are 0.81 for CCC and 11.41 for TDI. Note now that we do not have the situation of inter-method agreement being better than an intra-method agreement. Nonetheless, the closeness of intra- and inter-method agreement measures imply that the methods agree as well with themselves as with each other. This means we have no reason to prefer one method over the other on the basis of statistical considerations. However, the foregoing conclusions regarding modest agreement between the methods and their poor repeatability remain unchanged.

5.8   CHAPTER SUMMARY

1. Repeated measurements may be unlinked, linked, or longitudinal. This distinction affects how the data are modeled. Only the first two types are covered in this chapter.

2. The methodology developed here is appropriate for comparing methods with respect to their individual measurements rather than averages of the repeated measurements.

3. The models assume equal scales for methods and homoscedasticity for errors.

4. A subject × method interaction is incorporated in the models for both unlinked and linked data. The latter model additionally incorporates a subject × time interaction.

5. Repeated measurements data allow reliable estimation of error variances of the methods. This is not possible with paired measurements data.

6. With repeated measurements, one can also evaluate repeatability of a method, that is, intra-method agreement. If a method does not agree well with itself, it is unlikely to agree well with another method.

7. A measure of inter-method agreement can be easily adapted to measure intra-method agreement.

8. One normally expects the intra-method agreement of both methods to be higher than their inter-method agreement. But exceptions are possible, especially for linked data.

9. Lack of agreement between two methods is often due to poor repeatability of one of the methods.

10. Various measures of similarity, repeatability, and agreement are written as functions of model parameters, and the large-sample theory of ML estimators is used for inference on them.

11. The methodology requires the number of subjects to be large for standard error estimates and confidence intervals to be accurate.

5.9 TECHNICAL DETAILS

In this section, we represent the mixed-effects models (5.1) and (5.9) for unlinked and linked repeated measurements data in the matrix notation introduced in Chapter 3.

5.9.1 Unlinked Data

Define

$$\mathbf{Y}_{ij} = (Y_{ij1}, \ldots, Y_{ijm_{ij}})^T, \ \mathbf{e}_{ij} = (e_{ij1}, \ldots, e_{ijm_{ij}})^T,$$
$$\beta_1 = \mu_b, \ \beta_2 = \beta_0 + \mu_b, \ u_i = b_i - \mu_b, \ j = 1, 2, \ i = 1, \ldots, n,$$

and

$$\mathbf{Y}_i = \begin{pmatrix} \mathbf{Y}_{i1} \\ \mathbf{Y}_{i2} \end{pmatrix}, \ \mathbf{e}_i = \begin{pmatrix} \mathbf{e}_{i1} \\ \mathbf{e}_{i2} \end{pmatrix}, \ \mathbf{X}_i = \begin{pmatrix} \mathbf{1}_{m_{i1}} & \mathbf{0}_{m_{i1}} \\ \mathbf{0}_{m_{i1}} & \mathbf{1}_{m_{i2}} \end{pmatrix}, \ \mathbf{Z}_i = \begin{pmatrix} \mathbf{1}_{m_{i1}} & \mathbf{1}_{m_{i1}} & \mathbf{0}_{m_{i1}} \\ \mathbf{1}_{m_{i1}} & \mathbf{0}_{m_{i1}} & \mathbf{1}_{m_{i2}} \end{pmatrix}.$$
$$(5.38)$$

Let $\boldsymbol{\beta} = (\beta_1, \beta_2)^T$, $\mathbf{u}_i = (u_i, b_{i1}, b_{i2})^T$, and

$$\mathbf{R}_{ij} = \sigma_{ej}^2 \mathbf{I}_{m_{ij}}, \ \mathbf{R}_i = \text{diag}\{\mathbf{R}_{i1}, \mathbf{R}_{i2}\}, \ \mathbf{G} = \text{diag}\{\sigma_b^2, \psi^2, \psi^2\}. \quad (5.39)$$

The matrix $\mathbf{R}_i$ depends on i through m_{i1} and m_{i2}, the number of repeated measurements on subject i from the two methods. The matrix $\mathbf{G}$ is free of i. The model (5.1) can now be written as

$$\mathbf{Y}_i = \mathbf{X}_i \boldsymbol{\beta} + \mathbf{Z}_i \mathbf{u}_i + \mathbf{e}_i, \ i = 1, \ldots, n, \quad (5.40)$$

where

$$\mathbf{u}_i \sim \mathcal{N}_3(\mathbf{0}, \mathbf{G}), \ \mathbf{e}_i \sim \mathcal{N}_{M_i}(\mathbf{0}, \mathbf{R}_i).$$

It follows that

$$\mathbf{Y}_i \sim \mathcal{N}_{M_i}(\mathbf{X}_i \boldsymbol{\beta}, \mathbf{V}_i = \mathbf{Z}_i \mathbf{G} \mathbf{Z}_i^T + \mathbf{R}_i). \quad (5.41)$$

The elements of the mean vector $\mathbf{X}_i \boldsymbol{\beta}$ and the covariance matrix $\mathbf{V}_i$ are given earlier in (5.2)–(5.5) (Exercise 5.1). The vector of transformed parameters of this model is

$$\boldsymbol{\theta} = \left(\beta_0, \mu_b, \log(\sigma_b^2), \log(\psi^2), \log(\sigma_{e1}^2), \log(\sigma_{e2}^2)\right)^T.$$

5.9.2 Linked Data

Define $\mathbf{Y}_i$, $\mathbf{e}_i$, $\mathbf{X}_i$, and $\mathbf{R}_i$ as before but with $(m_{ij}, M_i) = (m_i, 2m_i)$. It is helpful to think of the times of measurement $k = 1, \ldots, m_i$, $i = 1, \ldots, n$ as the levels of a categorical time variable. Let $\tilde{m}$ be the number of its levels; only the first m_i of which, namely, $k = 1, \ldots, m_i$, are observed for subject i. Alternatively, one can take $\tilde{m} = \max_{i=1,\ldots,n} m_i$. Redefine $\mathbf{u}_i = (u_i, b_{i1}, b_{i2}, b_{i1}^*, \ldots, b_{i\tilde{m}}^*)^T$ as a $(3 + \tilde{m})$-vector; $\mathbf{G}$ as a $(3 + \tilde{m}) \times (3 + \tilde{m})$ diagonal matrix

$$\mathbf{G} = \text{diag}\{\sigma_b^2, \psi^2, \psi^2, \sigma_{b*}^2, \ldots, \sigma_{b*}^2\};$$

and $\mathbf{Z}_i$ as an $M_i \times (3 + \tilde{m})$ design matrix with the following characteristics:

- its first three columns are
$$\begin{pmatrix} \mathbf{1}_{m_i} & \mathbf{1}_{m_i} & \mathbf{0}_{m_i} \\ \mathbf{1}_{m_i} & \mathbf{0}_{m_i} & \mathbf{1}_{m_i} \end{pmatrix},$$

- the first and the last m_i rows of its last $\tilde{m}$ columns are identical, and

- each of them is an $m_i \times \tilde{m}$ matrix whose leading $m_i \times m_i$ submatrix is an identity matrix, and the rest of the elements are zeros.

As in the unlinked case, $\mathbf{G}$ is free of i, but $\mathbf{R}_i$ depends on i through m_i. We can now write the model (5.9) in the form (5.40) with

$$\mathbf{u}_i \sim \mathcal{N}_{3+\tilde{m}}(\mathbf{0}, \mathbf{G}), \ \mathbf{e}_i \sim \mathcal{N}_{M_i}(\mathbf{0}, \mathbf{R}_i),$$

implying

$$\mathbf{Y}_i \sim \mathcal{N}_{M_i}(\mathbf{X}_i \boldsymbol{\beta}, \mathbf{V}_i = \mathbf{Z}_i \mathbf{G} \mathbf{Z}_i^T + \mathbf{R}_i). \tag{5.42}$$

The elements of the mean vector and covariance matrix here are given in (5.10)–(5.14) (Exercise 5.3). The vector of transformed parameters of this model is

$$\boldsymbol{\theta} = \left(\beta_0, \mu_b, \log(\sigma_b^2), \log(\psi^2), \log(\sigma_{b*}^2), \log(\sigma_{e1}^2), \log(\sigma_{e2}^2)\right)^T.$$

The models (5.1) and (5.9) are fit by the ML method using a statistical software that fits mixed-effects models. Estimation of the various measures and standard errors of estimates and construction of confidence intervals and bounds proceed as described in Chapter 3.

5.10 BIBLIOGRAPHIC NOTE

A number of authors have discussed modeling and analysis of method comparison data with repeated measurements. Bland and Altman (1986, 1999, 2007) discuss computation of limits of agreement. They also present the intra-method counterpart of limits of agreement and term it the *repeatability coefficient*. However, they do not dwell on explicit modeling of data, which is the focus of Carstensen et al. (2008). Their models are similar but different from the ones in this chapter. This article is also the source of the oximetry data that we use for a case study. In addition, it introduces the terms *linked* and *unlinked* data that we adopt here. Such data were called *paired* and *unpaired* in an earlier paper by Chinchilli et al. (1996). Schluter (2009) presents a hierarchical Bayesian approach for analyzing repeated measurements data. Rather than modeling the individual measurements, Lai and Shiao (2005) directly model their differences using a mixed-effects model. Both Carstensen et al. (2008) and Lai and Shiao (2005) consider only the limits of agreement.

Several authors have considered variations of CCC for repeated measurements data. Chinchilli et al. (1996) propose a weighted CCC for both linked and unlinked scenarios. Their model is also a mixed-effects model, but they take a method of moments approach for estimation. Carrasco and Jover (2003) propose estimating CCC using the REML approach in a mixed-effects model framework, which is similar to ours. Barnhart et al. (2005) present intra-method, inter-method, and total-method versions of CCC for replicated data. Lin et al. (2007) also develop similar versions of various agreement measures, including CCC and TDI, under a mixed-effects model. Both articles use a GEE approach for estimation. Their definitions of inter- and intra-method agreement differs from ours. Quiroz (2005) develops equivalence tests based on CCC under a mixed-effects model for repeated measurements data. Chen and Barnhart (2008) compare CCC with various intraclass correlations under mixed-effects models. See also Carrasco et al. (2014).

The models in this chapter are special cases of those in Choudhary (2008). This article suggests bootstrap for inference if the number of subjects is not large, and also considers directly modeling differences of the paired measurements. Choudhary (2008), Quiroz and Burdick (2009), and Escaramis et al. (2010) discuss inference on TDI for repeated measurements data using mixed-effects models. Roy (2009) too considers such models but she focuses on inference on the measures of similarity.

Haber et al. (2005) introduce a new index based on inter-method and intra-method variability estimated from unlinked repeated measurements data. Haber and Barnhart (2008) introduce the notion of *disagreement functions* and use them to construct agreement measures that quantify inter-method agreement relative to intra-method agreement. They use a nonparametric approach for inference. Pan et al. (2012) propose a permutation-based agreement measure for unlinked data that compares observed disagreement between the methods to the agreement expected under *individual equivalence*—a condition under which the two methods have identical conditional distributions given a subject's characteristics. They consider a nonparametric and a parametric method based on model (5.1) for inference on their measure.

The models (5.1) and (5.9) are for basic repeated measurements data. Often, however, the data are more complex and require variations and extensions of these models that incorporate additional structures present in the data. One example is the neognathae data from Igic et al. (2010), the same study that collected the kiwi data. But unlike the kiwi data where all eggs are from birds of a single species, these data come from eggs of 18 birds, two birds from each of the nine species considered. To take into account that the birds are nested within species, the model (5.1) is extended to incorporate a random species effect. Further variations and extensions of (5.1) are employed in Brulez et al. (2014) to evaluate repeatability of visual scoring methods of eggshell patterns, for example, spot size and pigment intensity, of two passerines, great tits and blue tits.

Data Sources

The kiwi data are from Igic et al. (2010). They are presented in Table 5.3. Carstensen et al. (2008) is the source of the oximetry data. They are available in the R package MethComp of Carstensen et al. (2015).

ID	Micrometer	Microscope	ID	Micrometer	Microscope
1	300, 301, 296	318, 317, 322	9	250, 241, 241	272, 259, 276
2	315, 301, 304	318, 310, 312	10	315, 330, 329	336, 336, 352
3	356, 350, 350	385, 370, 380	11	268, 255, 270	283, 287, 275
4	435, 400, 421	431, 447, 447	12	301, 302, 300	306, 297, 291
5	296, 280, 270	298, 311, 316	13	220, 220, 200	229, 236, 244
6	320, 325, 310	331, 339, 305	14	325, 312, 310	318, 287, 289
7	320, 345, 310	335, 332, 331	15	355, 365, 353	360, 363, 371
8	358, 360, 359	332, 335, 324	16	311, 310, 302	327, 335, 337

Table 5.3   Kiwi data consisting of eggshell thickness measurements (in μm). They are provided by P. Cassey, see Igic et al. (2010).

EXERCISES

5.1 Show that the marginal distribution of the vector $\mathbf{Y}_i$ of unlinked observations on subject i $(i = 1, \ldots, n)$ is given by (5.41). Show also that the elements of the mean vector and covariance matrix of $\mathbf{Y}_i$ are given by (5.2)–(5.5).

5.2 Consider unlinked repeated measurements data associated with the model (5.1). The companion models for Y_j and Y_j^* $(j = 1, 2)$ are given by (5.6) and (5.23).

  (a) Show that the marginal distribution of (Y_1, Y_2) is given by (5.7). Deduce the distribution of D given in (5.8).

  (b) Show that the marginal distributions of (Y_j, Y_j^*) are given by (5.24) for $j = 1$ and (5.25) for $j = 2$. Deduce the distributions of D_j given in (5.26).

  (c) Verify the expressions for intra-method CCC and TDI given in (5.27).

  (d) What is the joint distribution of (Y_1, Y_1^*, Y_2, Y_2^*)?

5.3 Repeat Exercise 5.1 for the linked case. In particular, show that the marginal distribution of the vector $\mathbf{Y}_i$ of linked observations on subject i $(i = 1, \ldots, n)$ is given by (5.42). Show also that the elements of the mean vector and covariance matrix of $\mathbf{Y}_i$ are given by (5.10)–(5.14).

5.4 This is an analog of Exercise 5.2 for linked repeated measurements data that are modeled by (5.9). The companion models for Y_j and Y_j^* $(j = 1, 2)$ are given by (5.15) and (5.29).

  (a) Show that the marginal distribution of (Y_1, Y_2) is given by (5.16). Deduce the distribution of D given in (5.17).

  (b) Show that the marginal distributions of (Y_j, Y_j^*) are given by (5.30) for $j = 1$ and (5.31) for $j = 2$. Deduce the distributions of D_j given in (5.32).

  (c) Verify the expressions for intra-method CCC and TDI given in (5.33).

  (d) What is the joint distribution of (Y_1, Y_1^*, Y_2, Y_2^*)?

5.5 Can a method, say, method 1, agree more with another method than with itself? The answer depends on the data model and the agreement measure considered. This exercise explores this issue assuming model (5.1) for unlinked data and (5.9) for linked data, and TDI and CCC as agreement measures. With these measures, higher inter-method agreement than intra-method agreement of method 1 means $\text{TDI}(p) < \text{TDI}_1(p)$ and $\text{CCC} > \text{CCC}_1$. To simplify matters, assume that $\beta_0 = 0$ so that the inter-method agreement is solely determined by the variance components. It may be noted that a nonzero β_0 will lead to worse inter-method agreement than when $\beta_0 = 0$. The intra-method agreement is not affected by β_0.

  (a) In the unlinked case, show that

$$\text{TDI}(p) < \text{TDI}_1(p) \iff 2\psi^2 + \sigma_{e2}^2 < \sigma_{e1}^2;$$
$$\text{CCC} > \text{CCC}_1 \iff \text{var}(Y_1)\{\sigma_b^2 - \psi^2\} > \text{var}(Y_2)\{\sigma_b^2 + \psi^2\}.$$

  Argue that the conditions on the right are unlikely to hold in practice.

(b) In the linked case, show that

$$\text{TDI}(p) < \text{TDI}_1(p) \iff 2\psi^2 + \sigma_{e2}^2 < 2\sigma_{b*}^2 + \sigma_{e1}^2;$$

$$\text{CCC} > \text{CCC}_1 \iff \text{var}(Y_1)\{\sigma_b^2 + 2\sigma_{b*}^2 - \psi^2\} > \text{var}(Y_2)\{\sigma_b^2 + \psi^2\}.$$

(The conditions on the right hold for parameter estimates based on the original oximetry data; see Section 5.7.2.) When $\sigma_{e1}^2 = \sigma_{e2}^2$, these conditions are equivalent to the condition that $\psi^2 < \sigma_{b*}^2$.

5.6 Consider the kiwi data from Section 5.7.1.

(a) Fit model (5.1) to the data and verify the results in Table 5.1.

(b) Perform model diagnostics to verify the normality assumption for errors and random effects.

(c) Use the bootstrap approach described in Section 3.3.4 to compute analogs of the confidence intervals and bounds reported in Table 5.1. Compare the two sets of results.

5.7 Consider the oximetry data from Section 5.7.2.

(a) Fit model (5.9) to the data and verify the results in Table 5.2.

(b) Check the normality assumption for errors and random effects.

(c) How would the results change if these data were to be analyzed as unlinked repeated measurements data?

5.8 The knee joint angle (in degrees) in a joint position called "full passive extension" is measured three consecutive times in 29 subjects using each of two goniometers. One is a Lamoreux-type electrogoniometer and the other is a plastic manual goniometer. The data are presented in Table 5.4. Assume unlinked repeated measurements.

(a) Perform an exploratory analysis of the data. Do you notice any outliers?

(b) Fit model (5.1) and check its adequacy. In particular, does the homoscedasticity assumption seem appropriate, possibly after removing outliers, if any?

(c) Evaluate similarity and repeatability of the methods.

(d) Evaluate agreement between the methods. Is the agreement high enough to justify using the methods interchangeably, possibly after a recalibration?

(e) Assess the impact of outliers, if any, on your conclusions.

5.9 Cardiac ejection fraction (in %) is measured in 12 individuals using two methods— impedance cardiography (IC) and radionuclide ventriculography (RV). The data are presented in Table 5.5. Both methods have an equal number of repeated measurements on an individual, but this number varies between 3 and 6. Assume that the repeated measurements are paired over time, and they are taken in the order they appear in the table.

(a) Perform an exploratory analysis of the data.

(b) Fit model (5.9) and check its adequacy.

Subject	Electro	Manual	Subject	Electro	Manual
1	2, 1, 1	-2, 0, 1	16	-12, -12, -12	-13, -14, -14
2	12, 14, 13	16, 16, 15	17	-1, 0, 0	2, 1, 0
3	4, 4, 4	5, 6, 6	18	7, 6, 4	4, 4, 3
4	9, 7, 8	11, 10, 10	19	-10, -11, -10	-10, -9, -10
5	5, 6, 6	7, 8, 6	20	2, 8, 8	8, 9, 8
6	-9, -10, -9	-7, -8, -8	21	8, 7, 7	7, 6, 7
7	17, 17, 17	18, 19, 19	22	-5, -5, -5	-3, -2, -4
8	5, 5, 5	4, 5, 5	23	-6, -8, -7	-5, -5, -7
9	-7, -6, -5	0, -3, -2	24	3, 4, 4	5, 5, 5
10	1, 2, 1	0, 0, -2	25	-4, -3, -4	0, -1, -1
11	-4, -3, -3	-3, -2, -2	26	4, 4, 4	7, 6, 6
12	-1, -2, 1	3, -1, 1	27	-10, -11, -10	-8, -8, -8
13	4, 4, 2	7, 9, 9	28	1, -1, 0	1, 1, 2
14	-8, -10, -9	-6, -7, -6	29	-5, -4, -5	-3, -3, -3
15	-2, -2, -3	1, 1, 0			

Adapted from Eliasziw et al. (1994), ©1994 American Physical Therapy Association, with permission from American Physical Therapy Association.

Table 5.4   Knee joint angle (in degrees) data for Exercise 5.8.

Subject	IC	RV
1	6.57, 5.62, 6.9, 6.57, 6.35	7.83, 7.42, 7.89, 7.12, 7.88
2	4.06, 4.29, 4.26, 4.09	6.16, 7.26, 6.71, 6.54
3	4.71, 5.5, 5.08, 5.02, 6.01, 5.67	4.75, 5.24, 4.86, 4.78, 6.05, 5.42
4	4.14, 4.2, 4.61, 4.68, 5.04	4.21, 3.61, 3.72, 3.87, 3.92
5	3.03, 2.86, 2.77, 2.46, 2.32, 2.43	3.13, 2.98, 2.85, 3.17, 3.09, 3.12
6	5.9, 5.81, 5.7, 5.76	5.92, 6.42, 5.92, 6.27
7	5.09, 4.63, 4.61, 5.09	7.13, 6.62, 6.58, 6.93
8	4.72, 4.61, 4.36, 4.2, 4.36, 4.2	4.54, 4.81, 5.11, 5.29, 5.39, 5.57
9	3.17, 3.12, 2.96	4.48, 4.92, 3.97
10	4.35, 4.62, 3.16, 3.53, 3.53	4.22, 4.65, 4.74, 4.44, 4.5
11	7.2, 6.09, 7, 7.1, 7.4, 6.8	6.78, 6.07, 6.52, 6.42, 6.41, 5.76
12	4.5, 4.2, 3.8, 3.8, 4.2, 4.5	5.06, 4.72, 4.9, 4.8, 4.9, 5.1

Reprinted from Bland and Altman (1999) with permission from SAGE.

Table 5.5   Cardiac ejection fraction (in %) data for Exercise 5.9 (data provided by L. S. Bowling, see Bowling et al., 1993).

(c) Evaluate similarity and repeatability of the methods using appropriate measures.

(d) Evaluate agreement between the methods. Do the methods agree sufficiently well to be used interchangeably? If not, is there any recalibration that may bring them closer?

5.10 Table 5.6 provides measurements of peak expiratory flow rate (in l/min) made using a Wright peak flow meter and a mini Wright meter. Two measurements are taken by each meter on every subject. These data are from Bland and Altman (1986). They were collected to give a wide range of measurement, and are not representative of any population. Assume that the repeated measurements are unlinked. Analyze these data along the lines of the kiwi data case study discussed in Section 5.7 and Exercise 5.6.

Subject	Wright	Mini	Subject	Wright	Mini
1	494, 490	512, 525	10	433, 429	445, 432
2	395, 397	430, 415	11	417, 420	432, 420
3	516, 512	520, 508	12	656, 633	626, 605
4	434, 401	428, 444	13	267, 275	260, 227
5	476, 470	500, 500	14	478, 492	477, 467
6	557, 611	600, 625	15	178, 165	259, 268
7	413, 415	364, 460	16	423, 372	350, 370
8	442, 431	380, 390	17	427, 421	451, 443
9	650, 638	658, 642			

Reprinted from Bland and Altman (1986), ©1986 The Lancet, with permission from Elsevier.

Table 5.6   Peak expiratory flow rate (in l/min) data for Exercise 5.10.

5.11 Coronary artery calcium score is a measure of severity of arteriosclerosis, a risk factor for coronary heart disease. Two radiologists—A and B—make two replicate measurements of calcium score in 12 patients using the AJ-130 method. The data are given in Table 5.7. The repeated measurements are unlinked. Analyze these data.

Subject	A	B	Subject	A	B
1	7, 6	6, 6	7	53, 49	50, 51
2	29, 31	30, 30	8	23, 23	23, 24
3	1, 1	0, 0	9	70, 70	70, 70
4	5, 6	5, 5	10	16, 15	16, 16
5	38, 32	40, 40	11	114, 116	120, 120
6	40, 29	30, 29	12	43, 43	43, 43

Reprinted from Haber et al. (2005) with permission from M. Haber.

Table 5.7   Coronary artery calcium score data for Exercise 5.11.

5.12 Consider the visceral fat data from the R package MethComp of Carstensen et al. (2015). They consist of measurements of thickness of visceral fat layer (in cm) in 43 patients taken by two observers—KL and SL. Each measurement is replicated three times. The repeated measurements are unlinked. Analyze these data.

CHAPTER 6

HETEROSCEDASTIC DATA

6.1 PREVIEW

The methodologies of Chapters 4 and 5 allow the measurement methods to have different variances, but they are assumed to remain constant over the range of values being measured. In other words, the measurements are assumed to be *homoscedastic*. In practice, however, a method's variability often depends on the magnitude of measurement. This chapter is concerned with paired and unlinked repeated measurements data that exhibit such magnitude-dependent *heteroscedasticity*. We assume that the measurement methods have the same scale and extend the homoscedastic models of Chapters 4 and 5 to incorporate heteroscedasticity by letting the variances be functions of a suitably defined *variance covariate*. Two case studies illustrate this methodology.

6.2 INTRODUCTION

For homoscedastic data, the method comparison measures involve variances that are constant in that they do not depend on the values being measured. This assumption fails in many circumstances. In these cases, it is important to incorporate heteroscedasticity into the model. Otherwise, subsequent model-based inference on the measures may become unreliable. It may be possible to remove the heteroscedasticity altogether by a variance stabilizing transformation of data, such as the log transformation. Indeed, this transformation has been successful in removing the heteroscedasticity in vitamin D data (see Sections 1.13.3

and 4.4.3). But a transformation will not always be successful. Besides, a transformation other than the log is generally not recommended in method comparison studies because the differences of the transformed measurements may be difficult to interpret, rendering key agreement measures like TDI unusable. The VCF data in Exercises 1.10 and 6.9 provide an example where the log transformation is not quite successful in stabilizing the variance. Therefore, instead of attempting to remove the heteroscedasticity, we explicitly recognize it in the data modeling step as a function of the magnitude of measurement. This makes the method comparison measures that involve measurement's variability change with the measurement's magnitude.

As before, Y_{ij}, $j = 1, 2$, $i = 1, \ldots, n$ denote the paired measurements data with Y_{ij} as the measurement of the jth method on the ith subject. The $D_i = Y_{i2} - Y_{i1}$ denote the differences. Further, Y_{ijk}, $k = 1, \ldots, m_{ij}$, $j = 1, 2$, $i = 1, \ldots, n$, denote the unlinked repeated measurements data with Y_{ijk} as the kth repeated measurement of the jth method on the ith subject. We do not consider linked repeated measurements data in this chapter; they are discussed in Chapter 8 in a more general setting. We assume that the methods have the same scale.

6.2.1 Diagnosing Heteroscedasticity

It is possible to diagnose heteroscedasticity by examining a trellis plot, a Bland-Altman plot, or even a scatterplot of the data. See Section 5.3 for how the latter two plots may be constructed for the repeated measurements data. Heteroscedasticity is observed in a trellis plot when the within-subject spread of points changes with the measurement level. It is evident in a Bland-Altman plot when points have a nonconstant vertical scatter. Heteroscedasticity is often easier to detect in a variant of the Bland-Altman plot where absolute values of *centered differences*, that is, $|D_i - \overline{D}|$, are plotted on the vertical axis instead of the D_i themselves. One has to look for a trend in this plot, a simpler task than looking for a nonconstant scatter. A scatterplot also shows evidence of heteroscedasticity if the points have a nonconstant spread around the line or the curve that estimates the trend in the paired data.

With repeated measurements data, heteroscedasticity can also be diagnosed by examining plots of residuals obtained from fitting the homoscedastic mixed-effects model (5.1). A nonconstant vertical scatter in the plot of residuals against fitted values is suggestive of heteroscedasticity, and so is a trend in the plot of absolute residuals against the fitted values. The rationale behind these plots is that the expected value of the absolute value of a normal random variable with mean zero is a constant multiple of its standard deviation (Exercise 6.1). Therefore, if these plots show a trend, it indicates nonconstant variability. Although "residuals" may also be defined for paired measurements data following the homoscedastic bivariate normal model (4.6), their plots are generally not useful for diagnosing heteroscedasticity (see Section 6.5.2).

For both paired and repeated measurements data, one can also check for heteroscedasticity by conducting a test of null hypothesis of homoscedasticity. Such tests are provided later in this chapter.

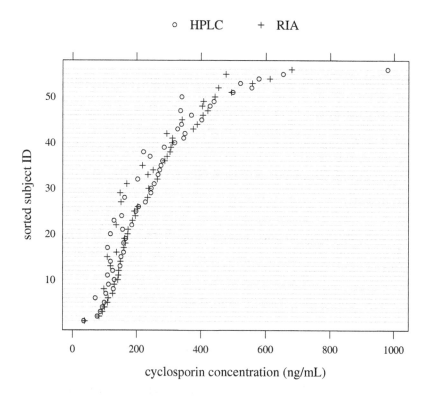

Figure 6.1   Trellis plot of cyclosporin data.

6.2.2   Example Datasets

Below we introduce two datasets that will be used for case studies in this chapter. We revisit them in Sections 6.4.6 and 6.5.6.

6.2.2.1 Cyclosporin Data   Cyclosporin is an immunosuppressant drug widely used to prevent rejection of transplanted organs. This dataset consists of concentrations of cyclosporin (ng/mL) measured by assaying an aliquot of each of $n = 56$ blood samples from organ transplant recipients using two methods: high performance liquid chromatography (HPLC, method 1), the standard method, and an alternative radio-immunoassay (RIA, method 2). These are paired measurements data, ranging from 35 to 980 ng/mL. Figure 6.1 displays their trellis plot. It shows that the within-subject spread of the measurements tends to increase with concentration level. The Bland-Altman plot and its variant with absolute values of centered differences on the vertical axis are displayed in Figure 6.2. The heteroscedasticity is also evident in both the Bland-Altman plot where the vertical scatter appears to increase with average and its variant where an increasing trend is clear. All the three plots show an outlier.

6.2.2.2 Cholesterol Data   These data come from a study in which two assays for serum cholesterol (mg/dL) are compared. One is Cobas Bio (method 1), a Centers for Disease Control standardized method that serves as the reference method. The other is

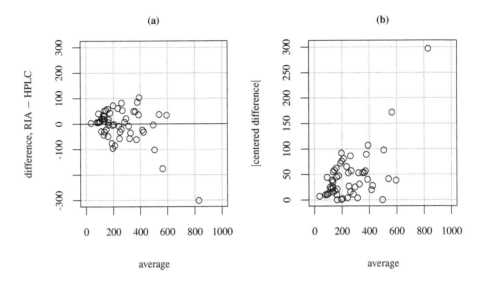

Figure 6.2   Plots for cyclosporin data. Panel (a): Bland-Altman plot with zero line. Panel (b): Plot of absolute values of centered differences against averages.

Ektachem 700 (method 2), a laboratory analyzer that is treated as the test method. These assays are labeled as cobasb and echem, respectively. There are $n = 100$ subjects in the study. Serum cholesterol of every subject is measured ten times using each assay. Thus, these data have a balanced design and there is a total of $M = 100 \times 2 \times 10 = 2000$ observations. The repeated measurements are unlinked because a subject's 20 measurements are obtained by subsampling the subject's original blood sample. The measurements range from 45 to 372 mg/dL. Figure 6.3 displays their trellis plot. It clearly shows that the within-subject variations of both methods tend to increase with cholesterol level.

6.3   VARIANCE FUNCTION MODELS

We need a variance covariate v to account for heteroscedasticity of measurements. Let v_i be the value of v for the ith subject. Since we would like to model variations of both measurement methods as functions of the magnitude of measurement, it is clear that the true measurement should be the covariate v. Note also that there is just one true value for each subject that both methods attempt to measure. Thus, this true value should be the common variance covariate for both methods. The measures of agreement will be functions of this covariate by definition, allowing us to evaluate how the extent of agreement changes with the magnitude of measurement.

A practical difficulty here is that the true values are not available in method comparison studies. We do, nevertheless, have error-free values of the methods, one from each method for every subject. (Recall from Section 1.3.1 that the true value of the subject and the error-free values of the methods are different quantities.) Let us denote the error-free values of the ith subject as μ_{i1} for method 1 and μ_{i2} for method 2. It is possible to model the variation

cobas ○   echem +

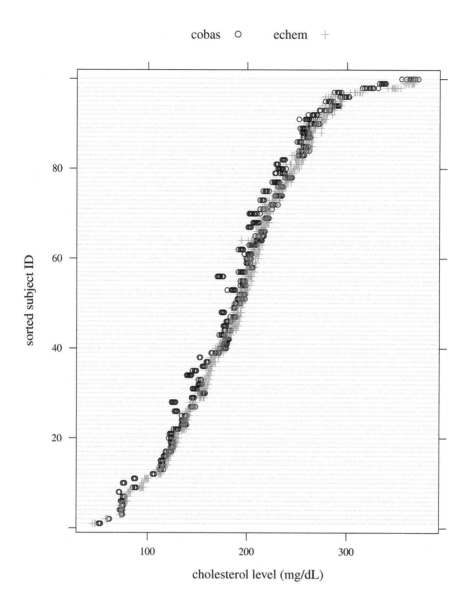

Figure 6.3   Trellis plot of cholesterol data.

for each method separately as a function of its own error-free value. But this will preclude us from evaluating agreement as a function of the magnitude of measurement, the common variance covariate. There are two obvious practical ways to get the common covariate as a function of the error-free values. One is to take $v_i = \mu_{i1}$ if there is an established method in the comparison serving as the reference, which if it exists, is taken to be method 1; otherwise, take $v_i = (\mu_{i1} + \mu_{i2})/2$, the average of the two error-free values. Another is to take $v_i = (\mu_{i1} + \mu_{i2})/2$ regardless of whether there is a reference in the comparison or not. More generally, we can think of the v_i as a *specified* function of the error-free values,

$$v_i = h(\mu_{i1}, \mu_{i2}), \tag{6.1}$$

denoting the magnitude of measurement for the purpose of modeling heteroscedasticity. The two v_i defined earlier are special cases of this h function. The error-free values and hence the v_i are unobservable random quantities. Generally they are non-negative as well.

Now that we have a working definition for the variance covariate v, we can define a *variance function* $g(v, \boldsymbol{\delta})$ that describes how the variation of a method changes with v and depends on a vector of *heteroscedasticity parameters* $\boldsymbol{\delta}$. More specifically, we will consider a model of the form $\sigma^2 g^2(v, \boldsymbol{\delta})$ for a variance. It may be noted that even though g is called a *variance* function, it is g^2 that actually models the variance. The function g modeling the standard deviation is necessarily non-negative. We assume that g has a *known* parametric form and, for simplicity, take the heteroscedasticity parameter to be a scalar δ (see Section 8.3.2 for an example with a vector $\boldsymbol{\delta}$). The function g is continuous in δ, and is defined in a way to ensure that $\delta = 0$ corresponds to homoscedasticity, that is, $g(v, 0) = 1$ for all v. Usually, it is also an increasing function in $|v|$.

We next introduce two simple, commonly used models for g. The first is the *power model*,

$$g(v, \delta) = |v|^\delta, \tag{6.2}$$

prescribing that g either increases or decreases as a power of the absolute value of the variance covariate. It increases in $|v|$ if δ is positive and decreases in $|v|$ if δ is negative. While the power δ may be any real number, large values for it in absolute value terms are rarely needed in practice. This model may not be appropriate if v can be zero or near zero because in this case the g function may also be zero or near zero, which may not be desirable. In particular, when $v = 0$, g is zero if $\delta > 0$ and is undefined if $\delta < 0$. If $v \neq 0$, the power model for g is equivalent to assuming that the log of standard deviation is a linear function of $\log(|v|)$ with intercept $\log(\sigma)$ and slope δ.

The second is the *exponential model*,

$$g(v, \delta) = \exp(\delta v), \tag{6.3}$$

Here both δ and v can be any real number, including zero. This model can also accommodate increasing and decreasing patterns of heteroscedasticity with v. In particular, if $v \geq 0$ and $\delta > 0$, which is commonly the case, the function increases exponentially in v. The exponential model is equivalent to assuming that the log of standard deviation is a linear function of v with intercept $\log(\sigma)$ and slope δ.

These models are obviously not exhaustive. However, it has been our experience that elaborate variance function models are generally not needed in method comparison studies. Our next task is to integrate the variance function models described here with the homoscedastic models of Chapters 4 and 5, yielding their heteroscedastic generalizations. We will first consider the repeated measurements data and then the paired measurements data.

6.4 REPEATED MEASUREMENTS DATA

In Chapter 5, under the assumption that the measurement methods have the same scale and the repeated measurements are unlinked, the data Y_{ijk}, $k = 1, \ldots, m_{ij}$, $j = 1, 2$,

$i = 1, \ldots, n$, are modeled using the homoscedastic mixed-effects model (5.1). This model makes the usual normality and independence assumptions (see Section 5.4.1), including that

$$e_{ijk} \sim \text{ independent } \mathcal{N}_1(0, \sigma_{ej}^2). \tag{6.4}$$

These errors are homoscedastic, that is, $\text{var}(e_{ijk})$ remains constant over the measurement range. From (5.1), the error-free values for methods 1 and 2 are, respectively,

$$\mu_{i1} = b_i + b_{i1}, \quad \mu_{i2} = \beta_0 + b_i + b_{i2}. \tag{6.5}$$

6.4.1 A Heteroscedastic Mixed-Effects Model

To let the error variances of the methods depend on the magnitude of measurement, consider the variance covariate v_i defined in (6.1). This v_i is a known function h of the error-free values (μ_{i1}, μ_{i2}) given by (6.5). It serves as the magnitude of measurement and being a function of the random effects (b_i, b_{i1}, b_{i2}), it is an unobservable random quantity. It also depends on the unknown intercept β_0.

The homoscedasticity assumption for the errors can be relaxed by letting their variances depend on the variance covariate v_i according to the variance function model

$$\text{var}(e_{ijk}|b_i, b_{i1}, b_{i2}) = \sigma_{ej}^2 \, g_j^2(v_i, \delta_j), \; v_i = h(\mu_{i1}, \mu_{i2}). \tag{6.6}$$

This model allows each method to have its own error variance function and heteroscedasticity parameter. But the covariate v_i remains common to both methods. Notice that (6.6) models the error variances conditional on the random effects. The errors and the random effects are not independent anymore because the latter appear in the variance function through the covariate v_i.

We obtain a heteroscedastic mixed-effects model by replacing the assumption (6.4) in the homoscedastic model (5.1) with the following assumption based on the variance function model in (6.6),

$$e_{ijk}|(b_i, b_{i1}, b_{i2}) \sim \text{ independent } \mathcal{N}_1\big(0, \sigma_{ej}^2 \, g_j^2(v_i, \delta_j)\big). \tag{6.7}$$

This model reduces to (5.1) when $\delta_1 = \delta_2 = 0$. It turns out that fitting this model poses computational difficulties (see Section 6.7). They arise from the fact that the random effects (b_i, b_{i1}, b_{i2}) appear in the error variances through the covariate v_i, preventing them from being explicitly averaged out to get a closed-form joint distribution for multiple measurements on a subject. This contrasts with the homoscedastic case where this distribution is multivariate normal.

One way to get around the computational difficulties is to approximate the variance covariate v_i by replacing the unobservable error-free values (μ_{i1}, μ_{i2}) that determine it by their known, observable proxies, say, $(\tilde{\mu}_{i1}, \tilde{\mu}_{i2})$. The proxies are chosen so that they are free of the subject's random effects and also are close to the error-free values. They are also held *fixed* during model fitting. This results in

$$\tilde{v}_i = h(\tilde{\mu}_{i1}, \tilde{\mu}_{i2}) \tag{6.8}$$

as the approximate variance covariate, and

$$\text{var}(e_{ijk}|\tilde{v}_i) = \sigma_{ej}^2 \, g_j^2\big(\tilde{v}_i, \delta_j\big) \tag{6.9}$$

as the corresponding variance function model. In contrast with (6.6), the $\tilde{v}_i$ here are fixed quantities, and the corresponding error variances are free of the random effects.

Now, upon replacing the variance function model (6.6) with (6.9), we obtain a heteroscedastic mixed-effects model. This model is formulated as follows:

$$Y_{i1k} = b_i + b_{i1} + e_{i1k}, \quad Y_{i2k} = \beta_0 + b_i + b_{i2} + e_{i2k}, \tag{6.10}$$

$k = 1, \ldots, m_{ij}, \, j = 1, 2, \, i = 1, \ldots, n$, where

- the true values b_i follow independent $\mathcal{N}_1(\mu_b, \sigma_b^2)$ distributions,

- the interactions b_{ij} follow independent $\mathcal{N}_1(0, \psi^2)$ distributions,

- for given $\tilde{v}_i$, the random errors e_{ijk} follow independent $\mathcal{N}_1\left(0, \sigma_{ej}^2 \, g_j^2(\tilde{v}_i, \delta_j)\right)$ distributions, and

- b_i, b_{ij}, and e_{ijk} are mutually independent.

This is the heteroscedastic model we will use for the repeated measurements data. The model (6.10) may be called "approximate" because the covariate $\tilde{v}_i$ involved herein is an approximation of the original variance covariate v_i. For a fixed $\tilde{v}_i$, the vectors of $M_i = m_{i1} + m_{i2}$ measurements on subject $i = 1, \ldots, n$ follow independent M_i-variate normal distributions with means (Section 6.7 and Exercise 6.2)

$$E(Y_{i1k}) = \mu_b, \quad E(Y_{i2k}) = \beta_0 + \mu_b \tag{6.11}$$

and variances

$$\mathrm{var}(Y_{ijk}) = \sigma_b^2 + \psi^2 + \sigma_{ej}^2 \, g_j^2(\tilde{v}_i, \delta_j). \tag{6.12}$$

Further,

$$\mathrm{cov}(Y_{ijk}, Y_{ijl}) = \sigma_b^2 + \psi^2, \quad k \neq l \tag{6.13}$$

is the common covariance between two replications of the same method, and

$$\mathrm{cov}(Y_{i1k}, Y_{i2l}) = \sigma_b^2 \tag{6.14}$$

is the common covariance between any two measurements from different methods on the same subject. Not surprisingly, the moments in (6.11)–(6.14) are identical to those in (5.2)–(5.5) derived for the homoscedastic model (5.1), with the obvious exception that the error variance σ_{ej}^2 has been replaced by $\sigma_{ej}^2 \, g_j^2(\tilde{v}_i, \delta_j)$ to incorporate heteroscedasticity. The unknown parameters in the model (6.10) are $(\beta_0, \mu_b, \sigma_b^2, \psi^2, \sigma_{e1}^2, \sigma_{e2}^2, \delta_1, \delta_2)$. All inferences based on this model are made by holding the covariate $\tilde{v}_i$ fixed. We will explain how to choose $\tilde{v}_i$ and the variance functions g_j in Section 6.4.2.

Next, we need the distribution of the "typical" measurement pair (Y_1, Y_2) induced by the model (6.10). This distribution is used to derive the model-based measures of similarity, repeatability, and agreement later in Section 6.4.5. Due to heteroscedasticity, this distribution now depends on the variance covariate. Paralleling the development in Section 5.4.1, we get the distribution of (Y_1, Y_2) for a given value $\tilde{v} \in \mathcal{V}$ of the covariate as (Exercise 6.3)

$$\begin{pmatrix} Y_1 \\ Y_2 \end{pmatrix} \Big| \, \tilde{v} \sim \mathcal{N}_2 \left(\begin{pmatrix} \mu_b \\ \beta_0 + \mu_b \end{pmatrix}, \right.$$
$$\left. \begin{pmatrix} \sigma_b^2 + \psi^2 + \sigma_{e1}^2 \, g_1^2(\tilde{v}, \delta_1) & \sigma_b^2 \\ \sigma_b^2 & \sigma_b^2 + \psi^2 + \sigma_{e2}^2 \, g_2^2(\tilde{v}, \delta_2) \end{pmatrix} \right). \tag{6.15}$$

In practice, $\mathcal{V}$ may be taken as the observed range of measurements. It follows that

$$D|\tilde{v} \sim \mathcal{N}_1\left(\beta_0, \tau^2(\tilde{v})\right), \tag{6.16}$$

where

$$\tau^2(\tilde{v}) = 2\psi^2 + \sigma_{e1}^2 g_1^2(\tilde{v}, \delta_1) + \sigma_{e2}^2 g_2^2(\tilde{v}, \delta_2). \tag{6.17}$$

6.4.2 Specifying the Variance Function

A key aspect of formulating the heteroscedastic model (6.10) is the specification of a model for the variance function in (6.9). This usually proceeds in three steps. First, we choose the proxies $(\tilde{\mu}_{i1}, \tilde{\mu}_{i2})$ of the error-free values (μ_{i1}, μ_{i2}) that determine $\tilde{v}_i$ through (6.8). By definition, the proxies need to be close to (μ_{i1}, μ_{i2}) while being free of the subject random effects. A simple choice is to take $\tilde{\mu}_{ij}$ as the sample mean of the replicate measurements of the jth method on the ith subject, that is,

$$\tilde{\mu}_{ij} = \overline{y}_{ij\cdot} = \sum_{k=1}^{m_{ij}} y_{ijk}/m_{ij}, \quad j = 1, 2. \tag{6.18}$$

It may be noted that $\overline{Y}_{ij\cdot}$ is a linear unbiased predictor of μ_{ij} and satisfies $E(\overline{Y}_{ij\cdot} - \mu_{ij}) = 0$. The model (6.10) with (6.18) as $\tilde{\mu}_{ij}$ can be fit by any statistical software capable of fitting heteroscedastic mixed-effects models with a known variance covariate.

An alternative possibility takes the BLUP of μ_{ij} as $\tilde{\mu}_{ij}$ (see Section 3.2.2). But the BLUPs themselves depend on unknown model parameters, calling for an *iterative reweighting* type of scheme for model fitting. It involves starting with an initial estimate of the model parameters, for example, using a homoscedastic fit, and cycling through the following steps until convergence:

- use the current parameter estimates to estimate the BLUPs,

- use the estimated BLUPs to compute the $\tilde{v}_i = h(\tilde{\mu}_{i1}, \tilde{\mu}_{i2})$ for an assumed h,

- update the parameter estimates by fitting the heteroscedastic model, treating the $\tilde{v}_i$ as known.

Obviously, the choice of BLUP as $\tilde{\mu}_{ij}$ makes the model fitting more computationally demanding than the previous alternative. But in our experience this additional cost does not pay off much in gaining higher accuracy of estimates (see Section 6.8 for a reference). Therefore, here we take the sample means $\overline{y}_{ij\cdot}$ in (6.18) as our $\tilde{\mu}_{ij}$.

The second step involves choosing the h function in (6.8) that determines the variance covariate $\tilde{v}_i$. As we have settled on using $\overline{y}_{ij\cdot}$ as $\tilde{\mu}_{ij}$, the two possibilities mentioned in Section 6.3 are

$$\tilde{v}_i = h(\overline{y}_{i1\cdot}, \overline{y}_{i2\cdot}) = \begin{cases} \overline{y}_{i1\cdot}, & \text{if method 1 is a reference method,} \\ (\overline{y}_{i1\cdot} + \overline{y}_{i2\cdot})/2, & \text{otherwise,} \end{cases} \tag{6.19}$$

and

$$\tilde{v}_i = h(\overline{y}_{i1\cdot}, \overline{y}_{i2\cdot}) = (\overline{y}_{i1\cdot} + \overline{y}_{i2\cdot})/2, \tag{6.20}$$

regardless of whether or not there exists a reference method. The two alternatives differ only when a reference method is present in the comparison. But even this distinction between them is not critical as the two tend to yield similar model fits. Nevertheless, here we work with the average (6.20) for the sake of concreteness. Note that the h function may also be a transformation of this average, for example, the log transformation.

The third step consists of choosing the actual variance functions g_j in (6.9). We are only interested in determining the forms of these functions; the coefficients involved in them constitute the unknown heteroscedasticity parameters δ_j that are estimated by the ML method together with all other model parameters. One way to come up with the desired functions is to fit the homoscedastic model (5.1) to the data, get the residuals, and analyze the absolute values of the residuals using ordinary regression. Under the model, these residuals are approximately normally distributed with mean zero, implying that the mean of the absolute residuals is approximately $\sqrt{(2/\pi)}$ times the standard deviations of the residuals (Exercise 6.1). These standard deviations in turn approximate the error standard deviations, which are precisely the functions g_j defined in (6.9) up to a multiplicative constant. This means we can determine the forms of the g_j functions by examining the trends in absolute residuals as a function of the variance covariate $\tilde{v}_i$ using ordinary regression techniques. For this, one may proceed as follows:

1. Plot the absolute residuals against $\tilde{v}_i$ for each method. Also plot the log of the absolute residuals against both $\tilde{v}_i$ and $\log(|\tilde{v}_i|)$.

2. Examine the trends in these scatterplots. Fit simple parametric functions, for example, linear or log-linear functions, via ordinary regression to describe the trends; superimpose the fitted curves on the scatterplots; and visually judge which functions provide the most reasonable fit. Take this function for the jth method as g_j, with coefficients in the function treated as unknown parameters. Consider simple linear regression fits of log of absolute residuals on either $\tilde{v}_i$, for the exponential model, or $\log(|\tilde{v}_i|)$, for the power model (see Section 6.3). The two methods may have altogether different g_j functions. Moreover, one may have more than one candidate for a g_j function.

6.4.3   Model Fitting and Evaluation

The model (6.10) treats the variance covariate $\tilde{v}_i$ as a known quantity that is held fixed during model fitting. Therefore, the model can be fit by the ML method using any mixed-effects model fitting software that can handle heteroscedasticity of errors in terms of known variance covariates. As before, upon fitting the model we get

$$(\hat{\beta}_0, \hat{\mu}_b, \hat{\sigma}_b^2, \hat{\sigma}_{bI}^2, \hat{\sigma}_{e1}^2, \hat{\sigma}_{e2}^2, \hat{\delta}_1, \hat{\delta}_2)$$

as the ML estimates of model parameters; $(\hat{b}_i, \hat{b}_{i1}, \hat{b}_{i2})$ as the predicted values of the random effects;

$$\hat{Y}_{i1k} = \hat{b}_i + \hat{b}_{i1}, \ \ \hat{Y}_{i2k} = \hat{\beta}_0 + \hat{b}_i + \hat{b}_{i2}$$

as the fitted values; $\hat{e}_{ijk} = Y_{ijk} - \hat{Y}_{ijk}$ as the residuals; and

$$\hat{e}_{ijk}/\{\hat{\sigma}_{ej}\, g_j(\tilde{v}_i, \hat{\delta}_j)\}$$

as the standardized residuals. When the heteroscedastic model (6.10) holds, these standardized residuals are approximately distributed as independent draws from a standard normal distribution. One can use these quantities to perform model diagnostics as described in Section 3.2.4 to validate the mixed-effects model assumptions.

Of particular interest is the adequacy of the assumed variance functions models. Obviously, if the residual plots for both methods pass the diagnostics, then the assumed g_j can be deemed adequate. Alternatively, if the number of replications m_{ij} is large enough for the sample standard deviations of measurements to be stable for each (i, j), then this adequacy can be judged directly. For this, one can examine the plot of the subject-specific sample standard deviations against $\tilde{v}_i$, separately for each method, superimposed with the model-based fitted error standard deviation curves. The latter are obtained by taking the square root of (6.9) and replacing the unknown parameters by their ML estimates. Naturally, if the assumed g_j functions do not fit well, one has to return to the step where absolute residuals from the homoscedastic model fit are analyzed by regression to come up with an alternative model that may provide a better fit. On the other hand, if there is more than one candidate model for the g_j functions then this adequacy checking can be repeated for each candidate to find the best fitting model with a natural preference for a simpler model.

6.4.4 Testing for Homoscedasticity

In applications, we need to supplement the visual assessment of the need for a heteroscedastic model by testing the null hypothesis of homoscedasticity,

$$H_0 : \delta_1 = \delta_2 = 0 \text{ versus } H_1 : \delta_j \neq 0 \text{ for at least one } j = 1, 2. \tag{6.21}$$

A likelihood ratio test can be used for this purpose. This involves fitting both the heteroscedastic model (6.10) and the homoscedastic model (5.1) that results when the null hypothesis is true. From (3.32), the likelihood ratio statistic is

$$2\{\log(L_2) - \log(L_1)\}, \tag{6.22}$$

where L_1 and L_2 are the maximum likelihoods under the models (5.1) and (6.10), respectively. Following Section 3.3.7, the p-value for testing H_0 can be approximated by the probability on the right of the observed value of the statistic under a χ^2 distribution with two degrees of freedom. The homoscedastic and heteroscedastic models can also be compared using model selection criteria such as AIC and BIC (Section 3.3.7). These can also be used to distinguish between multiple candidate models for the variance functions.

6.4.5 Evaluation of Similarity, Agreement, and Repeatability

We follow Sections 5.5 and 5.6 and adapt the methodology for evaluation of similarity, agreement, and repeatability developed there to handle the heteroscedastic model (6.10). The evaluation involves examining two-sided confidence intervals for measures of similarity and one-sided confidence bounds for measures of agreement and repeatability. When a measure depends on $\tilde{v} \in \mathcal{V}$, we get its pointwise confidence band over $\mathcal{V}$. A simultaneous confidence band over a grid in $\mathcal{V}$ can also be constructed (see Section 3.3.5).

Our task is to derive the various measures, focusing initially on the measures of similarity and agreement. Upon comparing the distributions of the "typical" measurement pair (Y_1, Y_2) that are used to develop these measures, we find that (6.15) is the same as (5.7) except that σ_{ej}^2 is replaced by $\sigma_{ej}^2 \, g_j^2(\tilde{v}, \delta_j)$. It follows that the same replacement in the measures based on (5.7) would give their heteroscedastic counterparts that are based on (6.15). The counterparts that involve the error variances are now functions of the variance covariate $\tilde{v}$.

The two measures of similarity considered in Section 5.5 are the fixed intercept β_0 and the precision ratio λ. The first remains the same and the heteroscedastic version of the second is

$$\lambda(\tilde{v}) = \frac{\sigma_{e1}^2 \, g_1^2(\tilde{v}, \delta_1)}{\sigma_{e2}^2 \, g_2^2(\tilde{v}, \delta_2)}. \tag{6.23}$$

The measures of agreement considered in Section 5.5 are the CCC and TDI. Using (5.19) and (5.21), we obtain

$$\mathrm{CCC}(\tilde{v}) = \frac{2\sigma_b^2}{\beta_0^2 + 2(\sigma_b^2 + \psi^2) + \sigma_{e1}^2 \, g_1^2(\tilde{v}, \delta_1) + \sigma_{e2}^2 \, g_2^2(\tilde{v}, \delta_2)}, \tag{6.24}$$

and

$$\mathrm{TDI}(p, \tilde{v}) = \tau(\tilde{v}) \left\{ \chi_{1,p}^2 \big(\beta_0^2 / \tau^2(\tilde{v}) \big) \right\}^{1/2}, \tag{6.25}$$

where $\tau^2(\tilde{v})$ is given $\tilde{v}$ in (6.17).

Consider next the measures of repeatability discussed in Section 5.6. These are derived from the distributions of (Y_j, Y_j^*), where Y_j^* is a replication of Y_j, $j = 1, 2$. Not surprisingly, these distributions under the heteroscedastic model (6.10) are the same as those given by (5.24) and (5.25) under the homoscedastic model (5.1) with the exception that σ_{ej}^2 is replaced by $\sigma_{ej}^2 \, g_j^2(\tilde{v}, \delta_j)$ (Exercise 6.4). The same replacement in the repeatability measures in (5.27) gives the heteroscedastic versions of CCC_j and TDI_j as

$$\mathrm{CCC}_j(\tilde{v}) = \frac{\sigma_b^2 + \psi^2}{\sigma_b^2 + \psi^2 + \sigma_{ej}^2 \, g_j^2(\tilde{v}, \delta_j)},$$

$$\mathrm{TDI}_j(p, \tilde{v}) = \left\{ 2\sigma_{ej}^2 \, g_j^2(\tilde{v}, \delta_j) \, \chi_{1,p}^2(0) \right\}^{1/2}, \quad j = 1, 2. \tag{6.26}$$

The heteroscedastic version of 95% limits of agreement can be obtained from (5.22) as

$$\hat{\beta}_0 \pm 1.96 \times \hat{\tau}(\tilde{v}), \tag{6.27}$$

with $\hat{\tau}^2(\tilde{v})$ denoting the ML estimator of $\tau^2(\tilde{v})$ given by (6.17); and its repeatability analogs can be obtained from (5.28) as

$$\pm 1.96 \times \sqrt{2} \, \hat{\sigma}_{ej} \, g_j(\tilde{v}, \hat{\delta}_j), \quad j = 1, 2. \tag{6.28}$$

6.4.6 Case Study: Cholesterol Data

These data, introduced in Section 6.2.2.2, consist of measurements of serum cholesterol (in mg/dL) obtained using Cobas Bio (method 1) and Ektachem assays (method 2) from $n = 100$ subjects. The data have a balanced design with $m = 10$ unlinked replications. Their trellis plot is displayed in Figure 6.3. Although considerable overlap is seen between the values of the two assays, it is also apparent that the Ektachem measurements tend to be larger and have higher within-subject variation than the Cobas Bio measurements. Moreover, for both assays, this variation seems to increase with the cholesterol level, implying magnitude-dependent heteroscedasticity. The within-subject variation remains substantially lower than the between-subject variation. There is also evidence of assay × subject interaction as the

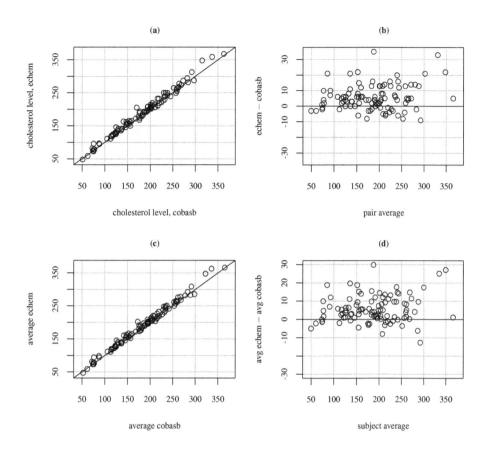

Figure 6.4   Plots for cholesterol data. Top panel (left to right): Scatterplot with line of equality and Bland-Altman plot with zero line based on 100 randomly formed measurement pairs. Bottom panel (left to right): Same as top panel but based on average measurements.

average difference between the assays does not appear constant over the subjects. Figure 6.4 shows scatterplots and Bland-Altman plots for these data based on both randomly formed measurement pairs (top panel) and averages over the replications (bottom panels). The two panels look nearly the same. The scatterplots show high correlation between the assays. The Bland-Altman plots are not centered at zero, suggesting a difference in fixed biases of the assays, but there is no trend in the plots, suggesting a common scale for the assays.

A distinguishing feature of these data, apparent from the trellis plot, is that it exhibits magnitude-dependent heteroscedasticity. To examine it further, we fit the homoscedastic mixed-effects model (5.1) and get the standardized residuals. In Figure 6.5, we plot them as well as their absolute values against the fitted values separately for each assay. The fan-shaped pattern in both residual plots confirms that the error variations of both assays increase with the magnitude of measurement. The increasing trends in both absolute residual plots lead to the same conclusion.

To fit the heteroscedastic model (6.10), we need to come up with models for the error variance functions of the two assays. From the discussion in Section 6.4.2, we take the

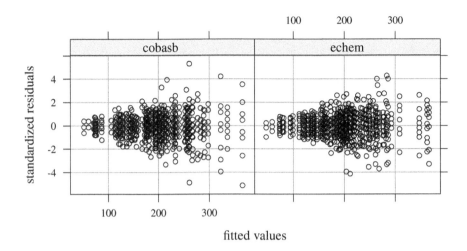

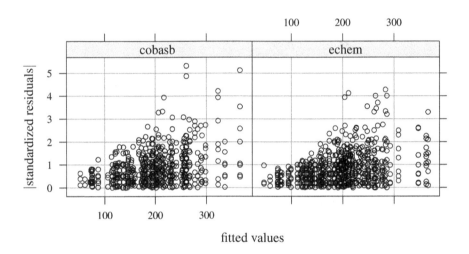

Figure 6.5   Plots of standardized residuals (top panel) and their absolute values (bottom panel) against fitted values from a homoscedastic fit to cholesterol data.

average (6.20) as the variance covariate $\tilde{v}_i$. As this is a positive quantity, there is no need to take its absolute value in the variance functions. Figure 6.6 displays plots of log of absolute values of residuals from the homoscedastic fit against both $\log(\tilde{v}_i)$ and $\tilde{v}_i$. These scatterplots are superimposed with fitted regression lines. It is apparent that the trend in each plot can be approximated by a straight line, at least as our first approximation. This suggests that both the power model (6.2) and the exponential model (6.3) seem reasonable choices for the variance function model. In addition, models of the same form can be used for both methods.

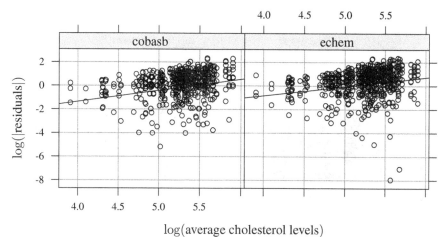

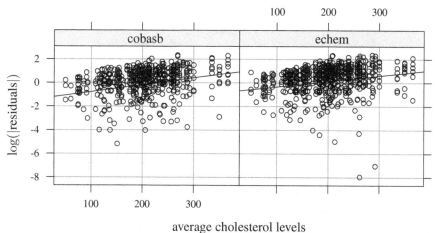

Figure 6.6 Plots of log of absolute residuals from a homoscedastic fit to cholesterol data against $\log(\tilde{v})$ (top panel) and $\tilde{v}$ (bottom panel) with $\tilde{v}$ as the average cholesterol level of a subject. A simple linear regression fit is superimposed on each plot.

Motivated by this finding, we first fit the heteroscedastic mixed-effects model (6.10) with the power variance function model, that is,

$$g_j(\tilde{v}_i, \delta_j) = \tilde{v}_i^{\delta_j}, \quad j = 1, 2,$$

for both assays. The resulting residual plot is shown in Figure 6.7. The residuals are centered at zero and their vertical scatter appears constant, suggesting that the power model is successful in explaining the heteroscedasticity in the data. However, the same is true for the exponential model as well (Exercise 6.5). Unable to distinguish between the two models on the basis of the residual plots alone, we turn to comparing the observed and the fitted

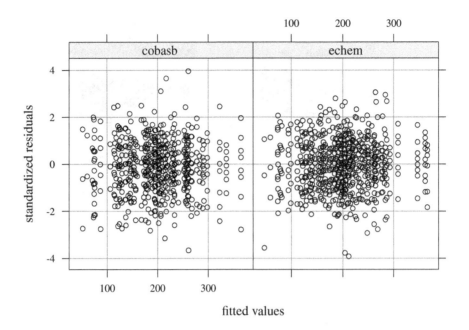

Figure 6.7 Residual plots from a heteroscedastic fit to cholesterol data using power variance function models.

within-subject standard deviations from the two models. Recall that $m = 10$ replications are available at each subject-method combination, enough to provide reasonably stable observed standard deviations. Figure 6.8 displays the observed and the fitted values. The fitted standard deviations from the power model for both assays appear linear because the estimated δ_1 and δ_2 are practically 1 (see Table 6.1). It is clear that both models provide comparable fits except near the right end of the measurement range where the power model appears to fit better than the exponential model. The two models can be further compared using the model comparison criteria AIC and BIC (Section 3.3.7). Their respective values are 9753 and 9798 for the power model, and 9767 and 9812 for the exponential model. Both criteria favor the power model as their values in this case are smaller than the exponential model. (The likelihood ratio test cannot be used to compare the two models because they are not nested.)

Further diagnostics for the power model, including the assessment of normality of random effects and errors, show some evidence of heavy tails for the residuals, but otherwise the fit is reasonably good (Exercise 6.5). This is not of serious concern, as in our experience, the overall conclusions of a method comparison data analysis based on mixed-effects models tend to be robust against error distributions with moderately heavy tails. Therefore, the power model is assumed for the rest of the analysis.

Table 6.1 presents estimates of the eight parameters in the model, their standard errors, and the 95% confidence intervals. Even though there is clear evidence of heteroscedasticity, it is useful nevertheless to test the null hypothesis of homoscedasticity, $\delta_1 = \delta_2 = 0$. The

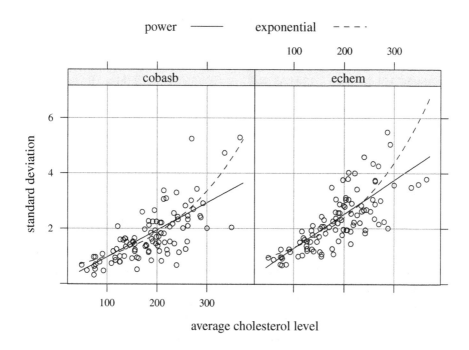

Figure 6.8 Observed versus fitted within-subject standard deviations from power (solid line) and exponential (broken curve) variance function models for cholesterol data. The covariate $\tilde{v}_i$, the subject average, is plotted on the horizontal axis. The observed values are represented by the points and the fitted values are represented by the curves.

Parameter	Estimate	SE	95% Interval
β_0	5.58	0.74	$(4.14, 7.02)$
μ_b	184.38	6.60	$(171.45, 197.31)$
$\log(\sigma_b^2)$	8.37	0.14	$(8.09, 8.65)$
$\log(\psi^2)$	3.28	0.14	$(3.00, 3.56)$
$\log(\sigma_{e1}^2)$	-9.43	0.57	$(-10.55, -8.31)$
$\log(\sigma_{e2}^2)$	-8.49	0.59	$(-9.64, -7.34)$
δ_1	1.02	0.06	$(0.91, 1.12)$
δ_2	0.98	0.06	$(0.86, 1.09)$

Table 6.1 Summary of parameter estimates for cholesterol data. Methods 1 and 2 refer to Cobas Bio and Ektachem, respectively.

log-likelihood for the fitted power model is -4868.6 and it is -5117.6 for the homoscedastic model (5.1) that corresponds to the null hypothesis. Thus, the value of the likelihood ratio statistic (6.22) is $2\{-4868.6 - (-5117.6)\} = 498$. The p-value for this test is practically zero, leading, as expected, to a strong rejection of the homoscedasticity hypothesis.

We substitute the ML estimates from Table 6.1 in (6.15) and (6.16) to obtain the fitted distribution of (Y_1, Y_2) given the cholesterol level $\tilde{v}$ as

$$\mathcal{N}_2\left(\begin{pmatrix}184.38\\189.96\end{pmatrix}, \begin{pmatrix}4351.14 + (8.0 \times 10^{-5})\,\tilde{v}^{2.03} & 4324.58\\4324.58 & 4351.14 + (2.06 \times 10^{-4})\,\tilde{v}^{1.95}\end{pmatrix}\right),$$

and of D given $\tilde{v}$ as

$$\mathcal{N}_1\left(5.58, 53.12 + (8.02 \times 10^{-5})\,\tilde{v}^{2.03} + (2.06 \times 10^{-4})\,\tilde{v}^{1.95}\right). \tag{6.29}$$

From Exercise 6.4, a similar substitution gives the fitted distributions of the intra-method differences D_j given $\tilde{v}$. It follows that

$$D_1|\tilde{v} \sim \mathcal{N}_1\left(0, (16.04 \times 10^{-5})\,\tilde{v}^{2.03}\right), \quad D_2|\tilde{v} \sim \mathcal{N}_1\left(0, (4.12 \times 10^{-4})\,\tilde{v}^{1.95}\right). \tag{6.30}$$

The range of $\tilde{v}$ is taken to be $\mathcal{V} = (45, 372)$, the observed measurement range. These distributions confirm several of our findings based on the various plots. In particular, the Cobas Bio assay has a smaller estimated mean and a smaller estimated error standard deviation than Ektachem. Cobas Bio's error standard deviation, $\{(8.0 \times 10^{-5})\,\tilde{v}^{2.03}\}^{1/2}$, increases from 0.59 to 4.62, whereas that of Ektachem, $\{(2.06 \times 10^{-4})\,\tilde{v}^{1.95}\}^{1/2}$, increases from 0.43 to 3.65. Both the error standard deviations are completely dominated by the between-subject standard deviation as measured by $\sqrt{\exp(8.37) + \exp(3.28)} = 65.9$. It is then not surprising that the overall standard deviations of both assays are nearly a constant around 66. Besides, the correlation between the assays is extremely high—around 0.99 throughout the range. The effect of nonconstant error variation is somewhat more apparent in the standard deviation of D; it increases from 7.32 to 9.37. Note from (6.17) that there are two components of variation in D—one due to the errors and the other due to subject $\times$ method interactions, a component of the between-subject variation. While the latter remains a constant, it dominates the former, making the standard deviation of D depend mildly on the magnitude of measurement.

Figure 6.9 plots the 95% limits of agreement for measurements between and within the methods. They are computed from (6.27) and (6.28), respectively. By definition, the inter-method limits are centered at $\hat{\beta}_0 = 5.58$ and the intra-method limits for both methods are centered at zero. The effect of error heteroscedasticity is clearly apparent in the intra-method limits but less so in the inter-method limits. This discrepancy occurs because the former limits are solely determined by the error variation, whereas the latter limits depend on the variation of D wherein the variation of the errors is dominated by that of the subject $\times$ method interactions.

Next, we examine similarity of the two assays. From Table 6.1, the 95% confidence interval for β_0 is $(4.15, 7.02)$. The entire interval is above zero. Recalling that β_0 represents the difference in means of the two assays under the equal scales assumption, this implies larger mean for Ektachem. Panel (a) of Figure 6.10 displays the estimate and two-sided 95% pointwise confidence band for the precision ratio $\lambda(\tilde{v})$ as a function of the cholesterol level. This measure is defined in (6.23). The entire band lies below one, leading to the conclusion that Cobas Bio is more precise than Ektachem. The estimated λ suggests that the former is about 40% more precise than the latter. On the whole, the two assays cannot be considered similar. Cobas Bio is clearly superior to Ektachem because of its higher precision. These findings are consistent with what we saw earlier in the plots.

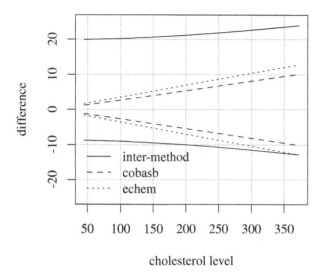

Figure 6.9   95% limits of inter- and intra-method agreement for cholesterol data as a function of magnitude of measurement. The inter-method limits, based on the distribution of D, are centered at 5.58. The intra-method limits, based on the distributions of D_1 and D_2, are centered at zero.

For evaluation of repeatability, panel (b) of Figure 6.10 presents one-sided 95% pointwise lower confidence bands for intra-method versions of CCC. Also presented in panel (c) of the figure are one-sided 95% pointwise upper confidence bands for the intra-method versions of TDI (0.90) and their reflections over a horizontal line at zero. These repeatability measures are defined in (6.26). We see that the CCC lower band for Cobas Bio is entirely above that of Ektachem and the converse is true for the TDI upper bands. This indicates that Cobas Bio has higher intra-method agreement than Ektachem. This conclusion is expected as our evaluation of similarity just showed that Cobas Bio has smaller error variation. More noteworthy is the fact that the CCC bands decrease and the TDI bands increase as the cholesterol level increases. This means that the extent of intra-method agreement for both assays becomes progressively worse as the magnitude of measurement increases. The intra-method CCC lower bands remain above 0.99 throughout the measurement range, implying that the CCC estimates clearly exceed 0.99. Because these are estimated reliabilities of the assays, such larges values essentially reflect that the within-subject variations for both assays are very small compared to the between-subject variation. The TDI bounds increase from 1 to about 9 for Cobas Bio and to about 12 for Ektachem as the cholesterol level increases from 45 to 372. The value of 12, for example, implies that, when the true cholesterol value is 372, 90% of the time the difference between two replications of Ektachem on the same subject falls within ±12. The TDI bounds are only about 2-3% of the magnitude of measurement, indicating a high degree of intra-method agreement for both assays.

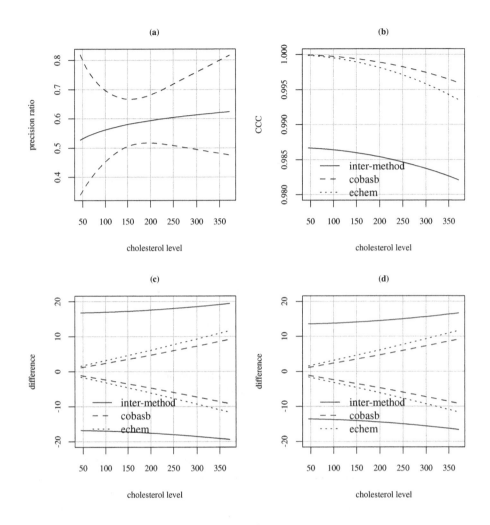

Figure 6.10   Plots for cholesterol data. (a) Estimate (solid curve) and 95% pointwise two-sided confidence band (broken curves) for precision ratio; (b) 95% lower confidence bands for inter- and intra-method versions of CCC; (c) 95% upper confidence bands for inter- and intra-method versions of TDI (0.90) as well as their reflections around the horizontal line at zero, giving the corresponding pointwise tolerance bands; and (d) same as panel (c) but with Ektachem recalibrated to have the same estimated mean as Cobas Bio.

Panels (b) and (c) of Figure 6.10 also present one-sided 95% pointwise confidence bands for CCC and TDI (0.90) for evaluation of agreement between the assays. Just like their intra-method counterparts, the CCC lower band decreases and the TDI upper band increases as the cholesterol level increases. Thus, in an absolute sense, the extent of agreement between the assays becomes progressively worse, albeit only by a small amount, with increasing cholesterol levels. The CCC lower bounds range between 0.982 and 0.987, suggesting excellent agreement between the assays over the entire measurement range. But this conclusion may be misleading because the between-subject variation in these data overwhelms the within-subject variation. A better view of agreement is given by the TDI whose estimate increases from 15.1 to 17.9 and upper bound increases from 17 to 19.5 as the cholesterol level increases from 45 to 372. For example, the bound of 17 shows that 90% of differences in measurements from the assays fall within ± 17 when the true value is 45. Such a difference is unacceptably large relative to the true value. On the other hand, a difference as large as ± 19.5 may be acceptable when the true value is 372. The bounds of 17 and 19.5 are, respectively, about 38% and 5% of the true value. It follows that we may conclude satisfactory agreement between the assays for large cholesterol values but not for very small values.

The similarity evaluation reveals that a difference in the means of the assays is a contributor to disagreement. Recalibration of Ektachem by subtracting $\hat{\beta}_0 = 5.58$ from its measurements makes the mean difference zero, but it improves the extent of agreement only slightly. The TDI bounds now range from 13.5 to 16.5 instead of 17 to 19.5 (compare panels (c) and (d) of Figure 6.10). The CCC bounds increase only slightly as they were already close to 1 (not shown).

Taken together, we find that the assays exhibit high intra-method agreement throughout the measurement range, especially at the low end of the range. But their inter-method agreement, although potentially satisfactory for the upper half of the measurement range, cannot be considered satisfactory at the low end. Even the recalibration of Ektachem does not help matters much. Thus, the assays cannot be used interchangeably. Cobas Bio remains the superior of the two assays because of its higher precision. The apparent mismatch in the conclusions regarding inter- and intra-method agreement can be explained by the fact that the variation in the errors is rather small while the variation in the subject × method interactions is relatively large. This results in small variation in D_1 and D_2 but not in D when considered relative to the true value—see (6.29) and (6.30). The relative variation is especially large at the low end of measurements. It also follows from this discussion that any further improvement in the extent of inter-method agreement would primarily involve reducing the interaction variation. This may not be a simple task.

It may be of interest to ask how the results would compare if the heteroscedasticity in the data is ignored and they are analyzed assuming the homoscedastic model (5.1). This is explored in Exercise 6.5. It turns out that the *overall* conclusions regarding similarity and repeatability are similar to the heteroscedastic case, with the obvious exception that these measures do not depend on the cholesterol value anymore. In addition, there is virtually no change in the inference on CCC as its 95% lower confidence bound is now 0.985, as opposed to ranging over 0.982 to 0.987 in the heteroscedastic case. The estimate of TDI (0.90) is 16 and its 95% upper confidence bound is 17.6. The bound of 17.6 is not terribly far from either endpoint of the interval $(17, 19.5)$ over which the heteroscedastic bound ranges (Figure 6.10, panel (c)). This is primarily because the effect of the error variation, the only entity that depends on the magnitude of measurement, is dominated by the between-subject variation. If this were not the case, the effect of heteroscedasticity on the overall conclusions would have been more prominent. In any case, it is clear that not taking account of heteroscedasticity leads to underestimation of the extent of agreement for small cholesterol levels and its overestimation for large ones.

Finally, recall that we chose the average in (6.20) as the variance covariate $\tilde{v}_i$ for modeling heteroscedasticity. We leave it for the reader to verify that choosing instead the average of either only the reference method measurements or all the measurements on the ith subject as the $\tilde{v}_i$ does not alter the results in any significant manner (Exercise 6.5).

6.5 PAIRED MEASUREMENTS DATA

In the previous section, replications of each measurement allowed us to model within-subject variations of the methods as functions of a variance covariate $\tilde{v}$ that served as a proxy for the magnitude of measurement. We then replaced the constant error variances in the homoscedastic mixed-effects model with variance function models to get a heteroscedastic model for the data. In principle, a similar approach can be used with the paired measurements data. It would model the error variations in the homoscedastic mixed-effects model (4.1) by variance function models. But this does not work in practice because the paired data do not have enough information to reliably estimate even the error variances in the homoscedastic model. Any addition of further parameters to model error heteroscedasticity will only make the matters worse. A more viable alternative in Chapter 4 was to model the data Y_{ij}, $j = 1, 2$, $i = 1, \ldots, n$ as a random sample of (Y_1, Y_2) following the bivariate normal distribution specified in (4.6). In particular, this model assumes that

$$\text{var}(Y_j) = \sigma_j^2, \quad j = 1, 2. \tag{6.31}$$

This model can be extended by directly letting these measurement variances, not the error variances of the methods, depend on the variance covariate $\tilde{v}$ through variance function models. We now provide the relevant details by paralleling the development of the previous section.

6.5.1 A Heteroscedastic Bivariate Normal Model

Let the variances of the measurement methods depend on a given value $\tilde{v}$ of the variance covariate as

$$\text{var}(Y_j|\tilde{v}) = \sigma_j^2 \, g_j^2(\tilde{v}, \delta_j), \quad j = 1, 2. \tag{6.32}$$

Here g_j is a variance function with heteroscedasticity parameter δ_j (Section 6.3), and $\tilde{v} \in \mathcal{V}$. Replacing the variances (6.31) in the bivariate normal model (4.6) with their heteroscedastic counterparts (6.32) gives the distribution of (Y_1, Y_2) given $\tilde{v}$ as

$$\begin{pmatrix} Y_1 \\ Y_2 \end{pmatrix} \bigg| \, \tilde{v} \sim \mathcal{N}_2 \left(\begin{pmatrix} \mu_1 \\ \mu_2 \end{pmatrix}, \begin{pmatrix} \sigma_1^2 g_1^2(\tilde{v}, \delta_1) & \sigma_{12}(\tilde{v}, \delta_1, \delta_2) \\ \sigma_{12}(\tilde{v}, \delta_1, \delta_2) & \sigma_2^2 g_2^2(\tilde{v}, \delta_2) \end{pmatrix} \right), \tag{6.33}$$

where

$$\sigma_{12}(\tilde{v}, \delta_1, \delta_2) = \rho \sigma_1 \sigma_2 \, g_1(\tilde{v}, \delta_1) g_2(\tilde{v}, \delta_2). \tag{6.34}$$

Notice that the covariance of this distribution depends on $\tilde{v}$ in such a way that the correlation ρ remains constant. This contrasts with the heteroscedastic model of previous section in which the covariance remained constant whereas the correlation depended on $\tilde{v}$, see (6.15). This switch is done for computational ease in model fitting (see Section 6.7). It follows from (6.33) that

$$D|\tilde{v} \sim \mathcal{N}_1 \big(\xi = \mu_2 - \mu_1, \tau^2(\tilde{v}) = \sigma_1^2 g_1^2(\tilde{v}, \delta_1) + \sigma_2^2 g_2^2(\tilde{v}, \delta_2) - 2\sigma_{12}(\tilde{v}, \delta_1, \delta_2) \big). \tag{6.35}$$

The model (6.33) for (Y_1, Y_2) suggests that given $\tilde{v}_i$, the value of $\tilde{v}$ for subject i, the observed measurement pairs (Y_{i1}, Y_{i2}) for $i = 1, \ldots, n$ can be modeled as

$$\begin{pmatrix} Y_{i1} \\ Y_{i2} \end{pmatrix} \bigg| \, \tilde{v}_i \sim \text{independent } \mathcal{N}_2 \left(\begin{pmatrix} \mu_1 \\ \mu_2 \end{pmatrix}, \begin{pmatrix} \sigma_1^2 g_1^2(\tilde{v}_i, \delta_1) & \sigma_{12}(\tilde{v}_i, \delta_1, \delta_2) \\ \sigma_{12}(\tilde{v}_i, \delta_1, \delta_2) & \sigma_2^2 g_2^2(\tilde{v}_i, \delta_2) \end{pmatrix} \right). \tag{6.36}$$

This is the heteroscedastic bivariate normal model we use for the paired measurements data. The pairs (Y_{i1}, Y_{i2}) are not identically distributed anymore because their variances depend on i through $\tilde{v}_i$. The model reduces to its homoscedastic counterpart (4.6) when $\delta_1 = \delta_2 = 0$.

6.5.2 Specifying the Variance Function

To complete the specification of the heteroscedastic model (6.36), we need to provide the variance functions g_j given by (6.32). For this, we follow the general three-step strategy outlined in Section 6.4.2 for repeated measurements data, but we need to make some changes necessitated by the fact that the data here are unreplicated. In the first step, we choose the proxies $\tilde{\mu}_{ij}$ for the error-free values of the methods. Even though there is no notion of "error-free" values in the bivariate normal model, we may still take $m_{ij} = 1$ in (6.18) leading to

$$\tilde{\mu}_{ij} = y_{ij}, \ j = 1, 2.$$

In the second step, we choose the specific function h of these (y_{i1}, y_{i2}) that determines the variance covariate $\tilde{v}_i = h(y_{i1}, y_{i2})$. From (6.19) and (6.20), the possibilities include $\tilde{v}_i = y_{i1}$ (if method 1 serves as our reference) and

$$\tilde{v}_i = (y_{i1} + y_{i2})/2. \tag{6.37}$$

As before, we mostly work with this average as the variance covariate. A function such as the log function of either y_{i1} or the average may also be taken as $\tilde{v}_i$, assuming that the measurements are positive.

In the third step, we choose functional forms for the g_j functions of the covariate $\tilde{v}_i$. For repeated measurements data, this was done by examining trends in the plots of absolute residuals from the corresponding homoscedastic fit against $\tilde{v}_i$ or functions thereof. But this approach fails for paired measurements data. To understand why this is so, consider the measurement pair (Y_{i1}, Y_{i2}). Under the homoscedastic bivariate normal model (4.6), we can write

$$Y_{ij} = \mu_j + e_{ij}, \ j = 1, 2,$$

where

$$\begin{pmatrix} e_{i1} \\ e_{i2} \end{pmatrix} \sim \mathcal{N}_2 \left(\begin{pmatrix} 0 \\ 0 \end{pmatrix}, \begin{pmatrix} \sigma_1^2 & \sigma_{12} \\ \sigma_{12} & \sigma_2^2 \end{pmatrix} \right).$$

These e_{ij} may be taken as the "errors." Recalling from (4.8) that $(\overline{Y}_{.j}, \hat{\sigma}_j^2)$ are ML estimators of (μ_j, σ_j^2), it follows that $\hat{e}_{ij} = (Y_{ij} - \overline{Y}_{.j})$ and $\hat{e}_{ij}/\hat{\sigma}_j$ can be taken as the raw and standardized residuals, respectively. Plots of these residuals against the averages $\tilde{v}_i$ in (6.37) exhibit linear trends even if the homoscedastic model (4.6) holds. This is caused by the simple fact that Y_{ij} and $(Y_{i1} + Y_{i2})/2$ are correlated (Exercise 6.7). Thus, examining trends in the plots of absolute residuals has limited usefulness for suggesting variance function models.

Instead of guessing the g_j functions from a visual assessment of residuals, we prefer to take the simple variance function models introduced in Section 6.4.2 and fit the resulting heteroscedastic models. Then, we examine the adequacy of the fitted g_j functions to see which one, if any, fits well. If none does, more complex models may be called for, but this is usually not necessary. If multiple models appear to fit equally well then the model comparison criteria such as AIC and BIC may be employed for model selection.

We now develop two graphical diagnostic tools based on differences to check the adequacy of the assumed g_j functions. Both utilize the fact that if the heteroscedastic model (6.36) with the assumed variance functions holds, it follows from (6.35) and Exercise 6.1 that $|D_i - \xi|$ has expectation $\sqrt{(2/\pi)}\,\tau(\tilde{v}_i)$. Therefore, if the model holds, the trend in the plot of a sample counterpart of $|D_i - \xi|$, for example, $|D_i - \overline{D}|$ or $|D_i - \hat{\xi}|$, against $\tilde{v}_i$ should be approximated by

$$\sqrt{(2/\pi)}\,\hat{\tau}(\tilde{v}_i). \tag{6.38}$$

Here $\hat{\xi}$ and $\hat{\tau}(\tilde{v}_i)$ are ML estimates of their population counterparts under the model.

The first diagnostic superimposes the plot of absolute values of centered differences $|D_i - \overline{D}|$ against $\tilde{v}_i$ with a curve of $\sqrt{(2/\pi)}\,\hat{\tau}(\tilde{v}_i)$. The assumed g_j functions may be adequate if the curve provides a reasonably good approximation to the trend in the main body of the plot. The second diagnostic plots absolute values of the standardized differences

$$|D_i - \hat{\xi}|/\hat{\tau}(\tilde{v}_i) \tag{6.39}$$

against $\tilde{v}_i$. The assumed g_j functions may be adequate if this plot is approximately centered at $\sqrt{(2/\pi)} \approx 0.8$. Otherwise, we need to consider other g_j functions in (6.32).

6.5.3 Model Fitting and Evaluation

As for the repeated measurements data, the variance covariate $\tilde{v}_i$ in the heteroscedastic model (6.36) is treated as a known quantity and is held fixed in model fitting. The model can be fit by the ML method using a numerical optimization routine (see Section 6.7) to get the ML estimates

$$(\hat{\mu}_1, \hat{\mu}_2, \hat{\sigma}_1^2, \hat{\sigma}_2^2, \hat{\rho}, \hat{\delta}_1, \hat{\delta}_2)$$

of the model parameters.

There are two aspects of evaluating the fitted model. One is checking the adequacy of the assumed variance functions, as discussed above. The other is checking the bivariate normal assumption. This can proceed as in Section 4.2.2; we now use the standardized pairs

$$\left(\frac{Y_{i1} - \hat{\mu}_1}{\hat{\sigma}_1\, g_1(\tilde{v}_i, \hat{\delta}_1)},\ \frac{Y_{i2} - \hat{\mu}_2}{\hat{\sigma}_2\, g_2(\tilde{v}_i, \hat{\delta}_2)} \right) \tag{6.40}$$

instead of the raw measurements (Y_{i1}, Y_{i2}). This guards against nonconstant variability interfering with the assessment of normality.

6.5.4 Testing for Homoscedasticity

Testing for the null hypothesis (6.21) of homoscedasticity against the assumed form for heteroscedasticity proceeds exactly as in Section 6.4.4 with L_1 and L_2, respectively, denoting the maximum likelihoods under the models (4.6) and (6.36).

6.5.5 Evaluation of Similarity and Agreement

This section adapts the methodology described in Section 4.3 for the homoscedastic model (4.6) to the heteroscedastic model (6.36). Evaluation of repeatability is not considered here as we do not have replicated data. Recall from Section 4.3 that the bivariate normal model does not allow inference on any measure of similarity in the sense of Section 1.7. We can, however, compare the means and the variances of the two methods. It follows from the conditional distribution of (Y_1, Y_2) given $\tilde{v}$ in (6.33) that the means can be compared through the mean difference $\xi = \mu_2 - \mu_1$, and the variances can be compared through the variance ratio

$$\frac{\sigma_2^2 \, g_2^2(\tilde{v}, \delta_2)}{\sigma_1^2 \, g_1^2(\tilde{v}, \delta_1)}. \tag{6.41}$$

In the absence of a scale difference in the methods, $\mu_2 - \mu_1$ can be interpreted as β_0, the difference in fixed biases of the methods. The heteroscedastic versions of CCC and TDI given in (4.10) can be obtained by replacing the moments by their counterparts from (6.33) and (6.35). This gives

$$\text{CCC}(\tilde{v}) = \frac{2\sigma_{12}(\tilde{v}, \delta_1, \delta_1)}{(\mu_2 - \mu_1)^2 + \sigma_1^2 \, g_1^2(\tilde{v}, \delta_1) + \sigma_2^2 \, g_2^2(\tilde{v}, \delta_2)}, \tag{6.42}$$

where the covariance function in the numerator is given by (6.34), and

$$\text{TDI}(p, \tilde{v}) = \tau(\tilde{v}) \left\{ \chi_{1,p}^2 \left(\xi^2 / \tau^2(\tilde{v}) \right) \right\}^{1/2}. \tag{6.43}$$

Inference on these measures proceeds as before. The heteroscedastic analog of the 95% limits of agreement in (4.12) is

$$\hat{\xi} \pm 1.96 \times \hat{\tau}(\tilde{v}), \tag{6.44}$$

with $\hat{\tau}^2(\tilde{v})$ denoting the ML estimator of $\tau^2(\tilde{v})$.

6.5.6 Case Study: Cyclosporin Data

These data, introduced in Section 6.2.2.1, consist of paired measurements of concentrations of cyclosporin (ng/mL) from HPLC (method 1) and RIA (method 2) in $n = 56$ blood samples. The HPLC method serves as the reference method. Figure 6.1 displays a trellis plot of the data. Although no method gives consistently higher measurements than the other, the RIA measurements do appear a bit higher on average than HPLC. The within-subject spread of the measurements has a tendency to increase with the measured concentration level. This variation, nevertheless, is small compared to the between-subject variation. Moreover, an outlier is clearly visible in the top right corner of the plot. Because of its location, the outlier serves to considerably increase the range of observed measurements, extending the upper limit from 653 to 980 while the lower limit is 35. Initially, we will include the outlier in the analysis because we would like the conclusions to hold over the wider range. Later, we will redo the analysis by dropping the outlier, and compare the conclusions.

A scatterplot of the data is displayed in Figure 6.11. It shows high correlation between the methods, and its funnel-like shape provides another view of heteroscedasticity in the data. The Bland-Altman plot shown in Figure 6.2 does not have any trend, implying that the methods may have the same scale. The vertical scatter in this plot tends to increase with the average, supporting heteroscedasticity inferred from other plots. A variation of the Bland-Altman plot where the absolute values of centered differences are plotted on the vertical axis is also displayed in Figure 6.2. The increasing trend in this plot provides yet another confirmation of the heteroscedasticity. The outlier in these plots accentuates the

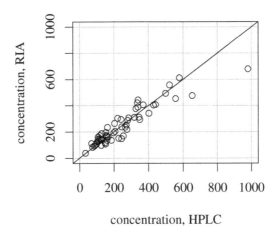

Figure 6.11   A scatterplot of cyclosporin data with line of equality.

pattern that the heteroscedasticity tends to increase with the magnitude of measurement, but this pattern is evident even without it.

Our next task is to fit the heteroscedastic bivariate normal model (6.36) with appropriate choices for the variance functions g_j. Following Section 6.5.2, we take the average (6.37) as the variance covariate $\tilde{v}_i$, and fit the model twice—once using power variance functions for both methods, and again using exponential variance functions for both methods. Figure 6.12 plots the absolute standardized differences (6.39) against $\tilde{v}_i$ for both variance functions. None of the plots show any prominent trend and both appear centered around 0.8, implying that both models may be a good fit. For further comparison, Figure 6.13 displays a plot of absolute centered differences $|D_i - \overline{D}|$ against $\tilde{v}_i$ superimposed with the curves of (6.38) under the two models. The curves are nearly identical till the concentration level of about 400, whereupon they quickly diverge. The curve in the exponential case appears to follow the outlier, suggesting that the exponential model may overestimate the variance for large values of $\tilde{v}_i$. In contrast, the power model does not have this issue and it appears to fit the trend quite well over the entire measurement range. Both AIC and BIC prefer the exponential model. Their respective values are 1297 and 1326 for power functions, and 1282 and 1301 for exponential functions. We, however, choose to work with the power model.

Bivariate normality for the standardized observations (6.40) under the power model also appears adequate, with the exception that the subject with paired measurements $(35, 38)$—the two smallest measurements in the data—has unusually small standardized values (around -3.5 for both methods; Exercise 6.8). This lack of fit at a single point on the boundary of the data space does not cause much concern. The reader is asked in Exercise 6.8 to redo the entire analysis with the exponential model and compare conclusions.

The model (6.36) with power variance functions $g_j(\tilde{v}_i, \delta_j) = \tilde{v}_i^{\delta_j}$ has seven parameters. Table 6.2 presents their estimates, standard errors, and 95% confidence intervals. The

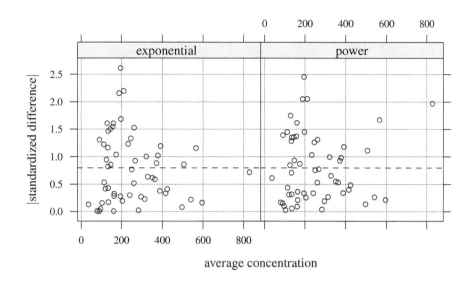

Figure 6.12 Plots of absolute standardized differences against averages for cyclosporin data with exponential and power variance function fits. A horizontal line at $\sqrt{(2/\pi)} \approx 0.8$ is superimposed on each plot.

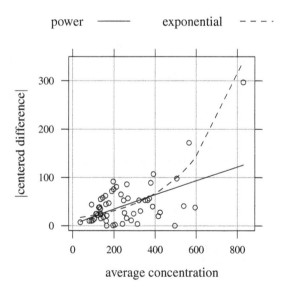

Figure 6.13 Plot of absolute centered differences against averages for cyclosporin data superimposed with $\sqrt{(2/\pi)}$ times fitted standard deviations of differences under power (solid line) and exponential (broken curve) variance function fits.

Parameter	Estimate	SE	95% Interval
μ_1	128.85	18.07	$(93.42, 164.28)$
μ_2	138.14	17.91	$(103.04, 173.23)$
$\log(\sigma_1^2)$	0.15	1.28	$(-2.36, 2.66)$
$\log(\sigma_2^2)$	0.77	1.30	$(-1.78, 3.33)$
$z(\rho)$	1.67	0.13	$(1.41, 1.93)$
δ_1	0.89	0.12	$(0.66, 1.12)$
δ_2	0.82	0.12	$(0.58, 1.06)$

Table 6.2   Summary of parameter estimates for cyclosporin data. Methods 1 and 2 refer to HPLC and RIA, respectively.

log-likelihood for the fitted heteroscedastic model is -641.5, and it is -669.4 for the homoscedastic model that corresponds to $\delta_1 = \delta_2 = 0$. From (6.22), the value of the likelihood ratio statistic for testing the null hypothesis of homoscedasticity is 56.2. The p-value is less than 0.001, suggesting a strong rejection of the null hypothesis and supporting the need for a heteroscedastic model.

Substitution of the ML estimates from Table 6.2 in (6.33) and (6.35), respectively, gives the fitted bivariate normal distribution for (Y_1, Y_2) given the concentration level $\tilde{v}$ as

$$\begin{pmatrix} Y_1 \\ Y_2 \end{pmatrix} \sim \mathcal{N}_2 \left(\begin{pmatrix} 128.85 \\ 138.14 \end{pmatrix}, \begin{pmatrix} 1.16\,\tilde{v}^{1.78} & 1.47\,\tilde{v}^{1.71} \\ 1.47\,\tilde{v}^{1.71} & 2.17\,\tilde{v}^{1.64} \end{pmatrix} \right),$$

and the fitted normal distribution of D given $\tilde{v}$ as

$$D \sim \mathcal{N}_1 \left(9.29, 1.16\,\tilde{v}^{1.78} + 2.17\,\tilde{v}^{1.64} - 2.95\,\tilde{v}^{1.71} \right).$$

Here $\tilde{v}$ ranges over the observed measurement range $\mathcal{V} = (35, 980)$. The fitted distributions confirm that RIA produces a higher mean than HPLC. Their correlation is 0.93. The standard deviation of HPLC increases from 25 to 494, and it increases from 27 to 421 for RIA. For concentrations above 100, HPLC's standard deviation is higher than that of RIA. The standard deviation of the difference increases from 10 to 184. From (6.44), it follows that the lower limit of the 95% limits of agreement decreases from -10 to -351, and its upper limit increases from 29 to 369. The limits of agreement become wider with the concentration level because of the heteroscedasticity.

For similarity evaluation, the estimate of the mean difference $\mu_2 - \mu_1$—which can be interpreted as the similarity measure β_0 (Section 1.7) because the methods seem to have the same scale—is 9.29 with a standard error of 5.64. Its 95% confidence interval is $(-1.77, 20.34)$. Although zero is contained in this interval, there is some indication that the mean of RIA may be greater than that of HPLC, corroborating the observation from the exploratory data analysis. Figure 6.14 presents the estimates and the 95% pointwise confidence band for the variance ratio defined in (6.41). The estimate slowly decreases from about 1.15 to 0.70, falling below 1 around 100. Thus, the estimated variability of HPLC is initially slightly less but gradually becomes more than that of RIA. Nevertheless, the value of 1 is covered in the pointwise band throughout the interval, suggesting that methods may have similar variabilities. Overall, this similarity evaluation does not offer conclusive evidence of a systematic difference in either the means or the variances of the two methods.

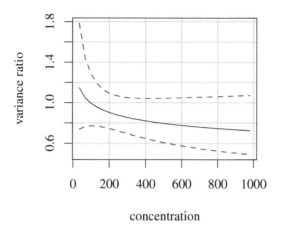

Figure 6.14   Estimate (solid curve) of the variance ratio for RIA over HPLC and its 95% pointwise confidence band (broken curves) for cyclosporin data.

Figure 6.15 displays appropriate one-sided 95% pointwise confidence bands for CCC and TDI (0.90) for agreement evaluation. The CCC lower bounds sharply increase from 0.70 to 0.89 and then decrease slowly to 0.87. The peak occurs around 200. A similar pattern holds for the estimated CCC as well. On the whole, the CCC values indicate a moderate level of agreement, especially for concentration levels above 100. A different picture emerges from TDI (0.90), whose estimated values increase from 22 to 302, and upper bounds increase from 36 to 426. The monotonic pattern in the agreement measure is in line with the pattern of heteroscedasticity seen in the Bland-Altman plot in Figure 6.2. The TDI bounds imply that the absolute difference can be as large as 36 when the true value is 35; and it can be up to 426 when the true value is 980. The bounds always remain over 40% of the corresponding cyclosporin level. Thus, they are too high for the level of agreement over any portion of the measurement range to be considered satisfactory.

The analysis thus far is based on all data, including the outlier in the top right corner of the trellis plot in Figure 6.1. To assess the outlier's impact on our conclusions, we redo the analysis by removing the associated subject. Thus, the new analysis is based on $n = 55$ subjects. The new estimate of mean difference $\mu_2 - \mu_1$ is 7.28, about 2 less than the old one, with confidence interval $(-4.37, 18.92)$. The estimate of variance ratio now decreases from 1.04 to 0.84, instead of from 1.15 to 0.70. As before, its pointwise confidence intervals cover 1 at all points. Taken together, the methods appear slightly more similar without the outlier. This finding, nevertheless, is not surprising as it is clear from the trellis plot (Figure 6.1) that the difference in measurements for the outlying subject is about 300. This is inconsistent with the pattern for the rest of the subjects where the differences are much smaller (below 180). The measurements from the outlying subject lead to a considerable increase in the between-subject variation of HPLC while not having that big of an impact on the between-subject variation of RIA. The slightly increased similarity of

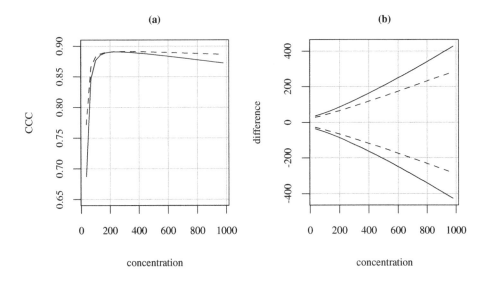

(a)   **(b)**

Figure 6.15   95% pointwise bounds for cyclosporin data with (solid curve) and without (broken curve) the outlier. Panel (a): Lower confidence bounds for CCC. Panel (b): Upper confidence bounds for TDI and their reflections around the horizontal line at zero, giving pointwise tolerance bands.

the methods translates into a slightly better agreement between them—see the confidence bands for CCC and TDI in Figure 6.15. However, the overall conclusion that the methods lack satisfactory agreement remains unchanged.

If we fit the homoscedastic mixed-effects model (5.1) to the complete data with $n = 56$, we obtain the lower bound for CCC as 0.88 and the upper bound for TDI (0.90) as 125 (Exercise 6.8). A comparison with their heteroscedastic versions in Figure 6.15 shows no practical difference in the CCC bounds except at the low end of the measurement range. However, the same cannot be said for the TDI bounds because the value of 125 falls in the middle of 36 to 426, the range of the heteroscedastic bounds. Clearly, ignoring heteroscedasticity leads to overestimation of TDI for small cyclosporin values and its underestimation for large cyclosporin values.

The sample means of HPLC and RIA values are 255 and 250.84, respectively. These ML estimates of the means under the homoscedastic model are considerably greater than their heteroscedastic counterparts in Table 6.2. This discrepancy is explained by the fact that the homoscedastic estimates are unweighted averages of the measurements, whereas the heteroscedastic estimates behave more or less like weighted averages with weights inversely related to their variances (Section 6.7). In the cyclosporin data, the variances of the measurements increase with magnitude. This means that, in the estimates from the heteroscedastic model, the large measurements have low weights and the small measurements have high weights, thus shrinking the estimates towards smaller values.

6.6 CHAPTER SUMMARY

1. The methodology for the analysis of homoscedastic data is generalized to incorporate magnitude-dependent heteroscedasticity in the measurement methods.

2. The approach differs depending upon whether the data have unlinked repeated measurements or simply paired measurements.

3. For unlinked repeated measurements data, the variances of the within-subject errors of the methods are modeled as functions of a variance covariate.

4. For paired measurements data, the variances of observed measurements of the methods are modeled as functions of a variance covariate.

5. The variance covariate is a function of the magnitude of measurement. It is treated as a fixed known quantity in model fitting. We have used the average of a subject's measurement as the variance covariate, but other choices are possible.

6. Each method may have its own variance function of the variance covariate.

7. To address heteroscedasticity, the measures of similarity and agreement that involve variances are modeled as functions of the variance covariate.

8. The methodology for repeated measurements assumes equal scales for the methods. This assumption is not necessary for paired measurements, but under this assumption the difference in the means can be interpreted as the difference in fixed biases.

9. The methodology requires a large number of subjects for the estimated standard errors and confidence intervals to be accurate.

6.7 TECHNICAL DETAILS

6.7.1 Repeated Measurements Data

The homoscedastic mixed-effects model (5.1) for unlinked repeated measurements data is written in the matrix notation in (5.40). This model assumes that the error vector

$$\mathbf{e}_i \sim \mathcal{N}_{M_i}(\mathbf{0}, \mathbf{R}_i), \quad \mathbf{R}_i = \text{diag}\{\mathbf{R}_{i1}, \mathbf{R}_{i2}\}, \quad \mathbf{R}_{ij} = \sigma_{ej}^2 \mathbf{I}_{m_{ij}}. \tag{6.45}$$

The heteroscedastic model with error distributions (6.7) amounts to replacing (6.45) with

$$\mathbf{e}_i | \mathbf{u}_i \sim \mathcal{N}_{M_i}\big(\mathbf{0}, \mathbf{R}_i(v_i)\big), \quad \mathbf{R}_i(v_i) = \text{diag}\{\mathbf{R}_{i1}(v_i), \mathbf{R}_{i2}(v_i)\},$$
$$\mathbf{R}_{ij} = \sigma_{ej}^2 \, g_j^2(v_i, \delta_j) \, \mathbf{I}_{m_{ij}}, \tag{6.46}$$

where the true variance covariate v_i is given by (6.6). By definition, $v_i = h(\mu_{i1}, \mu_{i2})$ is a function of the error-free values (μ_{i1}, μ_{i2}), given by (6.5), that are themselves functions of β and $\mathbf{u}_i$. This also explains the conditioning on $\mathbf{u}_i$ in the error distribution (6.46); $\mathbf{e}_i$ and $\mathbf{u}_i$ are not independent anymore. This heteroscedastic model can be written as

$$\mathbf{Y}_i | \mathbf{u}_i \sim \mathcal{N}_{M_i}\big(\mathbf{X}_i\beta + \mathbf{Z}_i\mathbf{u}_i, \mathbf{R}_i(v_i)\big), \quad \mathbf{u}_i \sim \mathcal{N}_3(\mathbf{0}, \mathbf{G}). \tag{6.47}$$

It reduces to the homoscedastic model when $\delta_1 = \delta_2 = 0$. The marginal density of $\mathbf{Y}_i$ under (6.47) can be obtained by integrating out $\mathbf{u}_i$ from the joint density of $(\mathbf{Y}_i, \mathbf{u}_i)$ as

$$f_\theta(\mathbf{y}_i) = \int f_\theta(\mathbf{y}_i, \mathbf{u}_i)\, d\mathbf{u}_i = \int f_\theta(\mathbf{y}_i|\mathbf{u}_i) f_\theta(\mathbf{u}_i)\, d\mathbf{u}_i, \tag{6.48}$$

where

$$\boldsymbol{\theta} = (\beta_0, \mu_b, \log(\sigma_b^2), \log(\psi^2), \log(\sigma_{e1}^2), \log(\sigma_{e2}^2), \delta_1, \delta_2)^T$$

is the vector of transformed model parameters, and $f_\theta(\mathbf{y}_i|\mathbf{u}_i)$ and $f_\theta(\mathbf{u}_i)$ are normal densities associated with the distributions in (6.47). However, the integral in (6.48) does not have a closed-form because $\mathbf{u}_i$ appears nonlinearly in the covariance matrix $\mathbf{R}_i(v_i)$ and cannot be integrated out explicitly. It is possible to numerically approximate this integral using, for example, Laplace approximation or Gauss-Hermite quadrature, thereby approximating the likelihood function, and using an optimization routine to get the ML estimate of $\boldsymbol{\theta}$.

An alternative to this approach of numerically approximating the likelihood is to approximate the model itself in a way that the resulting likelihood function has a closed form. This likelihood is then numerically maximized. This is the approach we use here. It involves replacing the unobservable error-free values (μ_{i1}, μ_{i2}) by their observable proxies $(\tilde{\mu}_{i1}, \tilde{\mu}_{i2})$ that are expected to be close to (μ_{i1}, μ_{i2}) but are free of $\mathbf{u}_i$ and are treated as known fixed quantities. From (6.8), it yields $\tilde{v}_i = h(\tilde{\mu}_{i1}, \tilde{\mu}_{i2})$ as the approximate variance covariate. One can also think of $\tilde{v}_i$ as the first term in the Taylor series expansion of v_i around $(\tilde{\mu}_{i1}, \tilde{\mu}_{i2})$. Replacing v_i in (6.9) with $\tilde{v}_i$ gives variance function models that are free of $\mathbf{u}_i$ and leads to the heteroscedastic mixed-effects model (6.10). This model can be written in the usual mixed-effects model form as

$$\mathbf{Y}_i = \mathbf{X}_i \boldsymbol{\beta} + \mathbf{Z}_i \mathbf{u}_i + \mathbf{e}_i, \ i = 1, \ldots, n, \tag{6.49}$$

where

$$\mathbf{e}_i|\tilde{v}_i \sim \mathcal{N}_{M_i}(\mathbf{0}, \mathbf{R}_i(\tilde{v}_i)), \ \mathbf{u}_i \sim \mathcal{N}_3(\mathbf{0}, \mathbf{G}),$$

and $\mathbf{R}_i(\tilde{v}_i)$ is from (6.46) with v_i replaced by $\tilde{v}_i$. In this formulation, $\tilde{v}_i$ is a known variance covariate, and the covariance matrix of $\mathbf{e}_i$ is free of $\mathbf{u}_i$, making $\mathbf{e}_i$ and $\mathbf{u}_i$ mutually independent. As a result, $\mathbf{u}_i$ in the integral given in (6.48) can be integrated out explicitly and we obtain

$$\mathbf{Y}_i|\tilde{v}_i \sim \mathcal{N}_{M_i}(\mathbf{X}_i\boldsymbol{\beta}, \mathbf{V}_i(\tilde{v}_i) = \mathbf{Z}_i\mathbf{G}\mathbf{Z}_i^T + \mathbf{R}_i(\tilde{v}_i)) \tag{6.50}$$

as the marginal density of $\mathbf{Y}_i|\tilde{v}_i$ (Exercise 6.2). Thus, the likelihood function $L(\boldsymbol{\theta})$ of the approximated model (6.49) is simply a product of normal densities associated with the distributions in (6.50). This model, being a mixed-effects model with normal marginal distributions, can be fit using any software that can handle mixed-effects models with a known variance covariate. All the inferences are based on the approximate model (6.49). Elements of the mean vector $\mathbf{X}_i\boldsymbol{\beta}$ and covariance matrix $\mathbf{V}_i$ in (6.50) were given earlier in (6.11)–(6.14). Guidelines for choosing the variance covariate and the variance functions were discussed in Section 6.4.2.

This approach for approximating the model to get a closed-form for the likelihood function is common in the literature on generalized linear mixed-effects models and nonlinear mixed-effects models. One may think of this as a *pseudo-likelihood approach*. It is also easier to implement than the approach based on likelihood approximation. Besides, the point and interval estimates of parameters in (6.47) obtained by model approximation approach tend to be at least as accurate and often more accurate than the likelihood approximation approach; see Section 6.8 for a reference.

6.7.2 Paired Measurements Data

The homoscedastic bivariate normal model (4.6) treats the vector of paired measurements $\mathbf{Y}_i, i = 1, \ldots, n$, as a random sample from a $\mathcal{N}_2(\boldsymbol{\mu}, \mathbf{V})$ distribution, where the mean vector $\boldsymbol{\mu}$ and the covariance matrix $\mathbf{V}$ are given by (4.17). Under the heteroscedastic bivariate normal model (6.36) with known variance covariate $\tilde{v}_i$, $\mathbf{Y}_i | \tilde{v}_i$ are independently distributed as $\mathcal{N}_2(\boldsymbol{\mu}, \mathbf{V}_i(\tilde{v}_i))$ random vectors, where $\boldsymbol{\mu}$ is same as before and $\mathbf{V}_i(\tilde{v}_i)$ is the covariance matrix in (6.36). This model reduces to the homoscedastic model when $\delta_1 = \delta_2 = 0$.

Letting $\boldsymbol{\theta} = (\boldsymbol{\theta}_1^T, \boldsymbol{\theta}_2^T)^T$ to be the vector of transformed model parameters, where

$$\boldsymbol{\theta}_1 = \boldsymbol{\mu}, \quad \boldsymbol{\theta}_2 = \left(\log(\sigma_1^2), \log(\sigma_2^2), z(\rho), \delta_1, \delta_2\right)^T,$$

the likelihood function can be written as

$$L(\boldsymbol{\theta}_1, \boldsymbol{\theta}_2) = (2\pi)^{-n} \left(\prod_{i=1}^{n} |\mathbf{V}_i(\tilde{v}_i)|\right)^{-1/2} \exp\left\{-\frac{1}{2}\sum_{i=1}^{n}(\mathbf{y}_i - \boldsymbol{\theta}_1)^T \mathbf{V}_i^{-1}(\tilde{v}_i)(\mathbf{y}_i - \boldsymbol{\theta}_1)\right\}.$$

One can directly maximize the log of this likelihood function to get the ML estimate of $\boldsymbol{\theta}$. Alternatively, the same can be obtained through an iteratively reweighting scheme, which involves starting with an initial estimate of $\boldsymbol{\theta}_2$ and iterating the following two steps until convergence is established:

Step 1. Use the current estimate of $\boldsymbol{\theta}_2$ to compute $\mathbf{V}_i(\tilde{v}_i)$ and update $\boldsymbol{\theta}_1$ as

$$\boldsymbol{\theta}_1 = \left(\sum_{i=1}^{n} \mathbf{V}_i^{-1}(\tilde{v}_i)\right)^{-1} \sum_{i=1}^{n} \mathbf{V}_i^{-1}(\tilde{v}_i)\mathbf{Y}_i.$$

Step 2. Update $\boldsymbol{\theta}_2$ by numerically maximizing $\log\{L(\boldsymbol{\theta}_1, \boldsymbol{\theta}_2)\}$ with respect to $\boldsymbol{\theta}_2$ with $\boldsymbol{\theta}_1$ set to its updated value in Step 1.

In Step 1, $\boldsymbol{\theta}_1$ is the solution of $\partial \log\{L(\boldsymbol{\theta}_1, \boldsymbol{\theta}_2)\}/\partial \boldsymbol{\theta}_1 = \mathbf{0}$ with $\boldsymbol{\theta}_2$ set to its current estimate. One can use the ML estimates (4.8) from the homoscedastic fit together with $\delta_1 = \delta_2 = 0$ to get an initial estimate of $\boldsymbol{\theta}_2$.

We need to explain why the correlation of the bivariate normal distribution in (6.36) is chosen to remain fixed rather than the covariance. The ML estimates are obtained by maximizing the log-likelihood function over the parameter space of the model. The parameters $(\mu_1, \mu_2, \delta_1, \delta_2)$ are unconstrained, but the remaining parameters are constrained so that the variances are positive and the correlation is in $(-1, 1)$. Constraining (σ_1^2, σ_2^2) to be positive is not an issue. Moreover, if the correlation is fixed, it can be taken as a parameter, and it is easy to ensure that it lies in $(-1, 1)$ during maximization. On the other hand, if the covariance is fixed, it needs to be a constrained in a way to ensure that the correlation, which now depends on $\tilde{v}_i$, remains in $(-1, 1)$ for all i. This is a harder task.

For both repeated and paired measurements data, once the ML estimate of the model parameter vector $\boldsymbol{\theta}$ is computed, the rest of the inference, including the construction of confidence bands, proceeds as described in Chapter 3.

6.8   BIBLIOGRAPHIC NOTE

Bland and Altman (1986, 1999) and Hawkins (2002) present real examples of heteroscedastic method comparison data. These authors perform a log transformation of the data to stabilize the variance. They are not interested in modeling heteroscedasticity as such. One may consult Carroll and Ruppert (1988) for an introduction to modeling of heteroscedasticity in linear regression models. Davidian and Giltinan (1995, Chapter 6) and Pinheiro and Bates (2000, Chapter 5) discuss heteroscedastic mixed-effects models. The latter authors describe the various variance function models available in their package `nlme`. The linearization strategy to approximate a likelihood function to get a closed-form expression can be found in Davidian and Giltinan (1995) and Stroup (2012). See also Rocke and Lorenzato (1995) for a two-component variance function model that yields a constant standard deviation at low magnitudes and allows the standard deviation to increase proportionally with magnitude when it is higher.

The material in Section 6.4 is based on Nawarathna and Choudhary (2013), although the model proposed therein differs slightly from ours. This article also compares four approaches for estimating parameters of the heteroscedastic model—two model approximation approaches, where one uses sample means as proxies for the error-free values and the other uses their estimated BLUPs; and two likelihood approximation approaches, where one uses Laplace approximation and the other uses Gauss-Hermite quadrature (Lange, 2010; and Liu and Pierce, 1994) to approximate the integral. It recommends the model approximation approach based on sample means as the overall best choice from the point of view of accuracy of inference and ease of computations. This is the approach we adopt in Section 6.4. The material in Section 6.5 is an adaptation of Choudhary and Ng (2006), who focus on modeling the variance of the difference in the paired measurements, not the measurements themselves that we consider here.

Data Sources

The cholesterol data are from Chinchilli et al. (1996) and the cyclosporin data are from Hawkins (2002). Both datasets can be obtained from the book's website.

EXERCISES

6.1 Suppose X follows a $\mathcal{N}_1(0, \sigma^2)$ distribution. Its absolute value $|X|$ is said to follow a *half-normal distribution*. Show that $E(|X|) = \sigma\sqrt{(2/\pi)}$.

6.2 Show that the marginal distribution of the observation vector $\mathbf{Y}_i$, $i = 1, \ldots, n$, under the heteroscedastic mixed-effects model (6.10) is given by (6.50). Show also that the elements of the mean vector and covariance matrix of $\mathbf{Y}_i$ are given by (6.11)–(6.14).

6.3 Verify that the companion model for (Y_1, Y_2) for a given variance covariate $\tilde{v}$ under the heteroscedastic mixed-effects model (6.10) is given by (6.15).

6.4 Show that, for a given variance covariate $\tilde{v}$, the joint distributions of two replications (Y_j, Y_j^*) of method $j = 1, 2$ under the heteroscedastic mixed-effects model (6.10) are, respectively,

$$\mathcal{N}_2\left(\begin{pmatrix}\mu_b\\\mu_b\end{pmatrix}, \begin{pmatrix}\sigma_b^2 + \psi^2 + \sigma_{e1}^2\, g_1^2(\tilde{v}, \delta_1) & \sigma_b^2 + \psi^2 \\ \sigma_b^2 + \psi^2 & \sigma_b^2 + \psi^2 + \sigma_{e1}^2\, g_1^2(\tilde{v}, \delta_1)\end{pmatrix}\right)$$

and

$$\mathcal{N}_2 \left(\begin{pmatrix} \beta_0 + \mu_b \\ \beta_0 + \mu_b \end{pmatrix}, \begin{pmatrix} \sigma_b^2 + \psi^2 + \sigma_{e2}^2 \, g_2^2(\tilde{v}, \delta_2) & \sigma_b^2 + \psi^2 \\ \sigma_b^2 + \psi^2 & \sigma_b^2 + \psi^2 + \sigma_{e2}^2 \, g_2^2(\tilde{v}, \delta_2) \end{pmatrix} \right).$$

6.5 Consider the cholesterol data from Section 6.4.6.

   (a) Fit the heteroscedastic mixed-effects model (6.10) with powers of $\tilde{v}_i$ in (6.20) as the variance functions. Verify the results in Table 6.1. Perform model diagnostics and check the normality assumption for errors and random effects.

   (b) Analyze the data by fitting the homoscedastic mixed-effects model (5.1), and compare conclusions with those based on the model fit in part (a).

   (c) Fit the model in part (a) with exponential variance function models instead of the power models. Which model provides a better fit? Justify your answer.

   (d) How do the estimates of model parameters and their standard errors in part (a) change if the variance covariate $\tilde{v}_i$ is taken as either $\overline{y}_{i1}$. or the average of all observations on subject i?

6.6 Consider the subcutaneous fat data from the R package MethComp of Carstensen et al. (2015). They consist of measurements of thickness of subcutaneous fat layer (in mm) in 43 patients taken by two observers—KL and SL. Each measurement is replicated three times. The repeated measurements are unlinked.

   (a) Perform an exploratory analysis of the data. Do they appear heteroscedastic?

   (b) Fit the homoscedastic model (5.1). Analyze the residuals from this fit to come up with candidate models for error variance functions of the two observers. Consider both the power and exponential models.

   (c) Fit the heteroscedastic model (6.10) using each of the candidate variance function models obtained in part (b). Check the adequacy of the fitted models, and find the one that fits best.

   (d) Test the null hypothesis of homoscedasticity using a likelihood ratio test.

   (e) Evaluate similarity and repeatability of the observers under the heteroscedastic model.

   (f) Evaluate agreement between the observers under the heteroscedastic model. Do the observers agree sufficiently well so that we can use them interchangeably over the entire measurement range? If not, is there a subset of the range where the agreement can be considered sufficient?

   (g) Evaluate agreement between the methods under the homoscedastic model that was fit in part (b). How do these conclusions compare with those in the previous part? What are the benefits, if any, of taking heteroscedasticity into account?

6.7 Consider the paired measurements data following the homoscedastic model (4.6).

   (a) Argue that $\text{cor}(Y_{ij} - \overline{Y}_{.j}, \{Y_{i1} + Y_{i2}\}/2) = \text{cor}(Y_{ij}, Y_{i1} + Y_{i2})$.

(b) Show that

$$\mathrm{cor}(Y_{ij}, Y_{i1} + Y_{i2}) = \frac{\sigma_j^2 + \sigma_{12}}{\{\sigma_j^2(\sigma_1^2 + \sigma_2^2 + 2\sigma_{12})\}^{1/2}}, \quad j = 1, 2.$$

6.8 Consider the cyclosporin data analyzed in Section 6.5.6.

(a) Fit the heteroscedastic bivariate normal model (6.36) with powers of the average as variance functions for the two methods. Verify the results in Table 6.2. Perform model diagnostics to assess the bivariate normality assumption for the standardized paired measurements (6.40).

(b) Analyze the data by fitting the homoscedastic bivariate normal model (4.6), and compare conclusions with those based on the model fit in part (a).

(c) Fit the model in part (a) with exponential variance function models.

(d) Compare the fitted bivariate distributions under the two variance function models. Which model provides a better fit? Why?

6.9 (Continuation of Exercise 1.10) Analyze the VCF data of Bland and Altman (1986) by fitting an appropriate heteroscedastic model. Be sure to justify the choice of variance functions and check the model assumptions. Do the methods agree well enough to be used interchangeably, perhaps on a subset of the measurement range? The data can be obtained from the book's website.

6.10 Consider the vitamin D data whose log-transformed version was analyzed in Section 4.4.3. Reanalyze these data on original scale by fitting an appropriate heteroscedastic model, and compare the conclusions with the analysis given there.

CHAPTER 7

DATA FROM MULTIPLE METHODS

7.1 PREVIEW

So far we have focussed on method comparison studies involving two measurement methods. Quite often, more than two methods are compared in the same study. It is of interest here to perform *multiple comparisons* of method pairs to evaluate the extent of similarity and agreement. This chapter generalizes the data models in Chapters 4 and 5 to accommodate multiple methods where we assume these methods are fixed rather than randomly chosen ones. It considers *simultaneous inference* on pairwise measures of similarity and agreement that adjusts for multiplicity. The measurements may or may not be repeated and the design may not be balanced. But it is assumed that the data are homoscedastic and the measurement methods have the same scale. Two case studies are used for illustration.

7.2 INTRODUCTION

Suppose there are $J (\geq 2)$ measurement methods under comparison. Here J is considered fixed and known. Two data designs are of interest. One is where the data are *unreplicated*, that is, there is only one measurement from each method on every subject. These data consist of $Y_{ij}, j = 1, \ldots, J, i = 1, \ldots, n$, with Y_{ij} representing the measurement from the jth method on the ith subject. There are a total of $N = Jn$ observations and they form an extension of the paired measurements data considered in Chapter 4.

Measuring Agreement: Models, Methods, and Applications. By P. K. Choudhary and H. N. Nagaraja
Copyright © 2017 John Wiley & Sons, Inc.

The other design is where the measurements are repeated. These data are denoted as Y_{ijk}, $k = 1, \ldots, m_{ij}$, $j = 1 \ldots, J$, $i = 1, \ldots, n$, with Y_{ijk} as the kth measurement of the jth method on the ith subject. This setup generalizes the one considered in Chapter 5. When $m_{i1} = \ldots = m_{iJ}$, the common value is denoted by m_i. Also, $M_i = \sum_{j=1}^{J} m_{ij}$ is the number of observations on subject i, and $N = \sum_{i=1}^{n} M_i$ is the total number of observations in the data. As before, the repeated measurements may be unlinked or linked. In the linked case, $m_{ij} = m_i$ for all $j = 1, \ldots, J$ by design, and $M_i = Jm_i$. As before, the steps in the analysis of data include displaying them, modeling them, and evaluation of similarity and agreement. First we explain how the last step calls for multiple comparisons as done in *analysis of variance* (ANOVA) models. Methods play the role of *treatments* in those models.

To understand the parallel between method comparison studies with multiple methods and ANOVA, it is helpful to recall that the ANOVA is concerned with comparison of more than two treatments, primarily through their means. The multiplicity of comparisons gives rise to the problem of *multiple comparisons*, which warrants *simultaneous inference* on the *contrasts* of interest in the treatment means. A contrast in the means is a linear combination of the means with the property that the coefficients add up to zero. A difference in two means is the simplest example of a contrast. More generally, if there are J treatments, then the $\binom{J}{2} = J(J-1)/2$ pairwise differences of treatment means may be the contrasts of interest. Alternatively, if one treatment serves as the control, then the differences in the means of the remaining $J-1$ treatments with the control mean may be the contrasts of interest. There are others that may also be of interest, for example, difference between the mean of a treatment and the average of all the treatments. For simultaneous inference on the contrasts, one can employ an appropriate set of simultaneous $100(1-\alpha)\%$ confidence intervals, guaranteeing that all the intervals *simultaneously* cover their respective contrasts with at least $1-\alpha$ probability. Because the simultaneous intervals adjust for the multiplicity of inferences, they are more relevant than the separate individual confidence intervals. If this adjustment is not made, the simultaneous coverage probability of the individual $100(1-\alpha)\%$ confidence intervals may be much less than $1-\alpha$ (Exercise 7.1).

In a method comparison study with two methods, there is only one method pair of interest. But if more than two methods are involved, there will be several such pairs. For example, if there is a reference method in the comparison, we may be interested in comparing each of the other methods with the reference method. This results in a total of $J-1$ method pairs. On the other hand, if the study does not have a reference method, we may be interested in comparing each method with every other method, resulting in a total of $\binom{J}{2}$ distinct method pairs. Thus, any inference we do for one method pair, viz., evaluation of agreement, has to be done multiple times. The comparisons with a reference and all-pairwise comparisons are akin to comparisons with a control and all-pairwise comparisons in an ANOVA setting. There is, however, one crucial difference. In ANOVA, the treatments are compared primarily through the contrasts in their means. But in method comparison studies, the measurement methods are compared through pairwise measures of similarity and agreement. In addition to the contrasts in the means, they also involve variances and covariances.

Despite the difference in the target parametric functions, the ANOVA analogy makes it clear that to evaluate similarity and agreement of the method pairs of interest, we need appropriate simultaneous confidence intervals, one-sided or two-sided, for the pairwise measures of similarity and agreement. The simultaneous intervals can, of course, be obtained by applying a Bonferroni adjustment to the individual intervals. It amounts to using $100(1 - \alpha/Q)\%$, with Q denoting the number of comparisons of interest, as the level of confidence for each individual interval (Exercise 7.1). But such an adjustment is known to be conservative in that the simultaneous coverage probability of the Q intervals may be much greater than the nominal level of $100(1 - \alpha)\%$. Further, the intervals may become too wide to be helpful for our purpose.

7.3 DISPLAYING DATA

The graphical tools for displaying data from two methods are easily adapted for multiple methods. For example, the trellis plot retains the same basic appearance as before except that each row now shows a subject's measurements from all methods, with different symbols, rather than two methods. The plot, however, may look cluttered if there are several methods and they have small within-subject variation, making it difficult to distinguish between the methods. Although the cluttering itself may be informative in that it may suggest similar characteristics for the methods, one may supplement the trellis plot with side-by-side boxplots of data from different methods to get a clearer comparison of their marginal distributions.

Besides the trellis plot, the scatterplot and the Bland-Altman plot are also used to display data from two methods. When there are more than two methods, we can make a "matrix" of the pairwise plots. In its standard form, a matrix of plots is an arrangement of scatterplots on a square grid, consisting of one plot for each pair of distinct variables. The panels in the diagonal either are left empty or contain the labels of the methods. Moreover, the same pairs of variables are plotted in the panels above and below the diagonal, but with variables on horizontal and vertical axes interchanged.

For method comparison data, we can devise a variation of the standard matrix to simultaneously display both scatterplots and Bland-Altman plots. To describe it, suppose each subject in the study is measured once using J methods, $Y_1, \ldots, Y_J$. The matrix consists of a $J \times J$ grid of boxes. The J boxes on the diagonal only contain the method labels from 1 to J. The $J(J - 1)/2$ boxes below and above the diagonal, respectively, contain the scatterplots and the Bland-Altman plots. The box in row i and column j below the diagonal (i.e., $i > j$) contains the scatterplot of (Y_j, Y_i). The box in row i and column j above the diagonal (i.e., $i < j$) contains the corresponding Bland-Altman plot—the scatterplot of $((Y_i + Y_j)/2, Y_j - Y_i)$. Of course, the positions of the scatterplots and the Bland-Altman plots can be interchanged. One can further embellish the matrix by displaying either histograms or boxplots of the variables on the diagonal. The preceding construction assumes unreplicated data. If the measurements are repeated, then as in Chapter 5, one can either use a randomly chosen measurement from a subject or the average of its multiple measurements.

7.4 EXAMPLE DATASETS

We now introduce two datasets with displays. Their detailed analysis is presented in Section 7.10.

7.4.1 Systolic Blood Pressure Data

These data were collected in a study to compare systolic and diastolic blood pressure measurements (in mm Hg) taken by three observers using a mercury sphygmomanometer and one observer using a digital sphygmomanometer. The digital one is cheaper and is easier to use than its mercury counterpart. The four observers in the comparison are as referred to as MS1, MS2, MS3, and DS, respectively. They are labeled as methods 1, 2, 3, and 4, respectively. It is of interest to compare the three MS observers among themselves and also with the DS observer, essentially implying all-pairwise comparisons. The measurements in this study are not replicated; each observer takes only one measurement on each subject. There are 228 subjects in the study. Here we focus only on the systolic measurements. They range from 82 to 236 mm Hg.

Figure 7.1 shows a trellis plot of the data. Each row in the plot has four observations, one per observer. The plot has a cluttered look, but the large overlap in the symbols implies that the measurements from the four observers tend to be close. It is also apparent that DS often has the largest measurement. The within-subject variation of the observations is small relative to the between-subject variation. There is no evidence of heteroscedasticity as the within-subject spread remains largely similar throughout the measurement range. The boxplots presented in Figure 7.2 show small differences in the marginal distributions of the observers. These distributions appear right-skewed.

Figure 7.3 displays a matrix of scatterplots and Bland-Altman plots for systolic blood pressure data. The scatterplots show high pairwise correlations among the four observers. The Bland-Altman plots do not exhibit any trend, implying a common scale for the observers, or nonconstant vertical scatter, confirming homoscedasticity of the data. The centers of the plots suggest small differences in the observers' means.

7.4.2 Tumor Size Data

These data consist of tumor sizes (in cm) of 40 lesions measured by five readers. The tumor sizes are "unidimensional" in that they are based on the longest diameter of the lesion. Each measurement is replicated twice. The replications are assumed to be unlinked. The measurements range from 1 to 9 cm.

Figure 7.4 presents a trellis plot of the data. Each row in this plot has ten observations, two per reader. The plot is not as cluttered as the plot of the previous dataset. The within-subject variation here is relatively large compared to what we have seen for other datasets presented in this book. But it does not seem to change with the magnitude of measurement. It is also evident that reader 2 is somewhat deviant compared to the rest as her/his measurements tend to be the smallest. Reader 3 often has the largest measurements. The boxplots presented in Figure 7.5 clarify these differences in the readers' marginal distributions. Both replications of measurements have been used in this plot. Alternatively, one can average the two replications or randomly select one of the replications without any qualitative change in the conclusions. The trellis plot shows considerable subject × reader interaction. It is confirmed by crossing of the line segments for different subjects in the interaction plot in Figure 7.6.

Figure 7.7 presents a matrix of scatterplots and Bland-Altman plots for tumor size data. The scatterplots show moderately high pairwise correlations among the five readers.

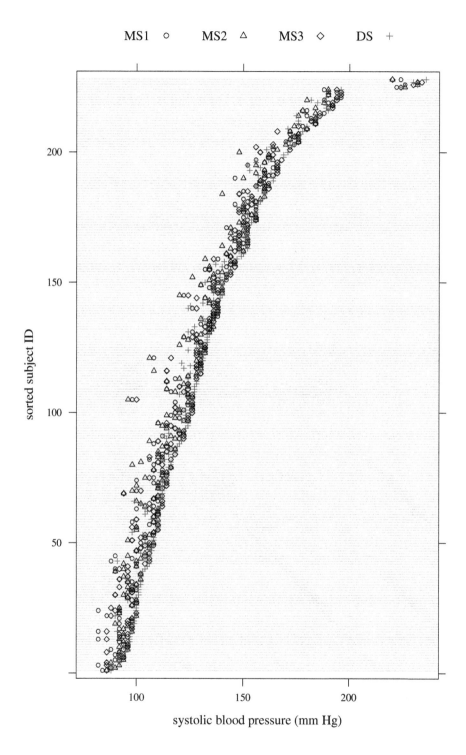

Figure 7.1   Trellis plot of systolic blood pressure data. The symbols for the four observers are given at the top of the plot.

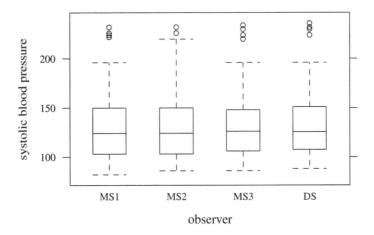

Figure 7.2   Side-by-side boxplots for systolic blood pressure data.

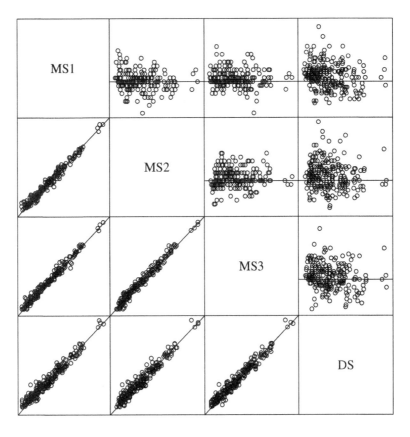

Figure 7.3   A matrix of scatterplots with line of equality (below the diagonal) and Bland-Altman plots with zero line (above the diagonal) for systolic blood pressure data. The measurements range from 82 to 236 mm Hg and their differences range from −16 to 30 mm Hg.

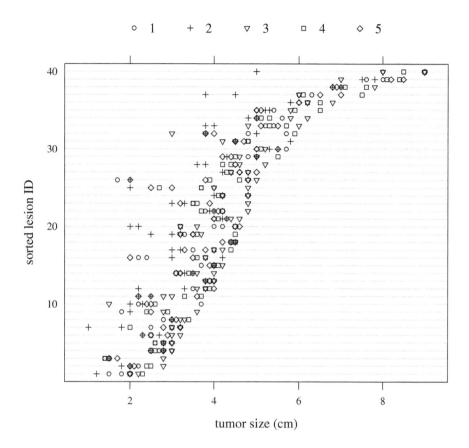

Figure 7.4   Trellis plot of tumor size data. The symbols for the five readers are given at the top of the plot.

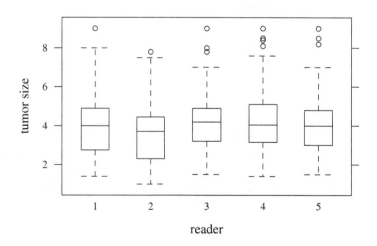

Figure 7.5   Side-by-side boxplots for tumor size data.

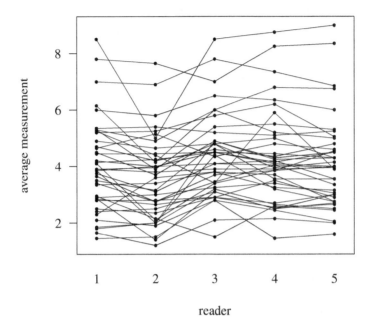

Figure 7.6   Interaction plot for tumor size data depicting lesion × reader interaction.

The Bland-Altman plots show that the readers, though on the same scale, have somewhat different means. The data appear homoscedastic.

7.5   MODELING UNREPLICATED DATA

Assuming that all the $J \, (\geq 2)$ methods have a common scale, the data Y_{ij}, $j = 1, \ldots, J$, $i = 1, \ldots, n$ can be modeled by the following straightforward extension of the mixed-effects model (4.1) for paired measurements data:

$$Y_{i1} = b_i + e_{i1}, \quad Y_{ij} = \beta_j + b_i + e_{ij}, \quad j = 2, \ldots, J.$$

Here β_j is the difference in the fixed biases of methods j and 1. The intercept β_0 in (4.1) is now denoted as β_2. As in (4.1), the true values b_i follow independent $\mathcal{N}_1(\mu_b, \sigma_b^2)$ distributions, the random errors e_{ij} follow independent $\mathcal{N}_1(0, \sigma_{ej}^2)$ distributions, and the b_i and e_{ij} are mutually independent. For notational convenience, we define $\beta_1 = 0$ as a known constant, allowing us to write the model as

$$Y_{ij} = \beta_j + b_i + e_{ij}, \quad j = 1, \ldots, J, \quad i = 1, \ldots, n. \tag{7.1}$$

This model allows each method to have its own error variance. The J measurements $(Y_{i1}, \ldots, Y_{iJ})$ on subject i share the same true value b_i. Consequently, we see that

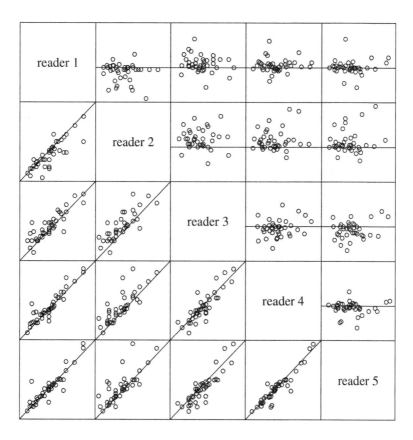

Figure 7.7   A matrix of scatterplots with line of equality (below the diagonal) and Bland-Altman plots with zero line (above the diagonal) for tumor size data. One measurement from each reader on every subject is randomly selected for this plot. The measurements range from 1 to 9 cm and their differences range from -3 to 4 cm.

(Exercise 7.2) these measurements are i.i.d. as $(Y_1, \ldots, Y_J)$, where

$$
\begin{pmatrix} Y_1 \\ Y_2 \\ \vdots \\ Y_J \end{pmatrix} \sim \mathcal{N}_J \left(\begin{pmatrix} \beta_1 + \mu_b \\ \beta_2 + \mu_b \\ \vdots \\ \beta_J + \mu_b \end{pmatrix}, \begin{pmatrix} \sigma_b^2 + \sigma_{e1}^2 & \sigma_b^2 & \cdots & \sigma_b^2 \\ \sigma_b^2 & \sigma_b^2 + \sigma_{e2}^2 & \cdots & \sigma_b^2 \\ \vdots & \vdots & \ddots & \vdots \\ \sigma_b^2 & \sigma_b^2 & \cdots & \sigma_b^2 + \sigma_{eJ}^2 \end{pmatrix} \right) . \tag{7.2}
$$

Thus, the means and variances of the measurements are

$$
E(Y_{ij}) = \beta_j + \mu_b, \quad \mathrm{var}(Y_{ij}) = \sigma_b^2 + \sigma_{ej}^2,
$$

and

$$
\mathrm{cov}(Y_{ij}, Y_{il}) = \sigma_b^2, \quad j \neq l,
$$

is the common covariance between measurements from any two methods on the same subject. The dependence in the measurements is induced by the sharing of the common true value b_i. This model has a total of $2J + 1$ unknown parameters,

$$(\beta_2, \ldots, \beta_J, \mu_b, \sigma_b^2, \sigma_{e1}^2, \ldots, \sigma_{eJ}^2).$$

When $J = 2$, the model (7.1) and the associated population distribution (7.2) reduce to their respective counterparts for paired measurements data in (4.1) and (4.2). Let $D_{jl} = Y_l - Y_j$ be the difference in measurements of the method pair $(j, l), j \neq l$. It follows from (7.2) that

$$D_{jl} \sim \mathcal{N}_1(\beta_l - \beta_j, \sigma_{ej}^2 + \sigma_{el}^2). \tag{7.3}$$

Moreover, the differences associated with different method pairs are independent.

7.6   MODELING REPEATED MEASUREMENTS DATA

As in Chapter 5, the modeling of repeated measurements data depends on whether the measurements are unlinked or linked. We consider these cases in turn, assuming as before that the methods have the same scale and $J > 2$. The models reduce to their counterparts with $J = 2$ provided an additional equal variance assumption is made.

7.6.1   Unlinked Data

To model the unlinked data Y_{ijk}, $k = 1, \ldots, m_{ij}$, $j = 1, \ldots, J (> 2)$, $i = 1, \ldots, n$, we can extend the mixed-effects model (5.1) as

$$Y_{ijk} = \beta_j + b_i + b_{ij} + e_{ijk}, \tag{7.4}$$

where, as in (7.1), $\beta_1 = 0$, and for $j > 2$, β_j represents the difference in the fixed biases of methods j and 1. Moreover, the intercept β_0 in (5.1) has been relabeled as β_2. As in (5.1), it is assumed that the true values b_i follow independent $\mathcal{N}_1(\mu_b, \sigma_b^2)$ distributions; the interactions b_{ij} follow independent $\mathcal{N}_1(0, \psi_j^2)$ distributions; the random errors e_{ijk} follow independent $\mathcal{N}_1(0, \sigma_{ej}^2)$ distributions; and b_i, b_{ij}, and e_{ijk} are mutually independent.

The model (7.4) for $J > 2$ allows the variance of the interaction effect to depend on the method, whereas in the model (5.1) for $J = 2$, the variance is assumed constant across the two methods. Thus, (7.4) reduces to (5.1) for $J = 2$ provided $\psi_1^2 = \psi_2^2 = \psi^2$. When $k = 1$, that is, the measurements are not replicated, the effect of the interaction term b_{ij} in (7.4) gets confounded with that of the error term and has to be removed from the model. Doing so yields the model (7.1) in Section 7.5 as a special case of (7.4).

Proceeding as in Section 5.4.1, we can average over the $J + 1$ mutually independent random effects $b_i, b_{i1}, \ldots, b_{iJ}$ in (7.4) to see that the vector of M_i measurements on subject i follows an independent M_i-variate normal distribution with means and variances (Exercise 7.3)

$$E(Y_{ijk}) = \beta_j + \mu_b, \quad \text{var}(Y_{ijk}) = \sigma_b^2 + \psi_j^2 + \sigma_{ej}^2. \tag{7.5}$$

The covariance between measurements depends on whether or not they come from the same method. Any two measurements of method j have the covariance

$$\text{cov}(Y_{ijk}, Y_{ijp}) = \sigma_b^2 + \psi_j^2, \quad k \neq p, \tag{7.6}$$

whereas any two measurements from different methods have the common covariance

$$\text{cov}(Y_{ijk}, Y_{ilp}) = \sigma_b^2, \quad j \neq l. \tag{7.7}$$

The subscripts k and p here may be equal or different. The model (7.4) has a total of $3J + 1$ unknown parameters,

$$(\beta_2, \ldots, \beta_J, \mu_b, \sigma_b^2, \psi_1^2, \ldots, \psi_J^2, \sigma_{e1}^2, \ldots, \sigma_{eJ}^2).$$

Our next task is to obtain the distribution of $(Y_1, \ldots, Y_J)$ induced by the model (7.4). Recall that this vector contains one measurement from each of the J methods on a randomly selected subject from the population. For this we proceed in the usual manner to drop the subscripts i and k in (7.4), getting its companion model as

$$Y_j = \beta_j + b + b_j + e_j, \quad j = 1, \ldots, J. \tag{7.8}$$

Here b, b_j, and e_j are identically distributed as b_i, b_{ij}, and e_{ijk}, respectively. Upon averaging over the distribution of $(b, b_1, \ldots, b_J)$, we get (Exercise 7.4)

$$\begin{pmatrix} Y_1 \\ Y_2 \\ \vdots \\ Y_J \end{pmatrix} \sim \mathcal{N}_J \left(\begin{pmatrix} \beta_1 + \mu_b \\ \beta_2 + \mu_b \\ \vdots \\ \beta_J + \mu_b \end{pmatrix}, \right.$$
$$\left. \begin{pmatrix} \sigma_b^2 + \psi_1^2 + \sigma_{e1}^2 & \sigma_b^2 & \cdots & \sigma_b^2 \\ \sigma_b^2 & \sigma_b^2 + \psi_2^2 + \sigma_{e2}^2 & \cdots & \sigma_b^2 \\ \vdots & \vdots & \ddots & \vdots \\ \sigma_b^2 & \sigma_b^2 & \cdots & \sigma_b^2 + \psi_J^2 + \sigma_{eJ}^2 \end{pmatrix} \right). \tag{7.9}$$

For the difference $D_{jl} = Y_l - Y_j$, $j \neq l$, it follows that

$$D_{jl} \sim \mathcal{N}_1(\beta_l - \beta_j, \psi_j^2 + \psi_l^2 + \sigma_{ej}^2 + \sigma_{el}^2). \tag{7.10}$$

The distribution in (7.9) is used to derive measures of similarity and agreement. The repeated measurements also allow evaluation of repeatability of each method. Following Section 5.6, to derive measures of repeatability, we need the distributions of the pairs (Y_j, Y_j^*), $j = 1, \ldots, J$, where $(Y_1^*, \ldots, Y_J^*)$ is a replication of $(Y_1, \ldots, Y_J)$ on the same subject. The companion model for $(Y_1^*, \ldots, Y_J^*)$ induced by the data model (7.4) is

$$Y_j^* = \beta_j + b + b_j + e_j^*, \quad j = 1, \ldots, J, \tag{7.11}$$

where $(e_1^*, \ldots, e_J^*)$ is an independent copy of $(e_1, \ldots, e_J)$ in (7.8). It follows from (7.8) and (7.11) that (Exercise 7.4)

$$\begin{pmatrix} Y_j \\ Y_j^* \end{pmatrix} \sim \mathcal{N}_2 \left(\begin{pmatrix} \beta_j + \mu_b \\ \beta_j + \mu_b \end{pmatrix}, \begin{pmatrix} \sigma_b^2 + \psi_j^2 + \sigma_{ej}^2 & \sigma_b^2 + \psi_j^2 \\ \sigma_b^2 + \psi_j^2 & \sigma_b^2 + \psi_j^2 + \sigma_{ej}^2 \end{pmatrix} \right). \tag{7.12}$$

For the difference $D_j = Y_j - Y_j^*$ in two replications of method j, from (7.12), we have

$$D_j \sim \mathcal{N}_1(0, 2\sigma_{ej}^2), \quad j = 1, \ldots, J. \tag{7.13}$$

7.6.2 Linked Data

As in Section 5.4.2, the model for the measurements $(Y_{i1k}, \ldots, Y_{iJk})$ linked by the common time $k = 1, \ldots, m_i$ for subjects $i = 1, \ldots, n$ is obtained by simply adding the random effect b_{ik}^* of time k to the model (7.4) for unlinked data. This yields

$$Y_{ijk} = \beta_j + b_i + b_{ij} + b_{ik}^* + e_{ijk}, \tag{7.14}$$

where the b_{ik}^*, also interpreted as subject $\times$ time interaction, follow independent $\mathcal{N}_1(0, \sigma_{b^*}^2)$ distributions. They are mutually independent of the other random terms in the model that continue to follow the same distributions as in (7.4). This model reduces to the model (5.1) for $J = 2$ if a common variance $\psi_1^2 = \psi_2^2 = \psi^2$ is assumed for the subject $\times$ method interactions.

Averaging over the $J + m_i + 1$ mutually independent random effects, namely,

$$b_i, b_{i1}, \ldots, b_{iJ}, b_{i1}^*, \ldots, b_{im_i}^*,$$

we see that the vector of $M_i = Jm_i$ observations on subject i follows an independent M_i-variate normal distribution with (Exercise 7.5)

$$E(Y_{ijk}) = \beta_j + \mu_b, \quad \text{var}(Y_{ijk}) = \sigma_b^2 + \psi_j^2 + \sigma_{b^*}^2 + \sigma_{ej}^2. \tag{7.15}$$

The covariance in any two measurements is induced by the common random effects they share. Therefore, the covariances depend on whether or not the measurements involved are taken by the same method and at the same time. For measurements taken by method j but at different times,

$$\text{cov}(Y_{ijk}, Y_{ijp}) = \sigma_b^2 + \psi_j^2, \quad k \neq p. \tag{7.16}$$

For measurements taken by different methods but at the same time,

$$\text{cov}(Y_{ijk}, Y_{ilk}) = \sigma_b^2 + \sigma_{b^*}^2, \quad j \neq l. \tag{7.17}$$

For measurements taken by different methods at different times,

$$\text{cov}(Y_{ijk}, Y_{ilp}) = \sigma_b^2, \quad j \neq l, \ k \neq p. \tag{7.18}$$

The model (7.14) has a total of $3J + 2$ unknown parameters,

$$(\beta_2, \ldots, \beta_J, \mu_b, \sigma_b^2, \psi_1^2, \ldots, \psi_J^2, \sigma_{b^*}^2, \sigma_{e1}^2, \ldots, \sigma_{eJ}^2).$$

Compared to the model (7.4), the additional parameter here is subject $\times$ time interaction variance $\sigma_{b^*}^2$.

Next, we need the distribution of $(Y_1, \ldots, Y_J)$ induced by the model (7.14) to derive measures of similarity and agreement. Proceeding along the lines of Section 5.4.2, it can be seen from Exercise 7.6 that this distribution is J-variate normal with mean vector

$$(\beta_1 + \mu_b, \beta_2 + \mu_b, \ldots, \beta_J + \mu_b) \tag{7.19}$$

and covariance matrix

$$\begin{pmatrix} \sigma_b^2 + \psi_1^2 + \sigma_{b^*}^2 + \sigma_{e1}^2 & \sigma_b^2 + \sigma_{b^*}^2 & \cdots & \sigma_b^2 + \sigma_{b^*}^2 \\ \sigma_b^2 + \sigma_{b^*}^2 & \sigma_b^2 + \psi_2^2 + \sigma_{b^*}^2 + \sigma_{e2}^2 & \cdots & \sigma_b^2 + \sigma_{b^*}^2 \\ \vdots & \vdots & \ddots & \vdots \\ \sigma_b^2 + \sigma_{b^*}^2 & \sigma_b^2 + \sigma_{b^*}^2 & \cdots & \sigma_b^2 + \psi_J^2 + \sigma_{b^*}^2 + \sigma_{eJ}^2 \end{pmatrix}. \tag{7.20}$$

This implies

$$D_{jl} = Y_l - Y_j \sim \mathcal{N}_1\left(\beta_l - \beta_j, \psi_j^2 + \psi_l^2 + \sigma_{ej}^2 + \sigma_{el}^2\right), \quad j \neq l. \tag{7.21}$$

As seen in Section 5.4.2 before, this distribution is identical to the one in (7.10) for unlinked data.

Analogous to Section 5.6.2, we also need the distributions of the pairs (Y_j, Y_j^*), $j = 1, \ldots, J$ to derive the measures of repeatability. Here $(Y_1^*, \ldots, Y_J^*)$ is another set of measurements taken on the same subject that produces $(Y_1, \ldots, Y_J)$. From Exercise 7.6, the desired distribution is

$$
\begin{pmatrix} Y_j \\ Y_j^* \end{pmatrix} \sim \mathcal{N}_2 \left(\begin{pmatrix} \beta_j + \mu_b \\ \beta_j + \mu_b \end{pmatrix}, \begin{pmatrix} \sigma_b^2 + \psi_j^2 + \sigma_{b*}^2 + \sigma_{ej}^2 & \sigma_b^2 + \psi_j^2 \\ \sigma_b^2 + \psi_j^2 & \sigma_b^2 + \psi_j^2 + \sigma_{b*}^2 + \sigma_{ej}^2 \end{pmatrix} \right). \quad (7.22)
$$

It follows that

$$
D_j = Y_j - Y_j^* \sim \mathcal{N}_1 \left(0, 2(\sigma_{b*}^2 + \sigma_{ej}^2) \right), \quad j = 1, \ldots, J. \quad (7.23)
$$

7.7 MODEL FITTING AND EVALUATION

All the three models—(7.1), (7.4), and (7.14)—can be fit by the ML method using any software that can fit mixed-effects models (see Section 7.12). The software would provide ML estimates of model parameters, predicted values of random effects, fitted values, and raw as well as standardized residuals. These quantities can be used as in Section 3.2.4 to perform model evaluation. We have used $\beta_1 = 0$ as a *known* parameter for notational convenience. Its "estimate" can be taken as $\hat{\beta}_1 = 0$.

Specifically, for the model (7.1) for unreplicated data, we get the ML estimates

$$
(\hat{\beta}_2, \ldots, \hat{\beta}_J, \hat{\mu}_b, \hat{\sigma}_b^2, \hat{\sigma}_{e1}^2, \ldots, \hat{\sigma}_{eJ}^2),
$$

the predicted true values $\hat{b}_i$, the fitted values $\hat{Y}_{ij} = \hat{\beta}_j + \hat{\mu}_b + \hat{b}_i$, the raw residuals $\hat{e}_{ij} = Y_{ij} - \hat{Y}_{ij}$, and the standardized residuals $\hat{e}_{ij}/\hat{\sigma}_{ej}$. Recall from Chapter 4 that the variance components in (4.1) for $J = 2$ are not estimated reliably with unreplicated data. No such difficulty arises when $J > 2$.

For the model (7.4) for unlinked repeated measurements data, we also have the ML estimates $(\hat{\psi}_1^2, \ldots, \hat{\psi}_J^2)$ and predicted subject $\times$ method interactions $\hat{b}_{ij}$; and the fitted values are $\hat{Y}_{ijk} = \hat{\beta}_j + \hat{\mu}_b + \hat{b}_i + \hat{b}_{ij}$. For the model (7.14) for linked repeated measurements data, we additionally have the ML estimate $\hat{\sigma}_{b*}^2$ and predicted subject $\times$ time interactions $\hat{b}_{ik}^*$; and the fitted values are $\hat{Y}_{ijk} = \hat{\beta}_j + \hat{\mu}_b + \hat{b}_i + \hat{b}_{ij} + \hat{b}_{ik}^*$. In both cases, the raw and the standardized residuals are $e_{ijk} = Y_{ijk} - \hat{Y}_{ijk}$ and $e_{ijk}/\hat{\sigma}_{ej}$, respectively.

Sometimes the default models (7.4) and (7.14) fail to provide reliable estimates of all the variance components. One remedy may be to simplify the model by assuming equal variances $\psi_j^2 = \psi^2$, $j = 1, \ldots, J$ for the subject $\times$ method interactions b_{ij} (see Exercise 7.11). Another may be to drop the b_i term from the model, assume that $(b_{i1}, \ldots, b_{iJ})$ follow independent multivariate normal distributions with zero mean and an unstructured covariance matrix, and take β_1 to be an unknown parameter (see Exercise 7.12). The models for both unreplicated and repeated measurements data also assume homoscedastic errors. If this assumption is in doubt, perhaps even after a log transformation of data, then the models can be extended as in Chapter 6 to allow heteroscedastic errors (see also Chapter 8). This chapter's methodology of evaluation of similarity and agreement can be easily adapted to work under the new models.

7.8 EVALUATION OF SIMILARITY AND AGREEMENT

In Chapters 4 and 5, measures of similarity and agreement were derived from the bivariate normal distribution of (Y_1, Y_2) induced by the model assumed for the data. Two measures of similarity were considered. One is the intercept β_0, representing the difference in fixed biases or the means of the two methods. This quantity is $\beta_2 - \beta_1$ in the notation of the present chapter (because $\beta_1 = 0$, by definition). The other is the ratio of precisions of the two methods, $\lambda = \sigma_{e1}^2 / \sigma_{e2}^2$. With repeated measurements, a modification of this precision ratio, $\lambda_1 = (\psi^2 + \sigma_{e1}^2)/(\psi^2 + \sigma_{e2}^2)$, is also considered to take the subject $\times$ method interactions into account. For measures of agreement, as usual we consider CCC and TDI.

When $J > 2$, we have multiple method pairs of interest, say, Q. For example, $Q = J - 1$ for comparisons with a reference, and $Q = \binom{J}{2}$ for all-pairwise comparisons. Associated with each of the Q method pairs, there is one value for every measure of similarity and agreement—all derived from the J-variate normal distribution of $(Y_1, \ldots, Y_J)$ induced by the assumed data model. The parameters of this distribution are given by (7.2) for unreplicated data, by (7.9) for unlinked repeated measurements data, and by (7.19) and (7.20) for linked repeated measurements data.

If the method pair (j, l) is of interest for some $j \neq l \in \{1, \ldots, J\}$, then the measures based on (Y_j, Y_l) can be obtained by essentially taking their counterparts based on (Y_1, Y_2) and replacing the subscripts $(1, 2)$ with (j, l). This leads to $\beta_l - \beta_j$ as the bias difference, $\lambda_{jl} = \sigma_{ej}^2 / \sigma_{el}^2$ as the precision ratio, and

$$\lambda_{1,jl} = (\psi_j^2 + \sigma_{ej}^2)/(\psi_l^2 + \sigma_{el}^2) \tag{7.24}$$

as the modified precision ratio that takes the subject $\times$ method interactions into account. Note that when only two methods are involved, equal interaction variances are assumed in (7.24). From (4.11) and (7.2), the two agreement measures for unreplicated data can be expressed as (Exercise 7.7)

$$\mathrm{CCC}_{jl} = \frac{2\sigma_b^2}{(\beta_l - \beta_j)^2 + 2\sigma_b^2 + \sigma_{ej}^2 + \sigma_{el}^2},$$

$$\mathrm{TDI}_{jl}(p) = \left\{ (\sigma_{ej}^2 + \sigma_{el}^2)\, \chi_{1,p}^2 \left(\frac{(\beta_l - \beta_j)^2}{\sigma_{ej}^2 + \sigma_{el}^2} \right) \right\}^{1/2}. \tag{7.25}$$

Likewise, for unlinked repeated measurements data, from (5.19), (5.21), and (7.9) they can be expressed as

$$\mathrm{CCC}_{jl} = \frac{2\sigma_b^2}{(\beta_l - \beta_j)^2 + 2\sigma_b^2 + \psi_j^2 + \psi_l^2 + \sigma_{ej}^2 + \sigma_{el}^2},$$

$$\mathrm{TDI}_{jl}(p) = \left\{ (\psi_j^2 + \psi_l^2 + \sigma_{ej}^2 + \sigma_{el}^2)\, \chi_{1,p}^2 \left(\frac{(\beta_l - \beta_j)^2}{\psi_j^2 + \psi_l^2 + \sigma_{ej}^2 + \sigma_{el}^2} \right) \right\}^{1/2}. \tag{7.26}$$

For linked repeated measurements data, from (5.20), (7.19), and (7.20) the CCC is

$$\mathrm{CCC}_{jl} = \frac{2(\sigma_b^2 + \sigma_{b*}^2)}{(\beta_l - \beta_j)^2 + 2(\sigma_b^2 + \sigma_{b*}^2) + \psi_j^2 + \psi_l^2 + \sigma_{ej}^2 + \sigma_{el}^2}, \tag{7.27}$$

and the TDI is the same as in (7.26). This happens because the difference D_{jl} has the same distribution for both unlinked and linked data—see (7.10) and (7.21). The expressions for these measures are verified in Exercise 7.7.

It is apparent from the ANOVA analogy in Section 7.2 that for similarity evaluation we need to examine two-sided simultaneous confidence intervals for the Q values of each similarity measure. Likewise, for agreement evaluation we need to examine one-sided simultaneous confidence bounds for the Q values of an agreement measure. These bounds, in addition to allowing us to infer which method pairs, if any, have sufficient agreement for interchangeable use, also allow us to compare the extent of agreement among the method pairs. As before, the ML estimators of the measures are obtained by replacing the unknown parameters in their expressions by their ML estimators, and the large-sample theory is used to get standard errors and simultaneous confidence bounds and intervals. The latter are of the same form as their individual counterparts,

$$\text{estimate} \pm \text{critical point} \times \text{SE(estimate)},$$

possibly on a transformed scale that makes the parameter range to be the entire real line. The critical point is now a percentile of an appropriate function of a Q-variate normal vector with standard normal marginals (see Section 3.3.2). One may also proceed as in Section 3.3.6 to perform a test of homogeneity to test the null hypothesis of equality of the Q values of the measure.

The 95% limits of agreement for (Y_j, Y_l) can be computed using the distributions of D_{jl} in (7.3), (7.10), and (7.21). These limits are

$$(\hat{\beta}_l - \hat{\beta}_j) \pm 1.96 \times \sqrt{\hat{\sigma}_{ej}^2 + \hat{\sigma}_{el}^2} \tag{7.28}$$

for unreplicated data, and are

$$(\hat{\beta}_l - \hat{\beta}_j) \pm 1.96 \times \sqrt{\hat{\psi}_j^2 + \hat{\psi}_l^2 + \hat{\sigma}_{ej}^2 + \hat{\sigma}_{el}^2} \tag{7.29}$$

for unlinked as well as linked repeated measurements data. Note that no multiplicity adjustment has been made in these limits.

7.9 EVALUATION OF REPEATABILITY

Section 5.6 discusses measures of repeatability that evaluate intra-method agreement when repeated measurements data are available. A measure of repeatability for method j is essentially a measure of agreement between (Y_j, Y_j^*)—two repeated measurements of method j on the same subject. From the distributions of (Y_j, Y_j^*) and the associated difference D_j in (7.12) and (7.13), the repeatability analogs of CCC and TDI for unlinked data can be found as (Exercise 7.8)

$$\text{CCC}_j = \frac{\sigma_b^2 + \psi_j^2}{\sigma_b^2 + \psi_j^2 + \sigma_{ej}^2},$$

$$\text{TDI}_j(p) = \left\{2\sigma_{ej}^2 \, \chi_{1,p}^2(0)\right\}^{1/2}, \quad j = 1, \dots, J. \tag{7.30}$$

For linked data, using (7.22) and (7.23) we obtain (Exercise 7.8)

$$\text{CCC}_j = \frac{\sigma_b^2 + \psi_j^2}{\sigma_b^2 + \psi_j^2 + \sigma_{b*}^2 + \sigma_{ej}^2},$$

$$\text{TDI}_j(p) = \left\{ 2(\sigma_{b*}^2 + \sigma_{ej}^2)\,\chi_{1,p}^2(0) \right\}^{1/2}, \quad j = 1, \ldots, J. \tag{7.31}$$

Recall from Section 5.6 that CCC_j represents the intraclass correlation between Y_j and Y_j^*. For unlinked data, it additionally represents the reliability of method j in the sense of (1.4).

One-sided confidence bounds for the repeatability measures are obtained in exactly the same manner as the agreement measures with the exception that the individual bounds suffice here. Although one can use simultaneous bounds, they are not really needed because the repeatability measures are primarily concerned with establishing a benchmark for how much agreement is possible, and not examining whether the methods have sufficiently high repeatability. The latter does not require adjustment for multiplicity of inferences.

One can use the distributions of D_j in (7.13) and (7.23) to get 95% limits of intra-method agreement for method $j = 1, \ldots, J$ for unlinked data as

$$\pm 1.96 \times \sqrt{2}\,\hat{\sigma}_{ej}, \tag{7.32}$$

and for linked data as

$$\pm 1.96 \times \sqrt{2(\hat{\sigma}_{b*}^2 + \hat{\sigma}_{ej}^2)}. \tag{7.33}$$

7.10 CASE STUDIES

7.10.1 Systolic Blood Pressure Data

The systolic blood pressure data introduced in Section 7.4 has measurements (in mm Hg) on $n = 228$ subjects taken by three observers—MS1, MS2, and MS3—using a mercury sphygmomanometer, and one observer—DS—using a digital sphygmomanometer. We call these observers methods 1, 2, 3, and 4, respectively. The measurements are not replicated. The interest is in comparing the MS observers among themselves and also with the DS observer. These are $\binom{4}{2} = 6$ pairwise comparisons. An exploratory data analysis based on the trellis plot in Figure 7.1, boxplots in Figure 7.2, and a matrix of scatterplots and Bland-Altman plots in Figure 7.3 shows that the observers are highly correlated and have a common scale, but small differences exist in their means. The data appear homoscedastic.

We fit the mixed-effects model (7.1) to the data. Figure 7.8 shows the resulting residual plot. It appears centered at zero and does not have any trend or nonconstant vertical scatter. Model diagnostics (not presented here) show that the normality assumption is adequate for the errors. But the random effects appear right-skewed, and this explains the right-skewness seen in the boxplots in Figure 7.2. We ignore this as usually a moderate departure from normality of random effects does not have much impact on the overall conclusions of a method comparison data analysis.

Table 7.1 summarizes ML estimates of the nine model parameters. Substituting the estimates in (7.2) gives the fitted multivariate normal distribution of (Y_1, Y_2, Y_3, Y_4), with means $(128.69, 128.98, 130.18, 131.45)$, variances $(938.30, 942.63, 937.21, 961.07)$, and common covariance 928.53. All pairwise correlations exceed 0.975. Both the mean and variance are largest for DS and smallest for MS1. It can also be seen that the pairwise

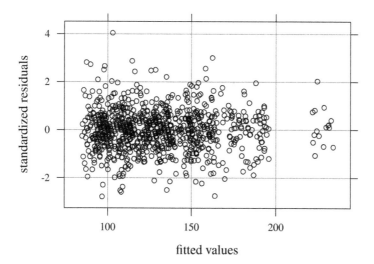

Figure 7.8 Residual plot for systolic blood pressure data.

Parameter	Estimate	SE	95% Interval
β_2	0.29	0.32	$(-0.34, 0.92)$
β_3	1.49	0.28	$(0.93, 2.05)$
β_4	2.75	0.43	$(1.91, 3.60)$
μ_b	128.69	2.03	$(124.72, 132.67)$
$\log(\sigma_b^2)$	6.83	0.09	$(6.65, 7.02)$
$\log(\sigma_{e1}^2)$	2.28	0.14	$(2.00, 2.56)$
$\log(\sigma_{e2}^2)$	2.65	0.12	$(2.41, 2.89)$
$\log(\sigma_{e3}^2)$	2.16	0.15	$(1.86, 2.46)$
$\log(\sigma_{e4}^2)$	3.48	0.10	$(3.28, 3.69)$

Table 7.1 Summary of parameter estimates for systolic blood pressure data. Methods 1, 2, 3, and 4 refer to the observers MS1, MS2, MS3, and DS, respectively.

differences among three MS observers have means between 0.3 and 1.2 and standard deviations between 4.3 and 4.9. Moreover, the differences between the MS observers and DS have means between 1.3 and 2.8 and standard deviations between 6.4 and 6.8. Neither the means nor the standard deviations are particularly large.

Table 7.2 presents estimates of similarity measures along with two-sided 95% simultaneous confidence intervals for the six pairwise bias differences and precision ratios. The critical point used in the intervals for the bias differences is 2.555, and it is 2.557 for the log of precision ratios. Although only one interval for bias difference contains zero and the rest lie to the right of zero, none of the interval endpoints is too far from zero. Thus, the biases and hence the means of the observers can be considered practically equal. The same,

Pair	Bias Difference $(\beta_l - \beta_j)$		Precision Ratio $(\sigma_{ej}^2/\sigma_{el}^2)$	
(j, l)	Estimate	95% Interval	Estimate	95% Interval
$(1, 2)$	0.29	$(-0.54, 1.12)$	0.69	$(0.42, 1.14)$
$(1, 3)$	1.49	$(0.76, 2.22)$	1.13	$(0.61, 2.08)$
$(2, 3)$	1.20	$(0.39, 2.01)$	1.63	$(0.95, 2.78)$
$(1, 4)$	2.75	$(1.65, 3.85)$	0.30	$(0.19, 0.48)$
$(2, 4)$	2.46	$(1.31, 3.62)$	0.43	$(0.28, 0.66)$
$(3, 4)$	1.26	$(0.18, 2.35)$	0.27	$(0.17, 0.43)$

Table 7.2   Estimates and 95% simultaneous confidence intervals for all-pairwise bias differences and precision ratios for systolic blood pressure data. Methods 1, 2, 3, and 4 refer to the observers MS1, MS2, MS3, and DS, respectively.

	CCC		TDI	
		95% Lower		95% Upper
Pair	Estimate	Bound	Estimate	Bound
$(1, 2)$	0.987	0.983	8.05	8.94
$(1, 3)$	0.989	0.985	7.48	8.29
$(2, 3)$	0.987	0.983	8.09	8.98
$(1, 4)$	0.974	0.966	11.62	12.84
$(2, 4)$	0.972	0.964	11.94	13.13
$(3, 4)$	0.977	0.970	10.76	11.92

Table 7.3   Estimates and one-sided 95% simultaneous confidence bounds for all-pairwise CCCs and TDIs (with $p = 0.90$) for systolic blood pressure data. Methods 1, 2, 3, and 4 refer to the observers MS1, MS2, MS3, and DS, respectively.

however, cannot be said for the precisions. The first three intervals for precision ratios contain 1 but the last three lie quite below 1. Thus, the MS observers can be considered equally precise, but DS is less precise than them. In fact, in the best case, DS may be about 70% as precise as an MS observer, but in the worst case, its precision may be less than 20% of an MS observer. Taken together, these findings suggest that the MS observers have similar characteristics among themselves, but DS differs from them by being less precise.

For agreement evaluation, Table 7.3 provides estimates and one-sided 95% simultaneous confidence bounds for the six pairwise CCCs and TDIs with $p = 0.90$. As usual, lower bounds are presented for CCCs and upper bounds for TDIs. The critical point used in the intervals for CCCs after a Fisher's z-transformation is -2.184, and the same for TDIs after a log transformation is 2.311. Interestingly, the bounds for both measures are practically identical for the three MS observer pairs, and the same can be said for three pairs involving DS. This means that the three MS observers agree equally well with each other and also with DS. The bounds also show that agreement between any two MS observers is higher than the agreement between an MS observer and DS. We see that all CCC bounds are close to one, indicating high agreement among all four observers. The TDI bounds are about 9 for the MS observer pairs and about 13 for the pairs involving DS. These values

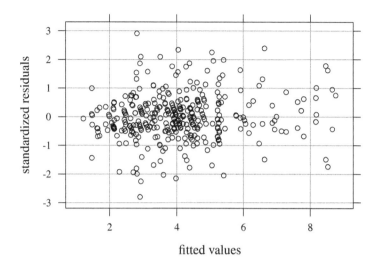

Figure 7.9 Residual plot for tumor size data.

are, respectively, about 7% and 10% of $\hat{\mu}_b = 129$ mm Hg. Given that the measurements themselves range from 82 to 236 mm Hg, the TDI bounds also indicate reasonably good agreement between all four observers, especially so among the MS observers.

7.10.2 Tumor Size Data

This dataset, introduced in Section 7.4, contains measurements of tumor sizes (in cm) of $n = 40$ lesions taken by five readers. Each measurement is repeated twice in an unlinked fashion. No reader serves as the reference and the interest is in all $\binom{5}{2} = 10$ pairwise comparisons of the readers. The graphical displays in Figures 7.4, 7.5, and 7.7 show that the readers have the same scale and their correlation is moderately high, but they have somewhat different means and have considerable within-subject variation. There is also subject × reader interaction and the data appear homoscedastic.

Figure 7.9 shows the residual plot that results from fitting the model (7.4). It does not show any trend and the vertical scatter appears constant. Besides, the normality of random effects and errors appear reasonable (Exercise 7.10). These suggest that the model fits well. Table 7.4 summarizes estimates of the 16 model parameters. From (7.9), we obtain the means and variances for the fitted normal distribution of $(Y_1, \ldots, Y_5)$ as $(4.03, 3.59, 4.34, 4.27, 4.11)$ and $(2.53, 2.96, 2.69, 2.49, 2.48)$, respectively, and 2.30 as the common covariance. The pairwise correlations range from 0.82 to 0.93. Reader 2 has the smallest mean and the largest variance.

Table 7.5 presents 95% simultaneous confidence intervals for the ten pairwise bias differences. The critical points for these intervals is 2.706. None of the four intervals involving reader 2 covers zero. The interval for reader pair (1, 2) lies below zero while the other three lie above zero. This confirms reader 2 to have the smallest mean. Her/his estimated mean difference is the smallest (0.43) with reader 1 and is the largest (0.74)

Parameter	Estimate	SE	95% Interval
β_2	-0.43	0.14	$(-0.71, -0.16)$
β_3	0.31	0.11	$(0.08, 0.54)$
β_4	0.24	0.09	$(0.07, 0.42)$
β_5	0.08	0.09	$(-0.09, 0.26)$
μ_b	4.03	0.25	$(3.54, 4.51)$
$\log(\sigma_b^2)$	0.83	0.23	$(0.39, 1.28)$
$\log(\psi_1^2)$	-1.97	0.39	$(-2.73, -1.21)$
$\log(\psi_2^2)$	-0.60	0.27	$(-1.13, -0.08)$
$\log(\psi_3^2)$	-1.22	0.30	$(-1.79, -0.64)$
$\log(\psi_4^2)$	-2.83	0.73	$(-4.26, -1.40)$
$\log(\psi_5^2)$	-2.59	0.57	$(-3.71, -1.47)$
$\log(\sigma_{e1}^2)$	-2.37	0.22	$(-2.81, -1.93)$
$\log(\sigma_{e2}^2)$	-2.22	0.22	$(-2.66, -1.79)$
$\log(\sigma_{e3}^2)$	-2.43	0.22	$(-2.86, -1.99)$
$\log(\sigma_{e4}^2)$	-2.04	0.22	$(-2.48, -1.60)$
$\log(\sigma_{e5}^2)$	-2.27	0.22	$(-2.71, -1.83)$

Table 7.4   Summary of parameter estimates for tumor size data.

Pair	Bias Difference $(\beta_l - \beta_j)$		Precision Ratio $\frac{(\psi_j^2 + \sigma_{ej}^2)}{(\psi_l^2 + \sigma_{el}^2)}$	
(j, l)	Estimate	95% Interval	Estimate	95% Interval
$(1, 2)$	-0.43	$(-0.81, -0.05)$	0.36	$(0.15, 0.84)$
$(1, 3)$	0.31	$(0.00, 0.62)$	0.61	$(0.24, 1.54)$
$(1, 4)$	0.24	$(0.01, 0.48)$	1.23	$(0.50, 3.06)$
$(1, 5)$	0.08	$(-0.16, 0.32)$	1.31	$(0.50, 3.39)$
$(2, 3)$	0.74	$(0.33, 1.16)$	1.70	$(0.72, 4.04)$
$(2, 4)$	0.67	$(0.31, 1.04)$	3.46	$(1.45, 8.30)$
$(2, 5)$	0.51	$(0.15, 0.88)$	3.67	$(1.41, 9.58)$
$(3, 4)$	-0.07	$(-0.36, 0.23)$	2.04	$(0.81, 5.12)$
$(3, 5)$	-0.23	$(-0.52, 0.07)$	2.16	$(0.89, 5.21)$
$(4, 5)$	-0.16	$(-0.38, 0.05)$	1.06	$(0.41, 2.74)$

Table 7.5   Estimates and 95% simultaneous confidence intervals for all-pairwise bias differences and modified precision ratios for tumor size data.

with reader 3. The remaining six intervals that do not involve reader 2 either cover zero or miss it by a whisker, implying that all other readers have practically the same means. The simultaneous intervals for precision ratios are not presented but the value of 1 is deep inside all the intervals. This suggests every reader has equal within-subject variations. However, a different picture emerges when we consider modified precision ratios given by (7.24) that include subject × reader interactions in the comparison. The 95% simultaneous confidence intervals are presented in Table 7.5. The critical point for these intervals on the log scale is 2.725. Three intervals involving reader 2 do not cover 1. They show that the modified

Reader	CCC$_j$		TDI$_j$	
j	Estimate	95% Lower Bound	Estimate	95% Upper Bound
1	0.963	0.939	0.71	0.86
2	0.963	0.941	0.77	0.92
3	0.967	0.947	0.69	0.83
4	0.948	0.914	0.84	1.01
5	0.958	0.931	0.75	0.90

Table 7.6 Estimates and one-sided 95% individual confidence bounds for repeatability versions of CCC and TDI (0.90) for tumor size data.

Pair	CCC$_{jl}$		TDI$_{jl}$	
(j, l)	Estimate	95% Lower Bound	Estimate	95% Upper Bound
(1, 2)	0.811	0.683	1.71	2.14
(1, 3)	0.866	0.770	1.39	1.71
(1, 4)	0.905	0.832	1.14	1.40
(1, 5)	0.917	0.852	1.06	1.30
(2, 3)	0.743	0.593	2.07	2.56
(2, 4)	0.780	0.640	1.87	2.33
(2, 5)	0.807	0.679	1.72	2.16
(3, 4)	0.888	0.807	1.25	1.53
(3, 5)	0.882	0.794	1.29	1.61
(4, 5)	0.921	0.859	1.03	1.26

Table 7.7 Estimates and 95% one-sided simultaneous confidence bounds for all-pairwise values of CCC and TDI (0.90) for tumor size data.

precision of reader 2 is substantially lower than those of readers 1, 4, and 5. The other intervals cover 1, implying similar pairwise precisions. On the whole, this similarity evaluation essentially confirms the deviant behavior of reader 2 in terms of both means and modified precisions.

Table 7.6 presents 95% one-sided individual confidence bounds for repeatability versions of CCC and TDI (0.90) for each reader. The critical point for the CCC intervals on the Fisher's z-scale is -1.645 and it is 1.645 for the TDI intervals on the log scale. Although on both measures reader 4 is the least and reader 3 is the most consistent, all readers have somewhat similar repeatability characteristic from a practical viewpoint. They have high reliabilities, as evidenced by the CCC estimates. However, the TDI bounds ranging from 0.8 to 1.0 are about 20–25% of $\hat{\mu}_b = 4.0$, indicating relatively weak intra-reader agreement.

Table 7.7 presents 95% one-sided simultaneous confidence bounds for all-pairwise values of CCC and TDI (0.90). The critical point used in the CCC intervals on the Fisher's z-scale is -2.250 and the same for the TDI intervals on the log scale is 2.464. The bounds range from 0.59 to 0.86 for CCC and from 1.26 to 2.56 for TDI. Remarkably, the bounds for both measures induce the same ordering of reader pairs on the basis of extent of agreement. In particular, the pair (2, 3) has the least agreement whereas the pair (4, 5) has the most. But even the highest level of agreement does not seem high enough to be deemed satisfactory. It is also apparent from the evaluation of similarity and repeatability that the relatively high error variation of the readers is a key cause of their poor agreement. It may be possible to reduce this error variation and hence improve the readers' agreement by providing uniform training in determining the tumor sizes. The training may also correct the deviant performance of reader 2.

7.11 CHAPTER SUMMARY

1. The methodology for data on two methods is extended to more than two methods.

2. It allows ANOVA-style multiple comparisons of method pairs, for example, all-pairwise comparisons or comparisons with a reference, on the basis of measures of pairwise similarity and agreement.

3. The approach involves extending models for data on two methods to allow J methods in a straightforward manner, and performing simultaneous inference on measures of pairwise similarity and agreement for method pairs of interest.

4. For unreplicated data, the model (4.1) is extended. In this extension, the usual problems in estimation of variance components do not arise.

5. For repeated measurements data, the models (5.1) and (5.9) for unlinked and linked data are generalized. By default, the variances for subject $\times$ method interactions are assumed to be unequal, but one can assume equal variances if needed.

6. The methodology can be further extended to allow heteroscedasticity of errors along the lines of Chapter 6.

7. As before, the methodology assumes that all the methods are on the same scale and the number of subjects is large.

7.12 TECHNICAL DETAILS

For paired measurements data, recall that the mixed-effects model (4.1) is written in the usual matrix form as (4.15). To write its extension (7.1) for unreplicated data on $J\ (\geq 2)$ methods in the same form, define

$$\beta_1 = \mu_b, \ \beta_j = \beta_j + \mu_b, \ j = 2, \ldots, J, \ \boldsymbol{\beta} = (\beta_1, \ldots, \beta_J)^T, \ u_i = b_i - \mu_b.$$

Expand the vectors and matrices in (4.14) as

$$\mathbf{Y}_i = (Y_{i1}, \ldots, Y_{iJ})^T, \ \mathbf{e}_i = (e_{i1}, \ldots, e_{iJ})^T, \ \mathbf{X} = \mathbf{I}_J, \ \mathbf{Z} = \mathbf{1}_J.$$

With this notation, the model (7.1) for $i = 1, \ldots, n$ can be written as

$$\mathbf{Y}_i = \mathbf{X}\boldsymbol{\beta} + \mathbf{Z}u_i + \mathbf{e}_i,$$
$$u_i \sim \mathcal{N}_1(0, G = \sigma_b^2), \ \mathbf{e}_i \sim \mathcal{N}_J\left(\mathbf{0}, \mathbf{R} = \text{diag}\{\sigma_{e1}^2, \ldots, \sigma_{eJ}^2\}\right). \tag{7.34}$$

As before, this implies $\mathbf{Y}_i \sim \mathcal{N}_J \left(\mathbf{X}\boldsymbol{\beta}, \mathbf{V} = \mathbf{Z}\mathbf{G}\mathbf{Z}^T + \mathbf{R} \right)$, where the mean vector $\mathbf{X}\boldsymbol{\beta}$ and the covariance matrix $\mathbf{V}$ yield the expressions in (7.2) upon using the fact that $\beta_1 = 0$. The vector of transformed parameters is

$$\boldsymbol{\theta} = \left(\beta_2, \ldots, \beta_J, \mu_b, \log(\sigma_b^2), \log(\sigma_{e1}^2), \ldots, \log(\sigma_{eJ}^2) \right)^T.$$

For unlinked repeated measurements data, we similarly expand the notation in (5.38) and (5.39) for two methods to accommodate $J\,(> 2)$ methods. This involves taking

$$\mathbf{u}_i = (u_i, b_{i1}, \ldots, b_{iJ})^T, \quad \mathbf{Y}_i = (\mathbf{Y}_{i1}, \ldots, \mathbf{Y}_{iJ})^T, \quad \mathbf{e}_i = (\mathbf{e}_{i1}, \ldots, \mathbf{e}_{iJ})^T,$$

$$\mathbf{X}_i = \begin{pmatrix} \mathbf{1}_{m_{i1}} & \cdots & \mathbf{0}_{m_{i1}} \\ \vdots & \ddots & \vdots \\ \mathbf{0}_{m_{iJ}} & \cdots & \mathbf{1}_{m_{iJ}} \end{pmatrix}, \quad \mathbf{Z}_i = \begin{pmatrix} \mathbf{1}_{m_{i1}} & \mathbf{1}_{m_{i1}} & \cdots & \mathbf{0}_{m_{i1}} \\ \vdots & \vdots & \ddots & \vdots \\ \mathbf{1}_{m_{iJ}} & \mathbf{0}_{m_{iJ}} & \cdots & \mathbf{1}_{m_{iJ}} \end{pmatrix},$$

$$\mathbf{R}_{ij} = \sigma_{ej}^2 \, \mathbf{I}_{m_{ij}}, \quad \mathbf{R}_i = \text{diag}\{\mathbf{R}_{i1}, \ldots, \mathbf{R}_{iJ}\}, \quad \mathbf{G} = \text{diag}\{\sigma_b^2, \psi_1^2, \ldots, \psi_J^2\}. \qquad (7.35)$$

The model (7.4) for $i = 1, \ldots, n$ can now be written as

$$\mathbf{Y}_i = \mathbf{X}_i\boldsymbol{\beta} + \mathbf{Z}_i\mathbf{u}_i + \mathbf{e}_i, \quad \mathbf{u}_i \sim \mathcal{N}_{J+1}(\mathbf{0}, \mathbf{G}), \quad \mathbf{e}_i \sim \mathcal{N}_{M_i}(\mathbf{0}, \mathbf{R}_i).$$

It follows that

$$\mathbf{Y}_i \sim \mathcal{N}_{M_i}(\mathbf{X}_i\boldsymbol{\beta}, \mathbf{V}_i = \mathbf{Z}_i\mathbf{G}\mathbf{Z}_i^T + \mathbf{R}_i), \qquad (7.36)$$

where the elements of the mean vector $\mathbf{X}_i\boldsymbol{\beta}$ and the covariance matrix $\mathbf{V}_i$ are given earlier in (7.5)–(7.7) (Exercise 7.3). The vector of transformed parameters of this model is

$$\boldsymbol{\theta} = \left(\beta_2, \ldots, \beta_J, \mu_b, \log(\sigma_b^2), \log(\psi_1^2), \ldots, \log(\psi_J^2), \log(\sigma_{e1}^2), \ldots, \log(\sigma_{eJ}^2) \right)^T.$$

For linked repeated measurements data, $\mathbf{Y}_i, \mathbf{e}_i, \mathbf{X}_i,$ and $\mathbf{R}_i$ are the same as for unlinked data with $(m_{ij}, M_i) = (m_i, Jm_i)$. But the random effects vector $\mathbf{u}_i$ is a $(1+J+\tilde{m})$-vector

$$\mathbf{u}_i = (u_i, b_{i1}, \ldots, b_{iJ}, b_{i1}^*, \ldots, b_{i\tilde{m}}^*)^T,$$

its covariance matrix $\mathbf{G}$ is a $(1 + J + \tilde{m}) \times (1 + J + \tilde{m})$ diagonal matrix

$$\mathbf{G} = \text{diag}\{\sigma_b^2, \psi_1^2, \ldots, \psi_J^2, \sigma_{b*}^2, \ldots, \sigma_{b*}^2\},$$

and the design matrix $\mathbf{Z}_i$ associated with $\mathbf{u}_i$ is an appropriately defined $M_i \times (1 + J + \tilde{m})$ matrix of ones and zeros, with $\tilde{m} = \max_{i=1,\ldots,n} m_i$ as in Section 5.9. Now the model (7.14) for $i = 1, \ldots, n$ can be written as

$$\mathbf{Y}_i = \mathbf{X}_i\boldsymbol{\beta} + \mathbf{Z}_i\mathbf{u}_i + \mathbf{e}_i, \quad \mathbf{u}_i \sim \mathcal{N}_{1+J+\tilde{m}}(\mathbf{0}, \mathbf{G}), \quad \mathbf{e}_i \sim \mathcal{N}_{M_i}(\mathbf{0}, \mathbf{R}_i), \qquad (7.37)$$

implying

$$\mathbf{Y}_i \sim \mathcal{N}_{M_i}(\mathbf{X}_i\boldsymbol{\beta}, \mathbf{V}_i = \mathbf{Z}_i\mathbf{G}\mathbf{Z}_i^T + \mathbf{R}_i). \qquad (7.38)$$

The elements of the mean vector and covariance matrix here are given in (7.15)–(7.18) (Exercise 7.5). The vector of transformed parameters of this model is

$$\boldsymbol{\theta} = \left(\beta_2, \ldots, \beta_J, \mu_b, \log(\sigma_b^2), \log(\psi_1^2), \ldots, \log(\psi_J^2), \log(\sigma_{b*}^2), \log(\sigma_{e1}^2), \ldots, \log(\sigma_{eJ}^2) \right)^T.$$

The models in this chapter can be fit by the ML method using a statistical software that handles mixed-effects models. We proceed as in Chapter 3 for the estimation of various measures, computation of standard errors of the estimates, and construction of individual as well as simultaneous confidence intervals and bounds.

7.13 BIBLIOGRAPHIC NOTE

Many of the papers cited in previous chapters for two methods, especially those dealing with CCC and modeling of data, actually contain extensions for multiple methods. The CCC-focussed articles include Lin (1989), King and Chinchilli (2001a), Barnhart et al. (2002), Carrasco and Jover (2003), Barnhart et al. (2005), and Lin et al. (2007). The modeling articles include Carstensen et al. (2008) and Schluter (2009). The papers on CCC summarize the overall level of agreement among the multiple methods in a single index by either taking a weighted average of the pairwise CCCs or replacing the moments in the definition of CCC by their weighted averages taken over the method pairs. In principle, such an approach can be used with other measures of similarity and agreement as well. However, we find such overall measures difficult to interpret and prefer to keep the pairwise measures separate and perform simultaneous inference on them. Unlike the overall measures, the separate pairwise measures allow us to directly compare the method pairs on the basis of extent of similarity or agreement and also to determine which pairs are similar or agree well, while adjusting for multiplicity of inferences.

The approach based on simultaneous inference on pairwise measures is inspired by the multiple comparisons of means in ANOVA for which the monograph by Hsu (1996) is a good reference. This approach has been taken by Hedayat et al. (2009) and Choudhary and Yin (2010). The first article works with unreplicated multivariate normal data and focuses on coverage probability as the agreement measure, which has one-to-one correspondence with TDI (Chapter 2). It develops simultaneous confidence bounds for pairwise values of the measure and a test of homogeneity for them. The second article works with unreplicated as well as repeated measurements data assumed to follow a mixed-effects model. It develops frequentist and Bayesian procedures for simultaneous bounds on pairwise values of any scalar agreement measure. This is also the basis for some of the material in this chapter. The models here are similar, but not identical, to those in Carstensen et al. (2008).

The critical points used in the simultaneous confidence bounds and intervals are computed using the `multcomp` package of Hothorn et al. (2008) in R.

St. Laurent (1998), Hutson et al. (1998), and Harris et al. (2001) assume a "gold standard" method in the comparison that serves as a reference. The comparisons with a reference can be accommodated in the multiple comparisons approach of this chapter.

Data Sources

The systolic blood pressure data are from Barnhart et al. (2002). Broemeling (2009, Chapter 6) is the source of the tumor size data and contains further details about them.

EXERCISES

7.1 (a) (Bonferroni Inequality) Let $A_1, A_2, \ldots, A_k$ be k events. Show that

$$P(\text{At least one of the } A_i \text{ occurs}) \leq \sum_{i=1}^{k} P(A_i).$$

(b) For the events in part (a), show that

$$P(\text{All occur}) = P(\cap_{i=1}^{k} A_i) \leq \min_{i=1,\ldots,k} P(A_i).$$

(c) For $i = 1, \ldots, k$, let I_i be a $100(1 - \alpha)\%$ confidence interval for parameter θ_i; and $E_i = \{\theta_i \in I_i\}$ be the event that the interval I_i covers the true parameter θ_i. Then, by definition, the coverage probability of the ith interval is $P(E_i) \geq 1 - \alpha$. Use parts (a) and (b) to show that the simultaneous coverage probability of the k intervals satisfies the inequalities

$$1 - k\alpha \leq P(\{\theta_1 \in I_1\} \cap \ldots \cap \{\theta_k \in I_k\}) = P(\cap_{i=1}^{k} E_i) \leq 1 - \alpha.$$

(d) Deduce from part (c) that if each I_i is a $100(1 - \alpha/k)\%$ confidence interval, then the k intervals together form a set of $100(1-\alpha)\%$ simultaneous confidence region for $\theta_1, \ldots, \theta_k$ that is generally conservative.

7.2 Under the model (7.1), show that the marginal distribution of $(Y_{i1}, \ldots, Y_{iJ})$ on subject i is given by (7.2) for $i = 1, \ldots, n$.

7.3 This is a generalization of Exercise 5.1 for $J \, (> 2)$ methods. Show that the marginal distribution of the vector $\mathbf{Y}_i$ of unlinked observations on subject i is given by (7.36) for $i = 1, \ldots, n$. Show also that the elements of the mean vector and covariance matrix of $\mathbf{Y}_i$ are given by (7.5)–(7.7).

7.4 This is a generalization of Exercise 5.2 for $J \, (> 2)$ methods. Consider the model (7.4) for unlinked repeated measurements data, and also the companion models for Y_j and $Y_j^* \, (j = 1, \ldots, J)$ given by (7.8) and (7.11).

(a) Show that the marginal distribution of $(Y_1, \ldots, Y_J)$ is given by (7.9). Verify the distribution of D_{jl} given in (7.10).

(b) Show that the marginal distribution of (Y_j, Y_j^*) is given by (7.12) for $j = 1, \ldots, J$. Deduce the distribution of D_j given in (7.13).

7.5 This analog of Exercise 7.3 for linked data is a generalization of Exercise 5.3 for $J \, (> 2)$ methods. Show that the marginal distribution of the vector $\mathbf{Y}_i$ of linked observations on subject i $(i = 1, \ldots, n)$ is given by (7.38). Show also that the elements of the mean vector and covariance matrix of $\mathbf{Y}_i$ are given by (7.15)–(7.18).

7.6 This analog of Exercise 7.4 for linked data is a generalization of Exercise 5.4 for $J \, (> 2)$ methods. Consider the model (7.14) for linked repeated measurements data.

(a) Show that the marginal distribution of $(Y_1, \ldots, Y_J)$ is a J-variate normal distribution with mean vector and covariance matrix given by (7.19) and (7.20). Verify the distribution of D_{jl} given in (7.21).

(b) Show that the marginal distribution of (Y_j, Y_j^*) is given by (7.22) for $j = 1, \ldots, J$. Deduce the distribution of D_j given in (7.23).

7.7 Confirm the expressions for agreement measures given in (7.25), (7.26), and (7.27).

7.8 Verify the expressions for repeatability measures given in (7.30) and (7.31).

7.9 Fractional area change is measured in 15 subjects in an echocardiographic imaging study using four methods—a fuzzy gold standard (FGS) derived from a consensus of experts, two distinct echocardiographers (EXP1 and EXP2), and an automatic

	Method			
Subject	FGS	EXP1	EXP2	ABD
1	41.25	26.96	45.96	26.78
2	37.95	39.87	36.95	26.88
3	37.23	31.69	31.72	39.08
4	40.62	36.41	30.58	24.63
5	34.67	44.77	40.55	39.82
6	32.31	31.46	33.03	28.53
7	28.53	35.13	10.97	28.84
8	39.25	40.69	33.10	39.06
9	35.37	33.93	34.85	30.24
10	40.17	43.99	38.72	34.77
11	38.53	22.86	31.07	42.43
12	36.39	40.99	26.34	34.48
13	40.82	32.78	34.61	34.21
14	37.52	24.09	29.65	25.69
15	42.01	51.99	42.00	37.03

Reprinted from Hutson (2010), ©2010 Elsevier, with permission from Elsevier.

Table 7.8   Fractional area change measurements (in %) for Exercise 7.9.

boundary detection (ABD) algorithm, which requires no observer input. Table 7.8 presents the data. As there is a reference method in the study, the comparisons with the reference are of interest.

(a) Perform an exploratory analysis. Do the methods appear to have the same scale? Do you notice any outliers? If yes, how would you deal with them?

(b) Fit model (7.1) to the data. Check adequacy of the model assumptions.

(c) Evaluate similarity between fuzzy gold standard and other methods.

(d) Evaluate agreement between fuzzy gold standard and other methods. Which of the methods can be used interchangeably with it?

(e) If outliers are seen, analyze the data again after removing them, and compare the conclusions.

7.10 Consider the tumor size data from Section 7.10.2.

(a) Fit model (7.4) to the data and verify the results in Tables 7.4–7.7.

(b) Perform model diagnostics to verify whether the normality assumption for errors and random effects appear reasonable.

7.11 Standardized uptake value, a measure of lesion size, is measured in 20 lung cancer patients by three readers with the help of CT-PET imaging. Each measurement is replicated twice in an unlinked manner. The data are presented on page 202 of Broemeling (2009).

(a) Perform an exploratory analysis of the data with summary measures and graphical displays.

(b) Fit model (7.4) to the data. Are the unequal variances for patient × reader interactions estimated reliably? If not, fit a simpler model that assumes equal variances for the interactions.

(c) Check adequacy of the simpler model. Does the homoscedasticity assumption appear reasonable? If not, is this assumption reasonable for the log-transformed data? Find an adequate model for the data either on the original scale or on the transformed scale.

(d) Evaluate repeatability of each reader.

(e) Evaluate similarity of all reader pairs.

(f) Evaluate pairwise agreement between all readers. Do the readers agree well?

7.12 Bland and Altman (1999) report a study where two observers and an automatic blood pressure measuring machine simultaneously measure systolic blood pressure. Each makes three observations in quick succession on 85 subjects. We assume the repeated measurements to be unlinked. The data can be obtained from the book's website.

(a) Fit model (7.4) to these data. Examine the estimates of variance components and judge whether they can be considered reliable.

(b) Fit the following modification of (7.4) to these data:

$$Y_{ijk} = \beta_j + b_{ij} + e_{ijk},$$

where β_j are unknown intercepts; the random effects (b_{i1}, b_{i2}, b_{i3}) are i.i.d. draws from a trivariate normal distribution with zero mean and an unstructured covariance matrix; and the errors follow independent $\mathcal{N}_1(0, \sigma_{ej}^2)$ distributions, independently of the random effects. Perform model diagnostics to check goodness of fit of the model. Comment specifically on the normality assumption for random effects and errors.

(c) Evaluate similarity and agreement using the model fit in part (b).

CHAPTER 8

DATA WITH COVARIATES

8.1 PREVIEW

So far the method comparison data were assumed to solely consist of observations from the measurement methods of interest on a number of subjects. Frequently, however, additional data on a number of influential covariates are also available. These covariates may be categorical or continuous quantities and may affect either the means or the variances of the methods. This chapter coalesces ideas from previous chapters to present a unified method that incorporates covariates in the analysis. Both unreplicated and repeated measurements data are considered. As before, our approach is to first model the data and then use the assumed model for evaluating similarity and agreement, and possibly repeatability as well. A case study illustrates the methodology.

8.2 INTRODUCTION

Quite often in a method comparison study, data are collected on a number of covariates in addition to the observations from the measurement methods of interest. The covariates may be categorical or continuous. They are fixed, known quantities and are assumed to be measured without error. They include subject-level covariates, for example, gender of the subject, and method-level covariates. Of course, we always have the "measurement method" itself as a method-level categorical covariate in the analysis. The other covariates may affect the means of the methods, thereby explaining a portion of the variability in

Measuring Agreement: Models, Methods, and Applications. By P. K. Choudhary and H. N. Nagaraja
Copyright © 2017 John Wiley & Sons, Inc.

the measurements. We refer to them as the *mean covariates*. Incorporating them in the analysis adjusts the extent of agreement between the methods to account for their effects. A subset of the covariates may also interact with the methods in that the difference between the means of two methods depends on the covariates. In this case, the extent of agreement depends on the covariates. It may also be that the variance of a measurement method, particularly its error variance, depends on covariates. Such covariates are called *variance covariates* (as we saw in Chapter 6). Even in this case, the extent of agreement depends on the covariates. Thus, there is a clear need for identifying covariates and incorporating them in the analysis.

Let the study have r mean covariates, $x_1, \ldots, x_r$, not including the effects of measurement methods. Each contributes one or more *explanatory* variables to the mean model. A categorical covariate with L levels is represented using $L-1$ indicator explanatory variables. A continuous covariate may be included either on the original scale or on a transformed scale. Let $\mathbf{x}$ be the vector of all explanatory variables contributed by the r covariates, including the main effects as well as the interactions of interest. Let $\tilde{v}$ be a variance covariate that may depend on the mean covariates. It is taken to be a scalar quantity that can be continuous or categorical. The ranges of the covariates are taken to be their observed ranges in the data.

We assume that the study involves $J\,(\geq 2)$ methods with single measurements or repeated measurements that may be linked or unlinked. The covariates do not change with time. Time-dependent covariates are discussed in Chapter 9 on longitudinal data. As before, let Y_{ij}, $j = 1, \ldots, J$, $i = 1, \ldots, n$ denote the unreplicated data, and Y_{ijk}, $k = 1, \ldots, m_{ij}, j = 1, \ldots, J, i = 1, \ldots, n$ denote the repeated measurements data. Here i is the subject index, j is the method index, and k indexes the order in which the repeated measurements are taken. We use M_i to denote the number of observations on subject i. It equals J for unreplicated data and $\sum_{j=1}^{J} m_{ij}$ for repeated measurements data. Let $N = \sum_{i=1}^{n} M_i$. Also, let $(x_{1i}, \ldots, x_{ri})$, $\mathbf{x}_i$, and $\tilde{v}_i$, respectively, denote for subject i the values of the vector of mean covariates $(x_1, \ldots, x_r)$, the vector of explanatory variables $\mathbf{x}$, and the variance covariate $\tilde{v}$.

As in previous chapters, we take a model-based approach. We include mean and variance covariates in the model and base our inferences on the expanded model.

8.3 MODELING OF DATA

We first discuss how the population means and variances of the methods can be modeled as functions of covariates.

8.3.1 Modeling Means of Methods

The population means of the methods have been assumed to be constants thus far. In particular, the mean μ_j of method j has the form

$$\mu_j = \beta_{0j}, \quad j = 1, \ldots, J,$$

where β_{0j} can be written in terms of model parameters (Exercise 8.1). We now let these means be functions of the explanatory variables $\mathbf{x}$ as in a linear regression analysis. The mean functions are linear in regression coefficients and are *parametric* in that they have specified functional forms. The forms are assumed to be the same for all the J methods to allow the data from different methods to have marginal distributions of the same form. As before, method 1 serves as the reference method. Two scenarios arise depending on whether or not covariates interact with the methods.

8.3.1.1 *No Method × Covariates Interaction*

When none of the covariates interacts with the methods, we can write the mean function for the jth method as

$$\mu_j(x_1,\ldots,x_r) = \beta_{0j} + \mathbf{x}^T\boldsymbol{\beta}_1, \tag{8.1}$$

where β_{0j} are intercepts and $\boldsymbol{\beta}_1$ is a vector of slope coefficients associated with $\mathbf{x}$. Only the intercepts here depend on j; the slopes are free of j because there is no interaction with the method. It follows that the difference in mean functions of methods j and l with identical covariate data is

$$\xi_{jl}(x_1,\ldots,x_r) = \mu_l(x_1,\ldots,x_r) - \mu_j(x_1,\ldots,x_r) = \beta_{0l} - \beta_{0j}, \quad j \neq l, \tag{8.2}$$

which does not depend on the covariates.

8.3.1.2 *Method × Covariates Interaction*

Suppose some of the r covariates interact with the methods. Let $\mathbf{x}_I$ be the $s \times 1$ vector of the interacting variables. The mean function for method j can be expressed as

$$\mu_j(x_1,\ldots,x_r) = \beta_{0j} + \mathbf{x}^T\boldsymbol{\beta}_1 + \mathbf{x}_I^T\boldsymbol{\beta}_{Ij}, \tag{8.3}$$

where $\boldsymbol{\beta}_{Ij}$ is the $s \times 1$ vector of regression coefficients associated with $\mathbf{x}_I$ and depends on j due to the interaction. Moreover, because method 1 serves as the reference, its coefficients for the interacting variables are assumed to be zero, that is,

$$\boldsymbol{\beta}_{I1} = \mathbf{0}.$$

This assumption is necessary to enforce identifiability. The difference in mean functions of methods j and l is

$$\xi_{jl}(x_1,\ldots,x_r) = (\beta_{0l} - \beta_{0j}) + \mathbf{x}_I^T(\boldsymbol{\beta}_{Il} - \boldsymbol{\beta}_{Ij}), \quad j \neq l. \tag{8.4}$$

The model (8.3) is a generalization of the model (8.1) and it reduces to the latter when there is no interaction, that is, $\boldsymbol{\beta}_{Ij} = \mathbf{0}$ for all j. In this case, the differences (8.2) and (8.4) are identical. The general form (8.3) is used in the subsequent sections.

8.3.2 Modeling Variances of Methods

Ideally, to model variances of the methods in terms of the variance covariate $\tilde{v}$, we model the error variances of the methods. However, we have seen earlier that reliable estimation of error variances requires either repeated measurements data or unreplicated data on more than two methods. In particular, the estimates are not reliable for paired measurements data in which case we can only model the overall variances. This suggests that we must consider the two scenarios separately.

Assume for now that we have repeated measurements data on $J \, (\geq 2)$ methods. If $\tilde{v}$ is continuous, we can proceed exactly as in Chapter 6 to model error variances as functions of $\tilde{v}$, that is,

$$\mathrm{var}(e_{ijk}) = \sigma_{ej}^2 \, g_j^2(\tilde{v}_i, \boldsymbol{\delta}_j), \tag{8.5}$$

where g_j is a specified variance function for method j that depends on the heteroscedasticity parameter vector $\boldsymbol{\delta}_j$ and has the property that $g_j(\tilde{v}, \mathbf{0}) = 1$. When $\boldsymbol{\delta}_1 = \ldots = \boldsymbol{\delta}_J = \mathbf{0}$, the model becomes homoscedastic. In practice, the variance functions g_j in (8.5) may be taken to be the same for all methods. In this case, it may also be reasonable to impose some structure on the heteroscedasticity parameters. For example, they may be assumed to identical, that is, $\boldsymbol{\delta}_1 = \ldots = \boldsymbol{\delta}_J$, but having a nonzero value. The model (8.5) is same as (6.9) except that J can be more than two here, and the covariate is not necessarily a proxy for the magnitude of measurement. Thus, the discussion in Section 6.4 about how to specify the variance functions and evaluate their adequacy is relevant here as well.

Suppose now that $\tilde{v}$ is a categorical variable with L levels and the error variance of method j changes with the level of $\tilde{v}$. The JL error variances can be written as

$$\text{var}(e_{ijk}) = \sigma_{ej}^2 \delta_{j\tilde{v}_i}^2. \tag{8.6}$$

However, this model has $J + JL$ parameters, implying the need to impose J constraints on the parameters to make the model identifiable. One can assume

$$\delta_{j1}^2 = 1, \ j = 1, \ldots, J,$$

which amounts to interpreting the heteroscedasticity parameters δ_{jl}^2 for $l = 2, \ldots, L$ as the ratio of error variances of method j under the lth and the first settings of the covariate $\tilde{v}$. The model is homoscedastic when all δ_{jl}^2 are one. Also, as in the continuous case, some structure may be imposed on these heteroscedasticity parameters. The model (8.6) can be seen to be a special case of the model (8.5) by taking

$$g_j(\tilde{v}_i, \boldsymbol{\delta}_j) = \delta_{j\tilde{v}_i}$$

as the variance function and

$$\boldsymbol{\delta}_j = (1 - \delta_{j2}^2, \ldots, 1 - \delta_{jL}^2)^T$$

as the vector of heteroscedasticity parameters. The general model (8.5) is used in the subsequent sections.

The above discussion has assumed repeated measurements data. Nonetheless, the model (8.5) can also be used for modeling error variances in the case of unreplicated data from $J\,(> 2)$ methods, provided, of course, that $\text{var}(e_{ijk})$ is replaced with $\text{var}(e_{ij})$. As seen in Section 6.5, upon replacing $\text{var}(e_{ijk})$ with $\text{var}(Y_{ij})$, it can also be used for modeling overall variances of measurements when we have paired measurements data.

8.3.3 Data Models

Our task now is to generalize the data models of previous chapters by integrating them with the mean function model (8.3) in terms of the covariates $x_1, \ldots, x_r$, and the variance function model (8.5) in terms of the covariate $\tilde{v}$. The specific models to be generalized are as follows: the bivariate normal model (4.6) for paired data; the mixed-effects model (7.1) for unreplicated data from $J > 2$ methods; the mixed-effects models (5.1) and (5.9) for unlinked and linked repeated measurements data from $J = 2$ methods; and the extensions (7.4) and (7.14) of (5.1) and (5.9) for $J > 2$ methods. The new models are formulated in general terms. In practice, one has to go through the usual model building exercise to find which covariates, if any, are significant for modeling either the means or the variances, and hence should be included in the model. Setting $\beta_{Ij} = 0$ for all j in the new models gives their versions without the method $\times$ covariate interaction. Homoscedastic versions are obtained by setting $\delta_j = 0$ for all j. Setting β_1 and β_{Ij} and δ_j for all j equal to 0 gives back the versions without the covariates.

In what follows, the mean function $\mu_j(x_{1i}, \ldots, x_{ri})$ is given by (8.3) with $\mathbf{x}$ and $\mathbf{x}_I$ replaced by their respective values $\mathbf{x}_i$ and $\mathbf{x}_{Ii}$ for subject i. Moreover, the mean difference function $\xi_{jl}(x_1, \ldots, x_r)$ is given by (8.4).

8.3.3.1 Repeated Measurements Data

Consider the model (7.4) for unlinked data from $J > 2$ methods. It assumes $\beta_1 = 0$ for identifiability. We make three changes to the model. First, we write the term $\beta_j + b_i$ in an equivalent form, $\beta_{0j} + u_i$, where $u_i = b_i - \mu_b$ and $\beta_{0j} = \beta_j + \mu_b$. The u_i represents the centered true value for subject i and β_{0j} represents the mean μ_j of method j. Next, we replace the constant mean with the mean function (8.3). Finally, the constant error variance σ_{ej}^2 is replaced by the variance function (8.5). Thus, the model (7.4) generalizes to

$$Y_{ijk} = \mu_j(x_{1i}, \ldots, x_{ri}) + u_i + b_{ij} + e_{ijk}, \tag{8.7}$$

where

$$u_i \sim \text{independent } \mathcal{N}_1(0, \sigma_b^2), \quad e_{ijk} \sim \text{independent } \mathcal{N}_1\big(0, \sigma_{ej}^2\, g_j^2(\tilde{v}_i, \delta_j)\big). \tag{8.8}$$

The other terms in (8.7) and the assumptions regarding them remain the same as in (7.4). The assumptions imply that the vector of M_i observations on subject i follows an independent M_i-variate normal distribution with

$$E(Y_{ijk}) = \mu_j(x_{1i}, \ldots, x_{ri}), \quad \text{var}(Y_{ijk}) = \sigma_b^2 + \psi_j^2 + \sigma_{ej}^2\, g_j^2(\tilde{v}_i, \delta_j), \tag{8.9}$$

and the covariances, free of the covariates, are given by (7.6) and (7.7); see Exercise 8.2. It also follows from this exercise that the joint distribution of the population vector $(Y_1, \ldots, Y_J)$ induced by the model (8.9) at covariate setting $(x_1, \ldots, x_r, \tilde{v})$ is a J-variate normal distribution with

$$E(Y_j) = \mu_j(x_1, \ldots, x_r), \quad \text{var}(Y_j) = \sigma_b^2 + \psi_j^2 + \sigma_{ej}^2\, g_j^2(\tilde{v}, \delta_j), \quad \text{cov}(Y_j, Y_l) = \sigma_b^2, \tag{8.10}$$

for $j \neq l$. Therefore, for the difference $D_{jl} = Y_l - Y_j$ we have

$$D_{jl} \sim \mathcal{N}_1\big(\xi_{jl}(x_1, \ldots, x_r), \tau_{jl}^2(\tilde{v})\big), \tag{8.11}$$

with

$$\tau_{jl}^2(\tilde{v}) = \psi_j^2 + \psi_l^2 + \sigma_{ej}^2\, g_j^2(\tilde{v}, \delta_j) + \sigma_{el}^2\, g_l^2(\tilde{v}, \delta_l). \tag{8.12}$$

These distributions are used to derive measures of similarity and agreement. Moreover, as in Section 7.6.1, the distribution of the measurement pair (Y_j, Y_j^*) from method j is bivariate normal with identical marginals (Exercise 8.2). Therefore, for $j = 1, \ldots, J$, the mean and variance of Y_j^* are same as those of Y_j given in (8.10). Further, we can see that

$$\text{cov}(Y_j, Y_j^*) = \sigma_b^2 + \psi_j^2, \tag{8.13}$$

and

$$D_j = Y_j - Y_j^* \sim \mathcal{N}_1\big(0, 2\sigma_{ej}^2\, g_j^2(\tilde{v}, \delta_j)\big). \tag{8.14}$$

These distributions are needed to derive measures of repeatability.

For linked data from $J (> 2)$ methods, we generalize the model (7.14) to write

$$Y_{ijk} = \mu_j(x_{1i}, \ldots, x_{ri}) + u_i + b_{ij} + b_{ik}^* + e_{ijk}, \tag{8.15}$$

where the distributions of u_i and e_{ijk} are given by (8.8), and the rest of the terms are from (7.14). Exercise 8.3 derives the marginal distribution of these data. It also shows that the joint distribution of $(Y_1, \ldots, Y_J)$ at $(x_1, \ldots, x_r, \tilde{v})$ is a J-variate normal distribution with $E(Y_j) = \mu_j(x_1, \ldots, x_r)$,

$$\mathrm{var}(Y_j) = \sigma_b^2 + \psi_j^2 + \sigma_{b*}^2 + \sigma_{ej}^2\, g_j^2(\tilde{v}, \boldsymbol{\delta}_j), \quad \mathrm{cov}(Y_j, Y_l) = \sigma_b^2 + \sigma_{b*}^2. \tag{8.16}$$

The distribution of the difference D_{jl} is the same as in unlinked data and is given by (8.11). Further, it can be seen that (Y_j, Y_j^*) follows a bivariate normal distribution with identical marginals and covariance given by (8.13). For the distribution of their difference D_j, we have

$$D_j \sim \mathcal{N}_1\big(0, 2\{\sigma_{b*}^2 + \sigma_{ej}^2\, g_j^2(\tilde{v}, \boldsymbol{\delta}_j)\}\big). \tag{8.17}$$

Thus far in this section we assumed $J > 2$. Under this assumption, the variance ψ_j^2 of subject × method interaction is allowed to depend on method (Section 7.6). All results hold for $J = 2$ as well, provided ψ_j^2 for all j is replaced by a common variance ψ^2 (Exercise 8.4). In particular, the model for unlinked repeated measurements data from $J = 2$ methods is

$$Y_{ijk} = \mu_j(x_{1i}, \ldots, x_{ri}) + u_i + b_{ij} + e_{ijk}, \tag{8.18}$$

and its counterpart for linked data is

$$Y_{ijk} = \mu_j(x_{1i}, \ldots, x_{ri}) + u_i + b_{ij} + b_{ik}^* + e_{ijk}, \tag{8.19}$$

where

$$b_{ij} \sim \text{independent } \mathcal{N}_1(0, \psi^2).$$

All other assumptions are same as in the $J > 2$ case. These models generalize the models (5.1) and (5.9) for unlinked and linked data, respectively. The model (8.18) also generalizes the heteroscedastic model (6.10) by not restricting the variance covariate to be a proxy for the true measurement and additionally allowing mean covariates in the model. The distributions of the various model-based quantities, for example, (Y_1, Y_2), D_{12}, Y_1^*, Y_2^*, D_1, and D_2, under (8.18) and (8.19) can be obtained from their counterparts for $J > 2$ by simply setting $\psi_1^2 = \psi_2^2 = \psi^2$.

8.3.3.2 Unreplicated Data from More Than Two Methods   The model (7.1) is extended as

$$Y_{ij} = \mu_j(x_{1i}, \ldots, x_{ri}) + u_i + e_{ij}. \tag{8.20}$$

The distributions of u_i and e_{ij} are given by (8.8) with e_{ij} replacing e_{ijk}. Marginal distribution of the data under this model is obtained in Exercise 8.5. It is also seen that the joint distribution of $(Y_1, \ldots, Y_J)$ at $(x_1, \ldots, x_r, \tilde{v})$ is a J-variate normal with $E(Y_j) = \mu_j(x_1, \ldots, x_r)$ and covariance structure described by

$$\mathrm{var}(Y_j) = \sigma_b^2 + \sigma_{ej}^2\, g_j^2(\tilde{v}, \boldsymbol{\delta}_j), \quad \mathrm{cov}(Y_j, Y_l) = \sigma_b^2. \tag{8.21}$$

The distribution of the difference D_{jl} is

$$D_{jl} \sim \mathcal{N}_1\big(\xi_{jl}(x_1, \ldots, x_r), \tau_{jl}^2(\tilde{v})\big), \tag{8.22}$$

where

$$\tau_{jl}^2(\tilde{v}) = \sigma_{ej}^2\, g_j^2(\tilde{v}, \boldsymbol{\delta}_j) + \sigma_{el}^2\, g_l^2(\tilde{v}, \boldsymbol{\delta}_l). \tag{8.23}$$

8.3.3.3 Paired Measurements Data Proceeding as before, but using the variance function in (8.5) to model $\text{var}(Y_j)$, the bivariate normal distribution (4.6) of (Y_1, Y_2) at covariate value $(x_1, \ldots, x_r, \tilde{v})$ is replaced by the assumption

$$\begin{pmatrix} Y_1 \\ Y_2 \end{pmatrix} \sim \mathcal{N}_2 \left(\begin{pmatrix} \mu_1(x_1, \ldots, x_r) \\ \mu_2(x_1, \ldots, x_r) \end{pmatrix}, \begin{pmatrix} \sigma_1^2 \, g_1^2(\tilde{v}, \boldsymbol{\delta}_1) & \sigma_{12}(\tilde{v}, \boldsymbol{\delta}_1, \boldsymbol{\delta}_2) \\ \sigma_{12}(\tilde{v}, \boldsymbol{\delta}_1, \boldsymbol{\delta}_2) & \sigma_2^2 \, g_2^2(\tilde{v}, \boldsymbol{\delta}_2) \end{pmatrix} \right). \tag{8.24}$$

Thus, the observed pairs (Y_{i1}, Y_{i2}) are independently distributed as

$$\begin{pmatrix} Y_{i1} \\ Y_{i2} \end{pmatrix} \sim \mathcal{N}_2 \left(\begin{pmatrix} \mu_1(x_{1i}, \ldots, x_{ri}) \\ \mu_2(x_{1i}, \ldots, x_{ri}) \end{pmatrix}, \begin{pmatrix} \sigma_1^2 \, g_1^2(\tilde{v}_i, \boldsymbol{\delta}_1) & \sigma_{12}(\tilde{v}_i, \boldsymbol{\delta}_1, \boldsymbol{\delta}_2) \\ \sigma_{12}(\tilde{v}_i, \boldsymbol{\delta}_1, \boldsymbol{\delta}_2) & \sigma_2^2 \, g_2^2(\tilde{v}_i, \boldsymbol{\delta}_2) \end{pmatrix} \right). \tag{8.25}$$

This model generalizes the heteroscedastic bivariate normal model (6.33) by letting the means depend on covariates. Here again the correlation ρ of the distribution is constant but the covariance depends on $\tilde{v}$ and heteroscedasticity parameters $(\boldsymbol{\delta}_1, \boldsymbol{\delta}_2)$. Further,

$$D_{12} \sim \mathcal{N}_1 \big(\xi_{12}(x_1, \ldots, x_r), \tau_{12}^2(\tilde{v}) \big), \tag{8.26}$$

where

$$\tau_{12}^2(\tilde{v}) = \sigma_1^2 \, g_1^2(\tilde{v}, \boldsymbol{\delta}_1) + \sigma_2^2 \, g_2^2(\tilde{v}, \boldsymbol{\delta}_2) - 2\sigma_{12}(\tilde{v}, \boldsymbol{\delta}_1, \boldsymbol{\delta}_2). \tag{8.27}$$

8.3.4 Model Fitting and Evaluation

The models introduced here need to be fit by the ML method using a statistical software package. For a given model, estimates of mean and variance functions are obtained by replacing the unknown parameters in them by their ML estimates. For the bivariate normal model, the estimated mean functions at the observed covariate values in the data also serve as the fitted values. For a mixed-effects model, the fitted values are obtained by adding the predicted values of the random effects to the estimated means. We obtain the residuals by subtracting the fitted values from the observed values and standardize them by dividing by their estimated standard deviations. These quantities are used for model evaluation (Section 3.2.4). It is important to check the adequacy of the assumed mean and variance function models. For the former, model diagnostics for a typical regression analysis can be carried out. For the latter, one can proceed as in Section 6.4.3 for a mixed-effects model and as in Section 6.5.3 for the bivariate normal model. The need for including a mean or a variance covariate in the model can be assessed using a likelihood ratio test or model comparison criterion (Section 3.3.7).

8.4 EVALUATION OF SIMILARITY, AGREEMENT, AND REPEATABILITY

For the evaluation of similarity and agreement, we proceed by combining ideas from Chapters 6 and 7. The distributions of $(Y_1, \ldots, Y_J)$ for $J \geq 2$ obtained in Section 8.3.3 at a covariate setting $(x_1, \ldots, x_r, \tilde{v})$ can be used in the usual manner to derive measures of similarity and agreement. They are adjusted for mean covariates in the model. They are also functions of covariates if either a covariate $\times$ method interaction or a variance covariate is included in the model. Among the similarity measures, the analog of the difference in fixed biases or means of methods j and l is $\xi_{jl}(x_1, \ldots, x_r)$, given by (8.4). It reduces to $\beta_{0l} - \beta_{0j}$, simply a difference in intercepts if none of the covariates interact with the methods. Further, as in Section 6.4.5, the precision ratio for a mixed-effects model is

$$\lambda_{jl}(\tilde{v}) = \frac{\sigma_{ej}^2 \, g_j^2(\tilde{v}, \boldsymbol{\delta}_j)}{\sigma_{el}^2 \, g_l^2(\tilde{v}, \boldsymbol{\delta}_l)}. \tag{8.28}$$

Such a ratio is not defined for the bivariate normal model. Instead, as in Section 6.5.5, we use the variance ratio,

$$\frac{\sigma_2^2 \, g_2^2(\tilde{v}, \boldsymbol{\delta}_2)}{\sigma_1^2 \, g_1^2(\tilde{v}, \boldsymbol{\delta}_1)}. \tag{8.29}$$

The measures of agreement between methods j and l under a model are obtained by replacing the features of distributions of (Y_j, Y_l) and D_{jl} used in their definitions by associated functions of model parameters (Exercise 8.6). However, the model depends on the study design, and hence we consider the various designs separately.

8.4.1   Measures of Agreement for Two methods

For unlinked repeated measurements data, the distributions of (Y_1, Y_2) and D_{12} are given by (8.10) and (8.11) with $\psi_1^2 = \psi_2^2 = \psi^2$. By substituting their moments in (2.6) and (2.29) we obtain $\mathrm{CCC}_{12}(x_1, \ldots, x_r, \tilde{v})$ as

$$\frac{2\sigma_b^2}{\xi_{12}^2(x_1, \ldots, x_r) + 2(\sigma_b^2 + \psi^2) + \sigma_{e1}^2 \, g_1^2(\tilde{v}, \boldsymbol{\delta}_1) + \sigma_{e2}^2 \, g_2^2(\tilde{v}, \boldsymbol{\delta}_2)} \tag{8.30}$$

and $\mathrm{TDI}_{12}(p_0, x_1, \ldots, x_r, \tilde{v})$ as

$$\tau_{12}(\tilde{v}) \left\{ \chi_{1,p_0}^2 \left(\frac{\xi_{12}^2(x_1, \ldots, x_r)}{\tau_{12}^2(\tilde{v})} \right) \right\}^{1/2}, \tag{8.31}$$

where

$$\tau_{12}^2(\tilde{v}) = 2\psi^2 + \sigma_{e1}^2 \, g_1^2(\tilde{v}, \boldsymbol{\delta}_1) + \sigma_{e2}^2 \, g_2^2(\tilde{v}, \boldsymbol{\delta}_2). \tag{8.32}$$

For linked repeated measurements data, the distribution of (Y_1, Y_2) is given by (8.16) with $\psi_1^2 = \psi_2^2 = \psi^2$. Using its moments in (2.6) we obtain $\mathrm{CCC}_{12}(x_1, \ldots, x_r, \tilde{v})$ as

$$\frac{2(\sigma_b^2 + \sigma_{b*}^2)}{\xi_{12}^2(x_1, \ldots, x_r) + 2(\sigma_b^2 + \psi^2 + \sigma_{b*}^2) + \sigma_{e1}^2 \, g_1^2(\tilde{v}, \boldsymbol{\delta}_1) + \sigma_{e2}^2 \, g_2^2(\tilde{v}, \boldsymbol{\delta}_2)}. \tag{8.33}$$

The distribution of D_{12} and hence the TDI function are identical to the unlinked case, given in (8.31).

For paired measurements data, the distributions of (Y_1, Y_2) and D_{12} are given by (8.24) and (8.26). Using their moments in the definitions of the agreement measures leads to

$$\mathrm{CCC}_{12}(x_1, \ldots, x_r, \tilde{v}) = \frac{2\sigma_{12}(\tilde{v}, \boldsymbol{\delta}_1, \boldsymbol{\delta}_2)}{\xi_{12}^2(x_1, \ldots, x_r) + \sigma_1^2 \, g_1^2(\tilde{v}, \boldsymbol{\delta}_1) + \sigma_2^2 \, g_2^2(\tilde{v}, \boldsymbol{\delta}_2)} \tag{8.34}$$

and $\mathrm{TDI}_{12}(p_0, x_1, \ldots, x_r, \tilde{v})$ as in (8.31), where $\tau_{12}^2(\tilde{v})$ is taken from (8.27).

8.4.2 Measures of Agreement for More Than Two Methods

For repeated measurements data, it follows directly from (2.6), (8.10), and (8.16) that $\text{CCC}_{jl}(x_1, \ldots, x_r, \tilde{v})$ for unlinked and linked data are, respectively, given by

$$\frac{2\sigma_b^2}{\xi_{jl}^2(x_1, \ldots, x_r) + 2\sigma_b^2 + \psi_j^2 + \psi_l^2 + \sigma_{ej}^2 \, g_j^2(\tilde{v}, \boldsymbol{\delta}_j) + \sigma_{el}^2 \, g_2^2(\tilde{v}, \boldsymbol{\delta}_l)} \tag{8.35}$$

and

$$\frac{2(\sigma_b^2 + \sigma_{b*}^2)}{\xi_{jl}^2(x_1, \ldots, x_r) + 2(\sigma_b^2 + \sigma_{b*}^2) + \psi_j^2 + \psi_l^2 + \sigma_{ej}^2 \, g_j^2(\tilde{v}, \boldsymbol{\delta}_j) + \sigma_{el}^2 \, g_l^2(\tilde{v}, \boldsymbol{\delta}_l)}. \tag{8.36}$$

It similarly follows from (2.29) and (8.11) that

$$\text{TDI}_{jl}(p_0, x_1, \ldots, x_r, , \tilde{v}) = \tau_{jl}(\tilde{v}) \left\{ \chi_{1,p_0}^2 \left(\frac{\xi_{jl}^2(x_1, \ldots, x_r)}{\tau_{jl}^2(\tilde{v})} \right) \right\}^{1/2} \tag{8.37}$$

for both unlinked and linked data with $\tau_{jl}^2(\tilde{v})$ given by (8.12).

For unreplicated data, we have

$$\text{CCC}_{jl}(x_1, \ldots, x_r, \tilde{v}) = \frac{2\sigma_b^2}{\xi_{jl}^2(x_1, \ldots, x_r) + 2\sigma_b^2 + \sigma_{ej}^2 \, g_j^2(\tilde{v}, \boldsymbol{\delta}_j) + \sigma_{el}^2 \, g_2^2(\tilde{v}, \boldsymbol{\delta}_l)} \tag{8.38}$$

from (2.6) and (8.21). We also see from (2.29) and (8.22) that $\text{TDI}_{jl}(p_0, x_1, \ldots, x_r, , \tilde{v})$ is given by (8.37), where $\tau_{jl}^2(\tilde{v})$ is taken from (8.23).

8.4.3 Measures of Repeatability

Measures of repeatability for evaluation of intra-method agreement for repeated measurements data are obtained using the distributions of (Y_j, Y_j^*) and D_j for $j = 1, \ldots, J$ given in Section 8.3.3.1. Proceeding as in Sections 6.4.5 and 7.9, we get the repeatability analogs for CCC and TDI for unlinked data from $J > 2$ methods. They are

$$\text{CCC}_j(\tilde{v}) = \frac{\sigma_b^2 + \psi_j^2}{\sigma_b^2 + \psi_j^2 + \sigma_{ej}^2 \, g_j^2(\tilde{v}, \boldsymbol{\delta}_j)},$$
$$\text{TDI}_j(p_0, \tilde{v}) = \left\{ 2\sigma_{ej}^2 \, g_j^2(\tilde{v}, \boldsymbol{\delta}_j) \chi_{1,p_0}^2(0) \right\}^{1/2}. \tag{8.39}$$

Their counterparts for linked data are

$$\text{CCC}_j(\tilde{v}) = \frac{\sigma_b^2 + \psi_j^2}{\sigma_b^2 + \psi_j^2 + \sigma_{b*}^2 + \sigma_{ej}^2 \, g_j^2(\tilde{v}, \boldsymbol{\delta}_j)},$$
$$\text{TDI}_j(p_0, \tilde{v}) = \left[2\{\sigma_{b*}^2 + \sigma_{ej}^2 \, g_j^2(\tilde{v}, \boldsymbol{\delta}_j)\} \chi_{1,p_0}^2(0) \right]^{1/2}. \tag{8.40}$$

These expressions are verified in Exercise 8.7. Expressions for the $J = 2$ case are obtained by replacing ψ_j^2 in (8.39) and (8.40) with the common value ψ^2. The resulting expressions are identical to (6.26) for unlinked data. Repeatability measures involve the variance covariate but not the mean covariates because their effects cancel out when Y_j is compared with Y_j^* at the same covariate setting.

8.4.4 Inference on Measures

The measures are estimated by the ML method, and inference on them proceeds as described in Chapter 3. As usual, we use two-sided confidence intervals for measures of similarity and appropriate one-sided confidence bounds for measures of agreement and repeatability. Depending upon the objectives of the study, the bounds and intervals may be pointwise or simultaneous over specified method pairs or covariate values (see Section 3.3.5). If a measure is a function of a categorical covariate, it may be of interest to examine whether it can be taken to remain constant over the levels of the covariate. One can perform this task either using two-sided simultaneous confidence intervals for appropriately defined differences of the values of the measure or using a test of homogeneity that tests the null hypothesis of equality of the measure's values (Section 3.3.6).

The 95% limits of agreement for comparing methods j and l in all cases have the form

$$\hat{\xi}_{jl}(x_1, \ldots, x_r) \pm 1.96 \times \hat{\tau}_{jl}^2(\tilde{v}), \tag{8.41}$$

where $\hat{\xi}_{jl}$ and $\hat{\tau}_{jl}^2$ are the ML estimators of the mean and variance of the difference D_{jl}. The repeatability analogs of this measure can be defined similarly.

8.5 CASE STUDY

The methodology developed in this chapter is illustrated using a blood pressure dataset. The dataset consists of systolic blood pressure measurements of $n = 384$ subjects measured using a mercury sphygmomanometer (method 1) and an automatic monitor, OMRON 711 (method 2). Each subject is measured twice using each method. Thus, there is a total of $384 \times 2 \times 2 = 1536$ blood pressure measurements. The replications are assumed to be unlinked. Three subject-level covariates—gender, age, and heart rate—are also recorded in the data. Gender is a categorical covariate with levels male and female. Age (in years) and heart rate (in beats per minutes) are continuous covariates. None of these covariates changes during replication. There are 196 female and 184 male subjects in the dataset and they are between 24 and 74 years of age. Their blood pressure ranges between 89 and 200 mm Hg. Their heart rate ranges between 43 and 160 beats per minute, with one subject at 160 and the rest at 121 or less.

Figure 8.1 presents separate trellis plots of data for each gender. The effect of gender is apparent at the low end of the measurement range where the males tend to have higher blood pressure than the females. Specifically, 99 is the smallest observation for the males, whereas 89 is the smallest for the females. There are 50 readings for females between 89 and 99. There are a handful of subjects with outlying observations. For example, among the four observations for the female in the topmost row, three are near 100 but one is near 200. We also see that the observations for the females from the mercury method tend to be a bit smaller than the automatic method. However, no such difference is apparent among the males. This provides evidence for a method × gender interaction. Next, the methods have comparable within-subject variations, but the variations appear to increase somewhat with the blood pressure level. Although these error variations appear small in relation to the between-subject variation, their magnitude is considerable. Figure 8.2 presents side-by-side boxplots of all measurements from the two methods for both genders. They corroborate the impressions regarding effect of gender and its interaction with method.

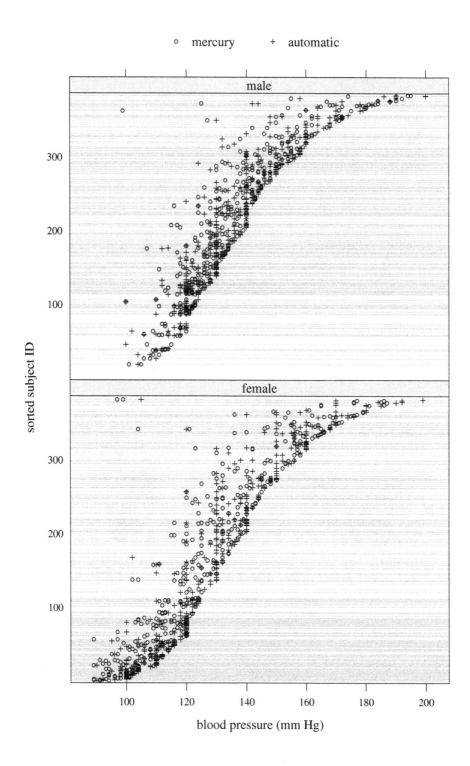

Figure 8.1 Trellis plots of blood pressure data by gender.

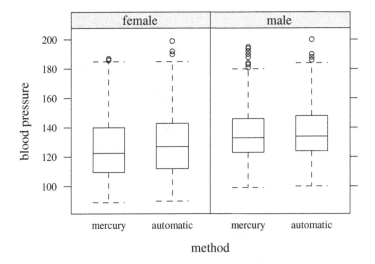

Figure 8.2   Side-by-side boxplots for blood pressure data by gender.

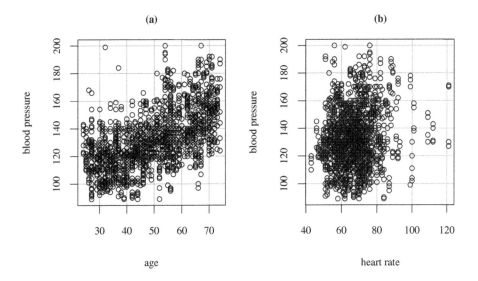

Figure 8.3   Scatterplots of blood pressure against age (left panel) and against heart rate (right panel).

Scatterplots of blood pressure against age and heart rate are presented in Figure 8.3. Blood pressure tends to increase with age. It also appears to have a mild positive correlation with heart rate. The latter plot excludes the subject with the unusually high heart rate of 160. The blood pressure readings for that subject, ranging from 146 to 155 mm Hg, are in the middle of the other values.

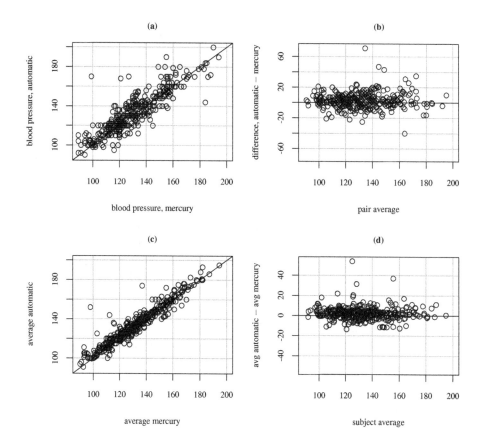

Figure 8.4   Plots for blood pressure data. Top panel (left to right): Scatterplot with line of equality and Bland-Altman plot with zero line based on randomly formed measurement pairs. Bottom panel (left to right): Same as top panel but based on average measurements.

Figure 8.4 displays scatterplots and Bland-Altman plots for the measurement pairs formed by randomly selecting one of the two replications of each method and also for the averages of the replications. The scatterplots show a moderately high correlation (0.87) between the measurements. The correlation is higher between the averages (0.95), but this is to be expected. Absence of any trend in the Bland-Altman plots suggest equal scales for the methods. All plots show a few outliers.

Our strategy is to first analyze the data without the covariates and then again with the covariates so that their impact on the results can be assessed. Therefore, first we fit the model (8.18) without any mean or variance covariates. This model is effectively the model (5.1). Evaluation of the fitted model reveals that the variance ψ^2 of the subject × method interaction b_{ij} is practically zero. Besides, there are four standardized residuals with absolute values between 5 and 10 and the corresponding observations exert some influence on the error variance estimates. Therefore, these observations are deleted from all analysis hereafter. Upon refitting the model, we find clear evidence of magnitude-dependent heteroscedasticity in the methods (see Chapter 6). To incorporate this heteroscedasticity, we follow Section 6.4 to take the variance covariate $\tilde{v}_i$ as the subject blood pressure average (6.20) and plot the log of the absolute residuals of the fitted model against $\log(\tilde{v}_i)$ separately for each method. The plots superimposed with fitted regression lines are displayed in Figure 8.5. The underlying trends in both plots can be approximated by a straight line, implying that the power model

$$g_j(\tilde{v}_i, \delta_j) = \tilde{v}_i^{\delta_j}, \quad j = 1, 2,$$

may be taken as the variance function models for both methods. Now these g_j functions are used to fit the model (8.18) without any mean covariates, which is effectively the heteroscedastic model (6.10). The p-value of less than 0.001 for the likelihood ratio test of the null hypothesis $\delta_1 = \delta_2 = 0$ (Section 6.4.4) confirms the need for incorporating heteroscedasticity. The residual plots for the fitted model, shown in Figure 8.6, points to the adequacy of the power model for describing heteroscedasticity. Finally, we refit the model by deleting the interaction term b_{ij} from the model. The p-value of 0.99 for the likelihood ratio test of the null hypothesis $\psi^2 = 0$ clearly justifies this deletion (Section 3.3.7). The ML estimates of parameters in the resulting model, called *Model A*, are presented in Table 8.1. They are virtually identical to the estimates for the previous model that includes the interaction (not shown).

Substituting the ML estimates in (8.3), (8.10), (8.11), and (8.12), we see that, under Model A, the fitted distributions of (Y_1, Y_2) and D_{12} at the blood pressure level $\tilde{v}$ are

$$\mathcal{N}_2\left(\begin{pmatrix} 130.93 \\ 133.10 \end{pmatrix}, \begin{pmatrix} 384.91 + (1.68 \times 10^{-5})\tilde{v}^{3.00} & 384.91 \\ 384.91 & 384.91 + (1.95 \times 10^{-2})\tilde{v}^{1.56} \end{pmatrix}\right),$$

$$\mathcal{N}_1\left(2.17, (1.68 \times 10^{-5})\tilde{v}^{3.00} + (1.95 \times 10^{-2})\tilde{v}^{1.56}\right), \tag{8.42}$$

respectively. Here $\tilde{v}$ ranges over $(89, 200)$ mm Hg, the observed measurement range in the data. The mercury method has a slightly smaller mean than the automatic method. The former's error standard deviation, given by $\{(1.68 \times 10^{-5})\tilde{v}^{3.00}\}^{1/2}$, increases from 3.4 to 11.5 and the same for the latter, given by $\{(1.95 \times 10^{-2})\tilde{v}^{1.56}\}^{1/2}$, increases from 4.6 to 8.6. The two functions cross near $\tilde{v} = 135$. These error standard deviations appear large relative to the magnitude of measurement. Nevertheless, they are dominated by the between-subject standard deviation of $\sqrt{384.91} = 19.6$. As a result, the overall standard deviations of both the methods show relatively little change over the measurement range— they vary between 20 and 23. Correlation between the methods, obtained using (8.42), decreases from 0.96 to 0.79. The mean of the difference in the measurements is 2.18 and its standard deviation increases from 5.7 to 14.4. Taken together, these results indicate somewhat weak intra- and inter-method agreement.

Our next task is to assess the effects of the three covariates—gender, age, and heart rate (labeled rate)—for inclusion in Model A as mean covariates. A standard model building exercise shows that the main effects of all three as well as gender × age and gender × method interactions are statistically significant, with p-values well under 0.05, and should be included. In the expanded model, called *Model B*, the mean functions (8.3) of the mercury (method 1) and automatic (method 2) methods are modeled as follows:

$$\mu_1(\text{gender, age, rate}) = \beta_{01} + \beta_1 I(\text{gender = male}) + \beta_2\,\text{age} + \beta_3\,\text{rate} +$$
$$\beta_4 I(\text{gender = male}) * \text{age},$$

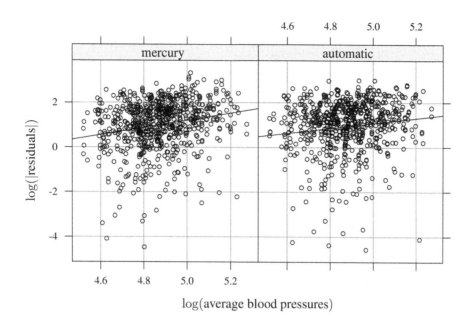

Figure 8.5   Plots of log of absolute residuals from a homoscedastic fit to blood pressure data against $\log(\tilde{v})$ with $\tilde{v}$ as subject average blood pressure. A simple linear regression fit is superimposed on each plot.

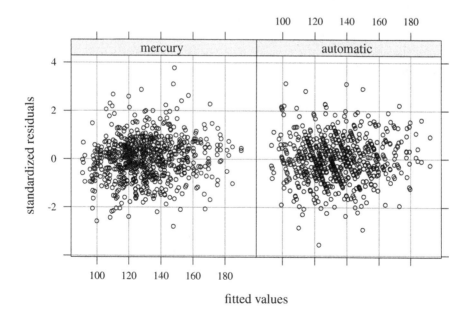

Figure 8.6   Residual plots from a heteroscedastic fit to blood pressure data using power variance function models.

	Model A			Model B		
Parameter	Estimate	SE	95% Interval	Estimate	SE	95% Interval
β_{01}	130.93	1.03	$(128.91, 132.94)$	60.42	5.81	$(49.04, 71.80)$
β_{02}	133.10	1.03	$(130.09, 135.11)$	63.61	5.81	$(52.22, 75.00)$
$\log(\sigma_b^2)$	5.95	0.07	$(5.81, 6.10)$	5.34	0.08	$(5.19, 5.49)$
$\log(\sigma_{e1}^2)$	-10.99	2.13	$(-15.16, -6.82)$	-11.61	2.09	$(-15.70, -7.52)$
$\log(\sigma_{e2}^2)$	-3.94	1.93	$(-7.73, -0.15)$	-4.61	1.94	$(-8.41, -0.82)$
δ_1	1.50	0.22	$(1.07, 1.93)$	1.56	0.21	$(1.14, 1.98)$
δ_2	0.78	0.20	$(0.39, 1.17)$	0.85	0.20	$(0.46, 1.24)$
β_1				31.88	5.57	$(20.97, 42.79)$
β_2				1.03	0.08	$(0.88, 1.19)$
β_3				0.21	0.07	$(0.08, 0.34)$
β_4				-0.42	0.11	$(-0.64, -0.21)$
β_{I2}				-2.30	0.61	$(-3.50, -1.10)$

Table 8.1 Summary of estimates of parameters of Models A (with variance covariate) and B (with mean and variance covariates) for blood pressure data. Methods 1 and 2 refer to mercury sphygmomanometer and automatic monitor, respectively.

$$\mu_2(\text{gender}, \text{age}, \text{rate}) = \beta_{02} + \beta_1 I(\text{gender} = \text{male}) + \beta_2 \, \text{age} + \beta_3 \, \text{rate} +$$
$$\beta_4 I(\text{gender} = \text{male}) * \text{age} + \beta_{I2} \, I(\text{gender} = \text{male}). \quad (8.43)$$

The rest of this model is identical to Model A. Table 8.1 provides estimates of the regression coefficients in (8.43) as well as other model parameters. The estimates of β_{01} and β_{02} show substantial change from Model A after accounting for variability in the blood pressure measurements due to the mean covariates. This also reduces the heterogeneity between the subjects vis-à-vis their blood pressure measurements, leading to a decrease in the estimate of $\log(\sigma_b^2)$. The estimates of $\log(\sigma_{e1}^2)$ and $\log(\sigma_{e2}^2)$ decrease somewhat, while the estimates of δ_1 and δ_2 increase slightly. In addition, there is a significant gender $\times$ method interaction effect β_{I2}.

A substitution of the estimates in (8.43) gives the fitted mean functions as

$$\hat{\mu}_1(\text{male}, \text{age}, \text{rate}) = 92.30 + 0.61 \, \text{age} + 0.21 \, \text{rate},$$
$$\hat{\mu}_2(\text{male}, \text{age}, \text{rate}) = 93.20 + 0.61 \, \text{age} + 0.21 \, \text{rate},$$
$$\hat{\mu}_1(\text{female}, \text{age}, \text{rate}) = 60.42 + 1.03 \, \text{age} + 0.21 \, \text{rate},$$
$$\hat{\mu}_2(\text{female}, \text{age}, \text{rate}) = 63.61 + 1.03 \, \text{age} + 0.21 \, \text{rate}. \quad (8.44)$$

The signs of the regression coefficients show that the mean blood pressure increases with age and also that blood pressure and heart rate are positively correlated. These findings are consistent with what we saw in Figure 8.3. To see the effect of gender, we can write the mean differences from (8.44) as

$$\hat{\mu}_1(\text{male}, \text{age}, \text{rate}) - \hat{\mu}_1(\text{female}, \text{age}, \text{rate}) = 31.88 - 0.42 \, \text{age},$$
$$\hat{\mu}_2(\text{male}, \text{age}, \text{rate}) - \hat{\mu}_2(\text{female}, \text{age}, \text{rate}) = 30.58 - 0.42 \, \text{age}.$$

These differences obviously depend on age because of the gender $\times$ age interaction. Over the observed age interval of 24 to 74 years, the first difference decreases from 21.8 to 0.8, and the second difference decreases from 19.5 to 0 until age 70; thereafter it falls slightly below 0 to -1.5. While this finding confirms the observation that males tend to have higher blood pressure than females (Figure 8.2), it additionally shows that their mean difference decreases with age and essentially vanishes around age 70. This is true regardless of the method used for measuring blood pressure.

As in (8.42), the fitted distributions of (Y_1, Y_2) and D_{12} under Model B are also normal distributions. But their means now depend on the covariates values. Mean functions of the bivariate distribution are given in (8.44). The covariance matrix of the distribution is

$$
\begin{pmatrix}
209.42 + (9.09 \times 10^{-6})\tilde{v}^{3.11} & 209.42 \\
209.42 & 209.42 + (9.92 \times 10^{-3})\tilde{v}^{1.69}
\end{pmatrix}.
\tag{8.45}
$$

The mean function of the difference in the methods is

$$
\begin{aligned}
\hat{\xi}_{12}(\text{gender, age, rate}) &= \hat{\beta}_{02} - \hat{\beta}_{01} + \hat{\beta}_{I2}\, I(\text{gender = male}) \\
&= 3.19 - 2.30\, I(\text{gender = male}).
\end{aligned}
\tag{8.46}
$$

Further, from (8.12), its variance function can be seen to be

$$
\hat{\tau}_{12}^2(\tilde{v}) = (9.09 \times 10^{-6})\tilde{v}^{3.11} + (9.92 \times 10^{-3})\tilde{v}^{1.69}.
\tag{8.47}
$$

The mean in (8.46) depends on gender because of the gender $\times$ method interaction, but is free of age and rate effects (see Section 8.3.1). Its value is 3.19 for females and 0.90 for males. The magnitudes and directions of these values are consistent with what we saw in Figures 8.1 and 8.2. The error standard deviation of the mercury method, given by $\{(9.09 \times 10^{-6})\tilde{v}^{3.11}\}^{1/2}$, increases from 3.3 to 11.7, and the same for the automatic method, given by $\{(9.92 \times 10^{-3})\tilde{v}^{1.69}\}^{1/2}$, increases from 4.5 to 8.9. The overall standard deviations of these methods range from 14.8 to 18.6 and 15.1 to 17.0, respectively, and their correlation decreases from 0.93 to 0.66. Furthermore, the standard deviation of the difference in the methods ranges from 5.6 to 14.7. The 95% limits of agreement as functions of $\tilde{v}$ can be computed using (8.41).

Upon comparing these Model B results with those under Model A, we see that the earlier mean difference $\hat{\xi}_{12}$ of 2.18 between the methods now falls between the values 0.90 for males and 3.19 for females. That said, the difference between the three values may not be considered practically important. The error variations of the methods, although given by seemingly different functions, remain very similar under the two models. However, the between-subject variation decreases from 384.9 to 209.4, causing notable reductions in the overall variances of the methods and also in their correlation.

We next proceed to the evaluation of similarity, agreement, and repeatability of the methods. For the measures that do not depend on the variance covariate $\tilde{v}$, we report 95% *individual* confidence bounds or intervals. For those that do, 95% *simultaneous* one- or two-sided confidence bands computed on a grid of 30 equally spaced points in $(89, 200)$ are reported. To evaluate similarity, we just recall that the estimates of the mean difference ξ_{12} are: 2.18 for Model A, and 0.90 for males and 3.19 for females in the case of Model B. The corresponding 95% confidence intervals are $(1.57, 2.78)$, $(0, 1.80)$, and $(2.39, 3.99)$, respectively. Although these differences are either clearly statistically significant or on the borderline, none of the confidence limits is large from a practical viewpoint. Figure 8.7 presents estimates and 95% confidence bands for the precision ratio function $\lambda_{12}(\tilde{v})$, defined by (8.28), under the two models. Estimates for Model B remain

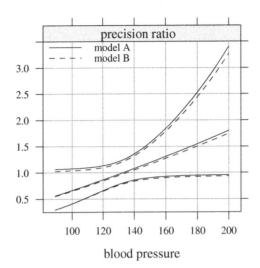

Figure 8.7   Estimates and two-sided 95% simultaneous confidence bands for the precision ratio λ_{12} under Models A and B.

at or below those for Model A, but there is little practical difference between them. The bands are widest near the edges, as is usually the case. The estimates range from 0.5 to 1.8 and exceed 1 near $\tilde{v} = 130$. Thus, the mercury method appears more precise than the automatic method at the low end of the measurement range, whereas the converse appears to hold at the opposite end. However, the difference is not statistically significant because 1 is contained within the bands throughout the range, albeit barely so near the edges. These findings appear to indicate that the methods can be considered to have similar means and precisions.

For agreement evaluation, we compute estimates and one-sided confidence bands for CCC_{12} and $TDI_{12}(0.90)$ as functions of $\tilde{v}$. The measures are obtained by setting $\psi^2 = 0$ in (8.30) and (8.31) (Exercise 8.8). Due to the nature of the heteroscedasticity, the CCC function is decreasing in $\tilde{v}$ whereas the TDI function is increasing in $\tilde{v}$. In the case of Model B, the measures are adjusted for the effects of the covariates age, gender, and heart rate. They remain a function of gender because of its interaction with method. The estimated CCC ranges from 0.78 to 0.95 for Model A; and from 0.66 to 0.93 and 0.65 to 0.91, respectively, for males and females in the case of Model B. Likewise, the estimated TDI ranges from 10.1 to 23.9 for Model A; and from 9.3 to 24.2 and 10.5 to 24.7, respectively, for males and females in the case of Model B. The methods exhibit higher agreement for males than females because their estimated mean difference is smaller for males. Although gender affects the extent of agreement, its actual effect is quite small because it is tied to the estimated gender $\times$ method interaction effect of $\hat{\beta}_{12} = -2.30$ (Table 8.1), which itself is relatively small. The estimated CCC functions under Model B remain below their Model A counterpart. This is due to the fact that the inclusion of covariates leads to a marked reduction in the between-subject variation, which in turn reduces the CCC. In contrast, the

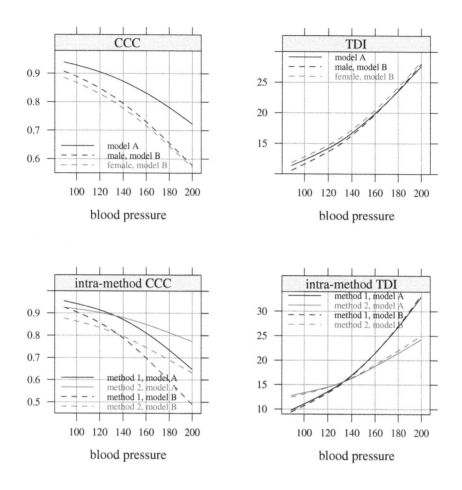

Figure 8.8   One-sided 95% simultaneous confidence bands for TDI(0.90) and CCC—lower bands for CCC and upper bands for TDI—and their intra-method versions for mercury (method 1) and automatic (method 2) methods.

estimated TDI functions remain similar under the two models because the covariates have no impact on the precisions of the methods.

Figure 8.8 presents simultaneous lower confidence bands for CCC and upper confidence bands for TDI under the two models. The covariates affect the bands in the same way as they affect the estimates. The CCC bands range from 0.7 to 0.95 for Model A and from 0.6 to 0.9 for Model B. The extent of agreement between the methods becomes progressively worse as the magnitude of measurement increases. Except possibly near the low end of the measurement range, the methods cannot be deemed to agree well enough to be used interchangeably. For both models, the same conclusion is provided by the TDI bands that increase from 11 to 28 as the blood pressure increases from 89 to 200.

For repeatability evaluation, Figure 8.8 presents simultaneous bands for intra-method CCC_j and $\text{TDI}_j(0.90)$, $j = 1, 2$. These measures are obtained by setting $\psi_j^2 = 0$ in (8.39);

see Exercise 8.8. The intra-method TDI band ranges from 10 to 35 for the mercury method and from 13 to 25 for the automatic method. The smallest value of 10 implies that, when the true measurement is near 90, two replicate measurements from the same method on the same subject may differ by as much as 10. Relative to the measurement's magnitude, this difference is too large to be considered acceptable. Therefore, it follows that none of the methods has acceptable repeatability. The same conclusion is reached on the basis of the CCC bands. In fact, when the true measurement is near 200, the mercury method agrees more with the automatic method than with itself on both measures (Exercise 8.8).

To conclude, the two methods under comparison do not agree well despite having similar characteristics. Further, the lack of agreement is driven by poor repeatability of the methods. Although the extent of agreement depends on gender, its actual effect is quite small. The inclusion of subject-level covariates in the model has different consequences for CCC and TDI. The covariates reduce the between-subject variation but have virtually no impact on the error variations of the methods. As a result, the CCC decreases but TDI remains practically unchanged. Thus, the adjusted CCC is smaller than its unadjusted counterpart, thereby making the agreement appear weaker after accounting for covariates. However, no such issue arises with TDI.

8.6 CHAPTER SUMMARY

1. The methodologies of previous chapters are generalized to incorporate covariates of two types. The mean covariates affect the means of the methods and the variance covariates affect their variances.

2. Covariates are assumed to be fixed, known quantities that are measured without error. They may be continuous or categorical.

3. The number of methods may be two or more. They are assumed to have the same scale.

4. Measurements may be unreplicated or repeated. In the latter case, they may be unlinked or linked.

5. The measures of similarity and agreement do not depend on mean covariates that do not interact with the methods. But they are functions of those that do and also of the variance covariates.

6. The measures of repeatability do not depend on mean covariates but depend on variance covariates.

7. The agreement measures are adjusted for covariates in the model.

8. Inclusion of subject-level mean covariates in the model tends to reduce between-subject variation, which in turn may reduce CCC. The same does not impact TDI unless the covariates interact with the methods or affect their error variations.

9. The methodologies for estimating standard errors and constructing confidence intervals are valid only for large number of subjects.

8.7   TECHNICAL DETAILS

This section essentially combines ideas from Sections 6.7 and 7.12 to express the models in Section 8.3.3 in matrix form. Except for the model (8.25) for paired measurements data, all others are mixed-effects models that can be represented in the general form (3.1),

$$\mathbf{Y}_i = \mathbf{X}_i\boldsymbol{\beta} + \mathbf{Z}_i\mathbf{u}_i + \mathbf{e}_i, \quad i = 1, \ldots, n.$$

Therefore, it suffices to consider the various design scenarios and identify the terms in this general formulation. Then, the properties such as means, variances, and covariances of measurements obtained in Section 8.3.3 can also be derived using the fact that, under the general formulation, the $\mathbf{Y}_i$ follow independent $\mathcal{N}_{M_i}(\mathbf{X}_i\boldsymbol{\beta}, \mathbf{V}_i = \mathbf{Z}_i\mathbf{G}\mathbf{Z}_i^T + \mathbf{R}_i(\tilde{v}_i))$ distributions.

For the repeated measurements data, define $\mathbf{Y}_i$ and $\mathbf{e}_i$ using (7.35), and assume that $\mathbf{e}_i \sim \mathcal{N}_{M_i}(\mathbf{0}, \mathbf{R}_i(\tilde{v}_i))$, where

$$\mathbf{R}_i(\tilde{v}_i) = \text{diag}\{\mathbf{R}_{i1}(\tilde{v}_i), \ldots, \mathbf{R}_{iJ}(\tilde{v}_i)\}, \quad \mathbf{R}_{ij}(\tilde{v}_i) = \sigma_{ej}^2 g_j^2(\tilde{v}_i, \boldsymbol{\delta}_j)\mathbf{I}_{m_{ij}}. \tag{8.48}$$

Define $\boldsymbol{\beta}$ and $\mathbf{X}_i$ as

$$\boldsymbol{\beta} = (\beta_{01}, \ldots, \beta_{0J}, \boldsymbol{\beta}_1^T, \boldsymbol{\beta}_{I2}^T, \ldots, \boldsymbol{\beta}_{IJ}^T)^T,$$

$$\mathbf{X}_i = \begin{pmatrix} \mathbf{1}_{m_{i1}} & \cdots & \mathbf{0}_{m_{i1}} & \mathbf{1}_{m_{i1}}\mathbf{x}_i^T & \mathbf{1}_{m_{i1}}\mathbf{x}_{I_i}^T & \cdots & \mathbf{0} \\ \vdots & \ddots & \vdots & \vdots & \vdots & \ddots & \vdots \\ \mathbf{0}_{m_{iJ}} & \cdots & \mathbf{1}_{m_{iJ}} & \mathbf{1}_{m_{iJ}}\mathbf{x}_i^T & \mathbf{0} & \cdots & \mathbf{1}_{m_{iJ}}\mathbf{x}_{I_i}^T \end{pmatrix}. \tag{8.49}$$

The general representation of model (8.7) for unlinked data from $J > 2$ methods now follows upon taking $\mathbf{Z}_i$ and $\mathbf{u}_i$ given by (7.35). Taking instead $\mathbf{Z}_i$ and $\mathbf{u}_i$ given by (7.37) yields the same representation of model (8.15) for linked data from $J > 2$ methods. These representations hold for models (8.18) and (8.19) for $J = 2$ as well, provided ψ_j^2 in the covariance matrix $\mathbf{G}$ of $\mathbf{u}_i$ is replaced by a common value ψ^2. The vector $\boldsymbol{\theta}$ of transformed parameters of these models consist of $\boldsymbol{\beta}$, $\log(\sigma_b^2)$, $\log(\sigma_{e1}^2), \ldots, \log(\sigma_{eJ}^2)$, $\boldsymbol{\delta}_1, \ldots \boldsymbol{\delta}_J$, and additionally, depending upon the model, $\log(\psi_1^2), \ldots, \log(\psi_J^2)$ or $\log(\psi^2)$, and $\log(\sigma_{b*}^2)$.

For unreplicated data from $J > 2$ methods, the representation for their model (8.20) is obtained by defining $\mathbf{Y}_i$, $\mathbf{u}_i$, $\mathbf{Z}_i$, and $\mathbf{e}_i$ as in (7.34); taking $\boldsymbol{\beta}$ as in (8.49); and substituting $m_{ij} = 1$ in (8.48) and (8.49) to get $\mathbf{R}_i(\tilde{v}_i)$ and $\mathbf{X}_i$, respectively. The resulting $\mathbf{u}_i$ and $\mathbf{G}$ are scalar quantities and the matrix $\mathbf{Z}_i = \mathbf{1}_J$ does not depend on the subject index i. The vector $\boldsymbol{\theta}$ in this case consists of $\boldsymbol{\beta}$, $\log(\sigma_b^2)$, $\log(\sigma_{e1}^2), \ldots, \log(\sigma_{eJ}^2)$, and $\boldsymbol{\delta}_1, \ldots \boldsymbol{\delta}_J$.

Finally, we consider the paired measurements data $\mathbf{Y}_i = (Y_{i1}, Y_{i2})^T$, $i = 1, \ldots, n$. These vectors follow independent bivariate normal distributions (8.25). The mean vector of this distribution can be written as $\mathbf{X}_i\boldsymbol{\beta}$ by taking $J = 2$ and $m_{ij} = 1$ in (8.49). Its covariance matrix is given in (8.25). In this case, $\boldsymbol{\theta} = (\boldsymbol{\beta}^T, \log(\sigma_1^2), \log(\sigma_2^2), z(\rho), \boldsymbol{\delta}_1^T, \boldsymbol{\delta}_2^T)^T$.

The models of this chapter are fit by the ML method. For the mixed-effects models, any statistical software capable of fitting such models with heteroscedasticity can be used. For the bivariate normal model, one can use the algorithm described in Section 6.7.2 by modifying it to show that the mean vector $\boldsymbol{\mu}$ for subject i is $\mathbf{X}_i\boldsymbol{\beta}$ and taking the vector $\boldsymbol{\theta}_1$ there to be $\boldsymbol{\beta}$.

8.8 BIBLIOGRAPHIC NOTE

A number of authors have considered incorporating covariates in the analysis of method comparison data. For paired measurements data, Bland and Altman (1999) use linear regression to model the trend in the Bland-Altman plot as a function of average measurement. The average serves as a proxy for the magnitude of the true measurement. The estimated trend is used to construct the limits of agreement as functions of the average. Geistanger et al. (2008) work with the same setup as Bland and Altman but use nonparametric regression to model the trend.

Barnhart and Williamson (2001) use a generalized estimating equations approach to model CCC as functions of covariates. They also provide a test of equality of CCCs over the covariate values. King and Chinchilli (2001a) develop a stratified CCC that adjusts for categorical covariates and provide a test of homogeneity of CCCs over the strata. Carrasco and Jover (2003) illustrate the importance of adjusting for covariates with a focus on CCC. Their approach involves including covariates in a mixed-effects model for data, but without the method × covariate interactions. They also assume homoscedasticity. Therefore, their CCC adjusted for covariates is a single index free of covariate values. Tsai (2015) recommends model selection to identify important covariates and suggests an estimator of CCC that is a weighted linear combination of the estimators proposed by Barnhart and Williamson (2001) and Carrasco and Jover (2003).

Choudhary and Ng (2006) work with paired measurements data and consider regression modeling of mean and variance of differences as functions of a covariate. Choudhary (2008) works with repeated measurements data and proposes a mixed-effects model that can incorporate covariates and heteroscedasticity. These articles also consider semiparametric modeling of mean functions using penalized splines, but they only focus on TDI as the measure of agreement. The model-based approach of this chapter is motivated by those of Carrasco and Jover (2003) and Choudhary (2008).

Data Source

The blood pressure data are from Carrasco and Jover (2003). They can be obtained from the book's website.

EXERCISES

8.1 Consider the models (7.1), (7.4), and (7.14) for data on $J\,(\geq 2)$ methods from Chapter 7. Argue that in each case the mean μ_j of the marginal distribution of a measurement from method j can be written as $\mu_j = \beta_j + \mu_b$, $j = 1, \ldots, J$.

8.2 Consider the model (8.7) for unlinked repeated measurements data from $J > 2$ methods.

   (a) Verify that the mean and variance of Y_{ijk} are given by (8.9) and the covariances are given by (7.6)–(7.7). Verify also that the same expressions are obtained if one uses the model's matrix representation from Section 8.7.

   (b) Write the companion models for Y_j and Y_j^* for $j = 1, \ldots, J$ at covariate setting $(x_1, \ldots, x_r, \tilde{v})$.

(c) Use part (b) to verify that the joint distribution of $(Y_1, \ldots, Y_J)$ is a J-variate normal distribution with moments given by (8.10). Deduce the distribution (8.11) for the difference D_{jl}.

(d) Use part (b) to show that for each $j = 1, \ldots, J$, (Y_j, Y_j^*) follows a bivariate normal distribution with identical univariate normal marginals and covariance given in (8.13). Deduce (8.14).

8.3 This is an analog of Exercise 8.2 for linked data. Consider the model (8.15) for linked repeated measurements data from $J > 2$ methods.

(a) Use this model's matrix representation in Section 8.7 to derive the marginal distribution of data.

(b) Write the companion models for Y_j and Y_j^* for $j = 1, \ldots, J$ at covariate setting $(x_1, \ldots, x_r, \tilde{v})$.

(c) Use part (b) to verify that the joint distribution of $(Y_1, \ldots, Y_J)$ is J-variate normal with moments given by (8.16). Verify also that the distribution of D_{jl} is given by (8.11).

(d) Use part (b) to deduce that for each $j = 1, \ldots, J$, (Y_j, Y_j^*) follows a bivariate normal distribution with identical univariate normal marginals and covariance given in (8.13). Verify (8.17).

8.4 Consider the models (8.18) and (8.19) obtained by taking $J = 2$ in (8.7) and (8.15), respectively, and setting $\psi_j^2 = \psi^2$ for $j = 1, 2$. By incorporating the mean function model (8.3) and the variance function model (8.5), show that they generalize, respectively, the models (5.1) and (5.9).

8.5 Obtain the marginal distribution of the data Y_{ij}, $j = 1, \ldots, J > 2$, $i = 1, \ldots, n$ under the model (8.20) using its matrix representation from Section 8.7. Also, verify the expressions in (8.21)–(8.23).

8.6 Verify the expressions for agreement measures given in Sections 8.4.1 and 8.4.2.

8.7 Verify the expressions for repeatability measures given in Section 8.4.3.

8.8 Consider the blood pressure data from Section 8.5.

(a) Fit Models A and B and verify the results in Table 8.1.

(b) Perform model diagnostics for both models. Are the model assumptions reasonable?

(c) Which model would you prefer? Why?

(d) Verify the expressions in (8.45)–(8.47).

(e) Obtain expressions for inter- and intra-method versions of CCC and TDI under Model B and verify the estimates reported in Section 8.5.

(f) Verify that the mercury method agrees more with the automatic method than with itself when $\tilde{v}$ is near 200. What explains this phenomenon?

8.9 Consider a study of eggshell thinning in black-headed gulls. The data are available at the book's website. The study involved ten eggs from each of two stages of development—embryo and feathered. From each egg, three replicate measurements of thickness (μm) were taken in two pigment areas—plain and speckled—at three different locations on the eggshell—blunt, pointy, and equator. Thus, there are $3 \times 2 \times 3 = 18$ observations from each egg, and there is a total of $10 \times 2 \times 18 = 360$ observations in the dataset. The investigators wanted to quantify agreement between the two pigment areas and also to see whether the agreement depends on the stage of development or the eggshell location. In the terminology of this chapter, we can think of this study a method comparison study with eggs as subjects, pigment areas as measurement methods, and stage and location as covariates.

Let Y_{ijkl} denote the kth repeated measurement in the jth pigment area of the lth location on the ith egg, $l = 1, 2, 3$, $k = 1, 2, 3$, $j = 1, 2$, $i = 1, \ldots, 20$. Assume that the three repeated measurements are unlinked. Take plain category of pigment area, embryo category of stage, and equator category of location as reference categories.

(a) Perform an exploratory analysis of data.

(b) Do stage and location appear to have an effect? Which interactions appear important?

(c) Fit the following model to the data:

$$Y_{ijkl} = \mu_j(\text{stage}_i, \text{location}_l) + u_i + b_{ij} + b_{il}^* + e_{ijkl},$$

where μ_j is the mean function of jth pigment area; u_i is the random effect of ith egg; b_{ij} and b_{il}^* are random interaction effects between egg and pigment area and location, respectively; and e_{ijkl} is the random error term. The random terms are independent for different indices and also independent of each other. Their distributions are as follows:

$$u_i \sim \mathcal{N}_1(0, \sigma_b^2), \; b_{ij} \sim \mathcal{N}_1(0, \psi^2), \; b_{il}^* \sim \mathcal{N}_1(0, \sigma_{b^*}^2), \; e_{ijkl} \sim \mathcal{N}_1(0, \sigma_{ej}^2).$$

In the mean function $\mu_j(\text{stage}, \text{location})$, include an intercept for jth pigment area, main effects for stage and location, and stage $\times$ location interaction effect.

(d) Evaluate goodness of fit of the assumed model.

(e) Define Y_j and Y_j^* as two replicate measurements of eggshell thickness in the jth pigment area of a given location on an egg of a given stage. Write the companion models for Y_j and Y_j^* induced by the assumed model. Find the distributions of (Y_j, Y_j^*), (Y_1, Y_2), $Y_j - Y_j^*$ and $Y_2 - Y_1$ at the given stage and location.

(f) Follow Section 8.4 to derive expressions for measures of similarity between the two pigment areas and also for CCC and TDI for measuring intra- and inter-method agreement between the areas.

(g) Perform appropriate inference on the measures derived in part (f) to evaluate similarity and repeatability of the two pigment areas and agreement between them. Explain your findings.

(h) Do the measurements from two pigment areas agree well? Does the extent of agreement depend on either stage or location?

CHAPTER 9

LONGITUDINAL DATA

9.1 PREVIEW

This chapter considers analysis of longitudinal data from two methods. It extends the methodology for linked repeated measurements data in Chapter 5 to allow systematic effects of time on the measurements. The within-subject errors of the methods may be correlated over time. Time may be treated as a discrete or continuous quantity. Its effect is captured primarily by letting the means of the methods depend on it. This in turn implies that the measures of similarity and agreement also depend on time. The methodology provides confidence bands for simultaneous evaluation of similarity and agreement over time. It does not require the measurements from both methods to be always observed together. It, however, assumes a common scale for the methods. A case study illustrates the methodology.

9.2 INTRODUCTION

Longitudinal data typically arise in method comparison studies when a cohort of subjects is followed over a period of time and the true value for a subject changes over time. Suppose there are n subjects in the study, labeled as $i = 1, \ldots, n$. The two methods being compared are labeled as $j = 1, 2$. Suppose also that the measurements are to be taken at prespecified time points $1, \ldots, \tilde{m}$. We think of these time points as the values of a discrete quantity called *measurement occasion*. The study design usually warrants that, for every subject,

Measuring Agreement: Models, Methods, and Applications. By P. K. Choudhary and H. N. Nagaraja
Copyright © 2017 John Wiley & Sons, Inc.

paired measurements by the two methods are taken on each occasion. In practice, however, there may be some subjects for whom on certain occasions either no measurements are available or a measurement is available from only one of the methods. In particular, suppose m_{ij} ($\leq \tilde{m}$) repeated measurements are available from method j on subject i. This number may depend on the subject index i as well as the method index j. We use $M_i = m_{i1} + m_{i2}$ to denote the total number of observations on the ith subject, and $N = \sum_{i=1}^{n} M_i$ to denote the total number observations in the dataset.

Let Y_{ijk} denote the kth repeated measurement from the jth method on the ith subject, and $o_{ijk} \in \{1, \ldots, \tilde{m}\}$ denote the actual occasion on which this measurement is taken, $k = 1, \ldots, m_{ij}$, $j = 1, 2$, $i = 1, \ldots, n$. Here k represents the order in which the measurements are taken. Each k is associated with a unique measurement occasion in $\{1, \ldots, \tilde{m}\}$. It is the value of the occasion index o_{ijk} that links the observations taken at the same time. For example, suppose the study design calls for taking four paired measurements from the two methods on each subject every three months, that is, $\tilde{m} = 4$. Consider a subject labeled 1 for whom only two measurements are available from method 1—at months 3 and 9, and only three measurements are available from method 2—at months 3, 6, and 9. Here $m_{11} = 2$ and $m_{12} = 3$. Moreover, $k = 1, 2$ for method 1 and $k = 1, 2, 3$ for method 2. Clearly, the index k incorrectly pairs the measurement of method 1 at 9 months with the measurement of method 2 at 6 months. In contrast, for the occasion index we have $(o_{111}, o_{112}) = (1, 3)$ for method 1 and $(o_{121}, o_{122}, o_{123}) = (1, 2, 3)$ for method 2, which implies correct pairings of the measurements.

We refer to a subject's sequence of measurements from a method as a "trajectory." The data may be called *paired* longitudinal data in that each subject contributes two dependent trajectories. However, the adjective "paired" here does not necessarily imply both methods are used on *each* measurement occasion. The modeling of these data generalizes that of linked repeated measurements data of Chapter 5 in two ways. It allows for systematic effect of time and random effect of measurement occasion, whereas only the latter was allowed for linked data. Further, linked data did not allow incomplete pairs of observations, whereas such a restriction is not imposed for longitudinal data.

The effect of time on measurements is taken into account by modeling the means of measurements as functions of time. This involves deciding in the beginning what to take as the "time" covariate because this choice guides how the mean functions are modeled. The time may be a discrete or a continuous covariate depending upon the available data and the interest of the investigator. In either case, let t denote the time covariate of interest and $\mathcal{T}$ be its domain. Also, let t_{ijk} denote the value of t associated with the measurement Y_{ijk}, $k = 1, \ldots, m_{ij}$, $j = 1, 2$, $i = 1, \ldots, n$. If t represents the measurement occasion, then $t_{ijk} \equiv o_{ijk}$ and $\mathcal{T} = \{1, \ldots, \tilde{m}\}$. On the other hand, if t represents a continuous quantity, for example, age of subject, then t_{ijk} and o_{ijk} are different, and $\mathcal{T}$ may be taken as the observed range of t in the data.

Our approach for modeling means as functions of time also allows the within-subject errors of the methods to be correlated over time. The difference in means—a measure of similarity—and measures of agreement that involve them are now functions of time. We assume that two methods are being compared and the errors are homoscedastic. This approach can be extended to deal with more than two methods and heteroscedastic errors along the lines of Chapters 6 and 7. But these extensions are not pursued here.

9.2.1 Displaying Data

The key distinguishing feature of longitudinal data is that the time of measurement has a significant effect. However, it cannot be seen in a trellis plot with one row per subject that we adopted in previous chapters. Therefore, we use method-specific plots of subjects' trajectories of measurements over time. These plots display all data, including the observations whose paired counterparts are missing. But they do not reveal how close the individual measurements from the two methods are. For this, we can take differences of the paired measurements and plot the trajectories of the differences. These plots can be supplemented with scatterplots, Bland-Altman plots and boxplots of differences for each measurement occasion. Naturally, the plots based on paired measurements use only the complete pairs in the data.

9.2.2 Percentage Body Fat Data

These data come from the Penn State Young Women's Health Study. They consist of percentage body fat measurements taken by two methods—skinfold caliper (method 1) and dual energy X-ray absorptiometry (DEXA, method 2)—on a cohort of $n = 112$ adolescent girls whose initial visit occurred around age 12. There are eight subsequent visits roughly six months apart. The visits do not occur at exactly six months for each subject. The measurement occasion variable here is the visit number with possible values $1, \ldots, 9$. The actual age of a subject (in years) is also recorded with each measurement. This age serves as the time covariate of interest. If all nine pairs of measurements were available for each subject, there would have been $112 \times 9 \times 2 = 2016$ observations in the dataset. However, we only have 1515 observations. Of these, 858 are from caliper and 657 are from DEXA. No DEXA observation is available at visit 1. This makes eight the maximum possible value for the number of complete pairs of observations on a subject. A total of 657 complete pairs from 91 subjects are available. Only 37 subjects provide all eight complete pairs. The remaining 75 subjects have observations from one or both methods missing on at least one of the visits. No complete pair is available from 21 subjects. The number of observations per subject averages 7.7 for caliper and 5.9 for DEXA. The ages of the subjects range from 10.7 to 17.3 years, with an average of 13.8 years. The percentage body fat measurements range from 12.7 to 37.4, with an average of 23.5.

Figure 9.1 displays the subjects' trajectories of body fat measurements over age for caliper and DEXA methods separately. Also superimposed on the plots are the estimated mean functions (see Section 9.5 for details regarding estimation). Both the mean functions fall mostly between 21 and 25, except near the endpoints where the estimates are not reliable, but the means behave differently over age. Roughly speaking, the caliper mean function increases from 22 at age 11 to 25 at age 13.5, decreases thereafter to about 23 at age 15, and increases again to 27 at age 17. On the other hand, the DEXA mean function decreases from 23 at age 11 to 21 at age 13, increases thereafter to just below 25 at age 16, and then shows a slight decline. Figure 9.2 displays the trajectories of DEXA minus caliper differences together with the difference of the fitted mean functions. It appears that, on average, the caliper measurement exceeds its DEXA counterpart except below age 11.5 and between ages 15 and 16 where the situation is slightly reversed. The mean difference decreases from above zero at age 11 to about -3 at age 13, increases thereafter to slightly above zero around age 15.5, and then decreases to about -2 at age 17. This

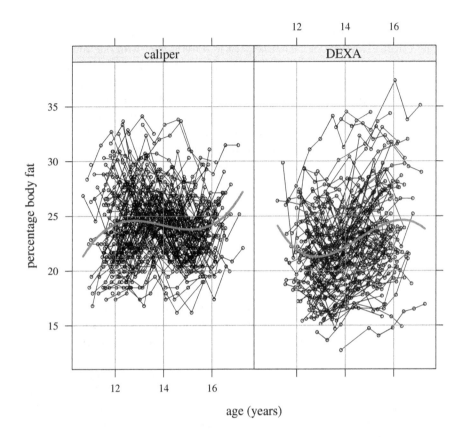

Figure 9.1   Trajectories of percentage body fat measurements for 112 girls. Lines connect the available time points from the same subject. The gray curves in the middle are the estimated mean functions.

pattern is also visible in the medians in boxplots of differences at visits two through nine given in Figure 9.3. Figures 9.4 and 9.5, respectively, display scatterplots and Bland-Altman plots of the available pairs at these visits. It is clear that the correlation between the methods remains moderate at all visits. A trend is visible in the Bland-Altman plot at some of the visits, implying potentially unequal scales of the methods, but there is no evidence of heteroscedasticity in the data. Overall, the exploratory analysis suggests that the discrepancy between the means of the methods varies with age. This in turn makes their agreement depend on age. The agreement, nevertheless, does not appear particularly strong. These data are further analyzed in Section 9.5.

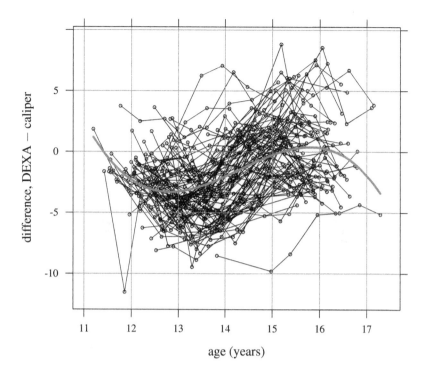

Figure 9.2 Trajectories of DEXA minus caliper differences in percentage body fat measurements for 91 girls with complete measurement pairs. Lines connect the available time points from the same subject. The gray curve in the middle is the estimated mean difference function.

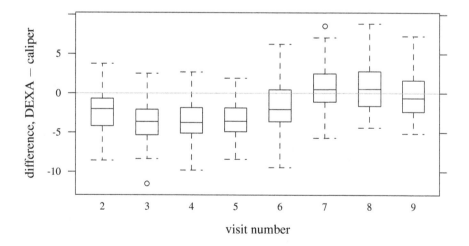

Figure 9.3 Side-by-side boxplots of DEXA minus caliper differences in percentage body fat measurements for visit numbers two through nine, with a reference line at zero.

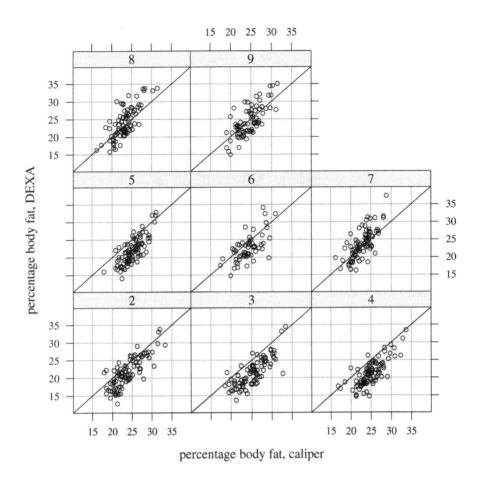

Figure 9.4 Scatterplots of percentage body fat measurements for visit numbers two (bottom left panel) through nine (top right panel). The line of equality is superimposed on each plot.

9.3 MODELING OF DATA

We start with the mixed-effects model (5.9) for linked repeated measurements data and extend it to incorporate effects of time. This involves writing (5.9) in the equivalent form

$$Y_{ijk} = \mu_j + u_i + b_{ij} + b^*_{ik} + e_{ijk}$$

where $u_i = b_i - \mu_b$ is the centered true value for subject i as well as method 1, now interpreted as a random effect of subject i common to all observations. Further, $(\mu_1, \mu_2) = (\mu_b, \beta_0 + \mu_b)$ are the population means of the two methods. We make three changes to the model while keeping the rest of the assumptions same as before.

First, we allow for the systematic effect of time by replacing the constant mean μ_j by the mean function $\mu_j(t)$, $t \in \mathcal{T}$. This makes $\mu_j(t) + u_i$ as the true value of method j

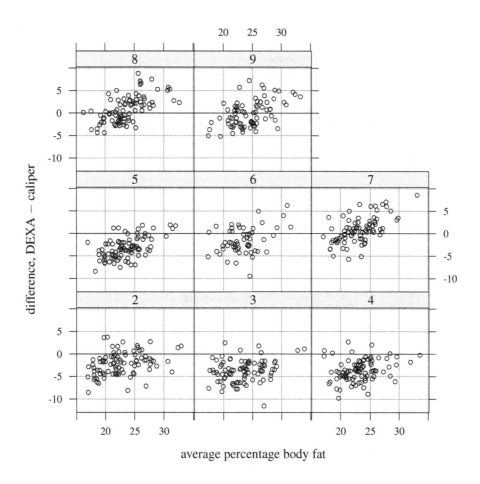

Figure 9.5 Bland-Altman plots of percentage body fat measurements for visit numbers two (bottom left panel) through nine (top right panel) for available pairs. A horizontal line at zero is superimposed on each plot.

for subject i at time t. The methods are still assumed to be on the same scale because the difference in their true values remains free of u_i; but it now depends on t.

Second, we replace the index k in the random effect b^*_{ik} of time of measurement with the index o_{ijk} to reflect that o_{ijk} is the measurement occasion of Y_{ijk}. Thus, $b^*_{io_{ijk}}$ is now the random effect of the measurement occasion.

Third, we allow for the possibility of dependence in the within-subject errors of each method while letting the errors arising from different methods or different subjects remain independent as before. Specifically, we assume that

$$\mathrm{cor}(e_{ijk}, e_{ijl}) = h(|t_{ijk} - t_{ijl}|, \boldsymbol{\omega}), \tag{9.1}$$

where h is a specified *correlation function*, t_{ijk} and t_{ijl} are the associated times of measurements, and $\boldsymbol{\omega}$ is a vector of correlation parameters. The correlation function $h(\cdot, \boldsymbol{\omega})$

is assumed to be continuous in $\boldsymbol{\omega}$, lies between -1 and 1, and satisfies the conditions that $h(0, \boldsymbol{\omega}) = 1$ and $h(\cdot, \mathbf{0}) = 0$. It depends on the measurement times only through their absolute difference, called *distance*. The time may be discrete, representing, for example, the measurement occasion, or continuous.

The correlation function in (9.1) does not depend on j, that is, the errors from both methods are assumed to follow the same correlation model. This assumption is made to keep the model fitting feasible with existing software capabilities. However, if the fitting is not an issue and the model remains identifiable, the assumption may be relaxed to let the methods have potentially different correlation functions with their own correlation parameters (Exercise 9.4).

9.3.1   The Longitudinal Data Model

The above changes to model (5.9) lead to the following mixed-effects model for longitudinal data:

$$Y_{ijk} = \mu_j(t_{ijk}) + u_i + b_{ij} + b^*_{io_{ijk}} + e_{ijk}, \tag{9.2}$$

for $i = 1, \ldots, n$, $j = 1, 2$, $k = 1, \ldots, m_{ij}$. Here $t_{ijk} \in \mathcal{T}$ are values of the time covariate t of interest and $o_{ijk} \in \{1, \ldots, \tilde{m}\}$ are the measurement occasions. The model makes the following assumptions:

- subject effects u_i follow independent $\mathcal{N}_1(0, \sigma_b^2)$ distributions,

- subject $\times$ method interactions b_{ij} follow independent $\mathcal{N}_1(0, \psi^2)$ distributions,

- subject $\times$ occasion interactions $b^*_{io_{ijk}}$ follow independent $\mathcal{N}_1(0, \sigma_{b*}^2)$ distributions,

- errors e_{ijk} follow $\mathcal{N}_1(0, \sigma_{ej}^2)$ distributions,

- errors associated with different subjects or methods are independent, but a method's errors on the same subject may be dependent following the correlation model (9.1), and

- $u_i, b_{ij}, b^*_{io_{ijk}}$ and e_{ijk} are mutually independent.

This model reduces to (5.9) for linked repeated measurements data when $\mu_j(t)$ is free of t, measurements from both methods are available on each occasion, and the correlation parameter $\boldsymbol{\omega} = \mathbf{0}$. Just as in Section 5.4.2, the marginal distributions of the vectors of M_i measurements on subject $i = 1, \ldots, n$ under (9.2) are independent M_i-variate normal distributions with means and variances

$$E(Y_{ijk}) = \mu_j(t_{ijk}), \quad \text{var}(Y_{ijk}) = \sigma_b^2 + \psi^2 + \sigma_{b*}^2 + \sigma_{ej}^2. \tag{9.3}$$

In addition, there are three types of covariances. One is between two measurements of the same method taken at different occasions,

$$\text{cov}(Y_{ijk}, Y_{ijl}) = \sigma_b^2 + \psi^2 + \sigma_{ej}^2 \, h(|t_{ijk} - t_{ijl}|, \boldsymbol{\omega}), \quad k \neq l. \tag{9.4}$$

The other two are between measurements from different methods taken at either the same occasion or different occasions. These can be collectively written as

$$\text{cov}(Y_{i1k}, Y_{i2l}) = \sigma_b^2 + I(o_{i1k} = o_{i2l})\sigma_{b*}^2, \tag{9.5}$$

where I is the indicator function, and $k, l = 1, \ldots, m_{ij}$. We need to specify models for the mean functions μ_j and the correlation function h to complete the specification of the model (9.2). These issues are discussed in the next two subsections.

Let $(Y_1(t), Y_2(t))$ be the paired measurements by the two methods at time $t \in \mathcal{T}$ on a randomly selected subject from the population. Also, let $D(t) = Y_2(t) - Y_1(t)$ denote their difference. We need their distributions under the model (9.2) to derive measures of similarity and agreement as functions of t. Proceeding exactly as in Section 5.4.2, we get the companion model for $(Y_1(t), Y_2(t))$ as

$$Y_1(t) = \mu_1(t) + u + b_1 + b^* + e_1, \quad Y_2(t) = \mu_2(t) + u + b_2 + b^* + e_2, \qquad (9.6)$$

where u, b_j, b^*, and e_j are identically distributed as u_i, b_{ij}, $b^*_{io_{ijk}}$, and e_{ijk}, respectively. It follows that (Exercise 9.3)

$$\begin{pmatrix} Y_1(t) \\ Y_2(t) \end{pmatrix} \sim \mathcal{N}_2 \left(\begin{pmatrix} \mu_1(t) \\ \mu_2(t) \end{pmatrix}, \begin{pmatrix} \sigma_b^2 + \psi^2 + \sigma_{b^*}^2 + \sigma_{e1}^2 & \sigma_b^2 + \sigma_{b^*}^2 \\ \sigma_b^2 + \sigma_{b^*}^2 & \sigma_b^2 + \psi^2 + \sigma_{b^*}^2 + \sigma_{e2}^2 \end{pmatrix} \right), \quad (9.7)$$

and

$$D(t) \sim \mathcal{N}_1 \left(\xi(t) = \mu_2(t) - \mu_1(t), \tau^2 = 2\psi^2 + \sigma_{e1}^2 + \sigma_{e2}^2 \right). \qquad (9.8)$$

The two distributions depend on t only through the mean functions.

9.3.2 Specifying the Mean Functions

As in Chapter 8, we model the mean functions $\mu_1(t)$ and $\mu_2(t)$ as functions of the same form but with different regression parameters. The models depend on whether t is discrete or continuous.

If t is discrete, representing the measurement occasion, then one possibility is to take

$$\mu_j(t) = \beta_{jt}, \quad t \in \mathcal{T} = \{1, \ldots, \tilde{m}\}, \quad j = 1, 2. \qquad (9.9)$$

It gives each combination of method and measurement occasion its own fixed intercept. This model is equivalent to a fixed-effects model that has a common intercept, main effects of methods and measurement occasions, and the method $\times$ occasion interaction effect.

If t is continuous, we proceed exactly as in a regression model and express $\mu_j(t)$ as a parametric function of t (or a suitable transformation thereof) that is linear in regression coefficients. For example, $\mu_j(t)$ may be taken as a polynomial in t of a given degree q,

$$\mu_j(t) = \beta_{0j} + \beta_{1j}t + \ldots + \beta_{pj}t^q, \quad t \in \mathcal{T}, \quad j = 1, 2, \qquad (9.10)$$

with unknown method-specific coefficients. Of course, other functional forms can be chosen. The choice is guided by the exploratory analysis of the data. Besides, one has to perform model diagnostics to justify the assumed form.

9.3.3 Specifying the Correlation Function

We now discuss some models for correlation function h of within-subject errors, defined by (9.1). If h is a nonzero constant, the errors are said to follow a model with *compound symmetry*. Under this model, each error has the same variance and each pair of errors has the same correlation regardless of the distance between the observations (Exercise 9.2).

This model may be reasonable if the study period is short. It may be unrealistic for long study periods because the correlation may wear out over time.

Besides the model with compound symmetry (or equal correlation), two classes of models are common within the framework of mixed-effects models—*time series* and *spatial correlation* models. They are, respectively, used in the analysis of time series and spatial data.

9.3.3.1 Time Series Correlation Models

The time series models generally require discrete times and work with data that are equally spaced in time. The associated correlation function is called the *autocorrelation function* and the distance is called *lag*—a discrete quantity. To specify a correlation function, one may examine the sample autocorrelation function of standardized residuals of the model fit assuming independent errors. Let $\hat{e}_{ijk}$ denote the residuals and let $\hat{e}^*_{ijk} = \hat{e}_{ijk}/\hat{\sigma}_{ej}$ denote their standardized counterparts. The sample autocorrelation at lag r for errors of method j can be defined as

$$\hat{h}_j(r) = \frac{\sum_{i=1}^{n} \sum_{o=1}^{\tilde{m}} a_{ijo}\, a_{ij(o+r)}\, \hat{e}^*_{ijo}\, \hat{e}^*_{ij(o+r)}/M_j(r)}{\sum_{i=1}^{n} \sum_{o=1}^{\tilde{m}} a_{ijo}\, \hat{e}^{*2}_{ijo}/M_j(0)}, \quad r = 0, 1, \ldots, \tilde{m}-1, \quad (9.11)$$

where

$$a_{ijo} = \begin{cases} 1, & \text{if a measurement on subject } i \text{ by method } j \text{ is available on occasion } o, \\ 0, & \text{otherwise,} \end{cases}$$

and

$$M_j(r) = \sum_{i=1}^{n} \sum_{o=1}^{\tilde{m}} a_{ijo}\, a_{ij(o+r)}$$

is the number of nonzero terms in the sum in the numerator. The autocorrelation at lag zero is 1 by definition. If the features of $\hat{h}_1$ and $\hat{h}_2$ are similar to those of the autocorrelation function h of a known correlation model, this h can be used to specify the autocorrelation.

A simple but especially useful time series correlation model is the *autoregressive model* of order one, denoted as AR(1). It has a single correlation parameter ω. If the time is discrete, its autocorrelation function at lag r is

$$h(r, \omega) = \omega^r, \ r = 0, 1, \ldots, \quad (9.12)$$

where ω represents the lag-1 correlation and lies between -1 and 1. This correlation function also happens to have a simple analog for continuous times,

$$h(r, \omega) = \omega^r, \ r \geq 0, \quad (9.13)$$

where the distance r is continuous, and ω is between 0 and 1. In either case, this model's characteristic feature is that in absolute terms its correlation function decreases at an exponential rate as the distance r increases. Time series models other than the AR(1) usually do not have simple continuous time analogs for autocorrelation.

9.3.3.2 Spatial Correlation Models

The spatial correlation models are generally specified in terms of *semivariograms*. Let $e^*_{ijk} = e_{ijk}/\sigma_{ej}$ denote the standardized errors of a model. These have zero means and unit standard deviations. Their *semivariogram* is defined as $\text{var}(e^*_{ijk} - e^*_{ijl})/2$. It can be expressed as

$$\text{var}(e^*_{ijk} - e^*_{ijl})/2 = E\{(e^*_{ijk} - e^*_{ijl})^2\}/2 = 1 - \text{cor}(e^*_{ijk}, e^*_{ijl}), \qquad (9.14)$$

relating it with correlation between the standardized errors. Letting s denote a semivariogram function, we can write from (9.1) that

$$s(|t_{ijk} - t_{ijl}|, \boldsymbol{\omega}) = 1 - h(|t_{ijk} - t_{ijl}|, \boldsymbol{\omega}). \qquad (9.15)$$

Thus, it follows that a model for the correlation function h may be specified in terms of a model for the semivariogram function s. The properties of h imply that s is continuous in the correlation parameter $\boldsymbol{\omega}$, equals 1 when $\boldsymbol{\omega} = \mathbf{0}$, and satisfies $s(0, \boldsymbol{\omega}) = 0$. The distances $|t_{ijk} - t_{ijl}|$ in (9.15) can be discrete but they are usually continuous. Although we are using the same correlation parameter $\boldsymbol{\omega}$ on both sides of (9.15), it may not have the same interpretation under the two models.

A spatial correlation model for errors in a longitudinal data model may be specified by examining the semivariograms estimated using the standardized residuals $\hat{e}^*_{ijk}$ of the model fit assuming independent errors. The semivariogram function for method j can be estimated by

$$\hat{s}_j(r) = \frac{1}{2M_j(r)} \sum_{i=1}^{n} \sum_{(k,l) \in A_{ij}(r)} (\hat{e}^*_{ijk} - \hat{e}^*_{ijl})^2, \qquad (9.16)$$

where $M_j(r)$ is the number of terms in the triple sum in the numerator, and

$$A_{ij}(r) = \{k, l = 1, \ldots, m_{ij} : |t_{ijk} - t_{ijl}| = r\}$$

is the index set that identifies the residual pairs associated with subject i and method j that are apart by distance r. The estimates in (9.16) may not be stable if r is a continuous quantity. In this case, we obtain more stable estimates by splitting the range of r into, say, 20 intervals using the quantiles of r, and averaging the semivariogram values over each interval. Just like the time series case, the features of these estimated semivariogram functions may be matched to those of the semivariogram function of a known model to come up with an adequate spatial correlation model.

A popular spatial correlation model is the *exponential model*, whose semivariogram function is

$$s(r, \omega) = 1 - \exp(-r/\omega), \ r \geq 0, \qquad (9.17)$$

where $\omega > 0$. In this case, $s(r, 0)$ is not defined, but $s(r, \omega)$ converges to 1 as ω tends to 0. By taking $\tilde{\omega} = \exp(-1/\omega)$ in (9.17), we get

$$s(r, \omega) = 1 - \tilde{\omega}^r,$$

and from (9.15), we have $h(r, \tilde{\omega}) = \tilde{\omega}^r$. It follows from (9.13) that the exponential model with correlation parameter ω is equivalent to the continuous AR(1) model with correlation parameter $\tilde{\omega}$.

Now that we are familiar with some basic correlation models for errors, a natural question is whether to opt for a time series or a spatial correlation model. The answer is dictated by the time covariate t of interest and whether the data are equally spaced in time. If t

represents the measurement occasion, a discrete quantity, and the data are equally spaced, a time series model may be used. If t is a continuous quantity or the data are unequally spaced, a spatial correlation model would be appropriate. Regardless of how a model is chosen, its adequacy must be verified using model diagnostics.

We note from (9.4) that there is an interplay between the correlation structure of the errors and the subject $\times$ method interaction effect b_{ij} because both induce correlations between a method's repeated measurements on a subject. Specifying a correlation structure for errors may obviate the need for the b_{ij} term in the model, which can be assessed using a test of hypothesis or a model selection criterion (see Section 9.3.4). Alternatively, if the b_{ij} term is kept in the model, there may not be any need to model dependence in errors (Exercise 9.2).

9.3.4 Model Fitting and Evaluation

Fitting the model (9.2) involves computing the log-likelihood function of the data and maximizing it numerically with respect to the model parameters using a statistical software package (see Section 9.7 for some technical details). This yields ML estimates of parameters and predicted values of random effects. The fitted values are

$$\hat{Y}_{ijk} = \hat{\mu}_j(t_{ijk}) + \hat{u}_i + \hat{b}_{ij} + \hat{b}^*_{iO_{ijk}},$$

where $\hat{\mu}_j(t)$ is the estimated mean function. In particular, when the means are modeled as the polynomial in (9.10), the estimated mean functions are

$$\hat{\mu}_j(t) = \hat{\beta}_{0j} + \hat{\beta}_{1j}t + \ldots + \hat{\beta}_{pj}t^q, \quad t \in \mathcal{T}, \quad j = 1, 2. \tag{9.18}$$

The raw and standardized residuals of the fitted model are $\hat{e}_{ijk} = Y_{ijk} - \hat{Y}_{ijk}$ and $\hat{e}_{ijk}/\hat{\sigma}_{ej}$, respectively. These quantities can be used in the usual manner for model checking if the within-subject errors are not correlated. If they are, the *normalized residuals* are used for model checking instead of the standardized residuals (Section 3.2.4).

The independence assumption for within-subject errors of the two methods can be verified using plots of the sample autocorrelation functions (9.11) and the estimated semi-variogram functions (9.16). If the errors of method j are independent, then approximately $100(1 - \alpha)\%$ of their sample autocorrelations for $r > 0$ should fall within the bounds

$$\pm z_{1-\alpha/2}/\sqrt{M_j(r)}. \tag{9.19}$$

Thus, the independence assumption may not be reasonable if quite a few of the sample autocorrelations fall outside these bounds. The same conclusion is reached if the estimated semivariogram functions do not appear to be a constant. To judge the adequacy of the fitted correlation model, we can use the same approach but with normalized instead of standardized residuals.

A likelihood ratio test can also be performed to test for independence of errors. Under the correlation model (9.1), independence amounts to setting the correlation parameter $\omega = 0$. Therefore, the hypotheses to be tested are

$$H_0 : \omega = 0 \text{ versus } H_1 : \omega \neq 0. \tag{9.20}$$

The test statistic (3.32) is obtained by fitting the model with and without the correlation. The degrees of freedom for the test is the number of elements in ω. Alternatively, the two models can be compared with AIC or BIC (Section 3.3.7). These criteria can also be used to compare candidate correlation function models.

As mentioned at the end of Section 9.3.3.2, incorporating a correlation structure in the errors may render the random interaction effect b_{ij} in model (9.2) unnecessary. Removing it from the model is equivalent to setting its variance $\psi^2 = 0$. Thus, we can assess the need for an interaction term by testing

$$H_0 : \psi^2 = 0 \text{ versus } H_1 : \psi^2 \neq 0, \tag{9.21}$$

using a likelihood ratio test. The test statistic (3.32) is obtained by fitting the model with and without the random effect and it has 1 degree of freedom. This test, however, is conservative (see Section 3.3.7).

9.4 EVALUATION OF SIMILARITY AND AGREEMENT

The longitudinal data counterparts of the measures of similarity and agreement are obtained by using the distributions $(Y_1(t), Y_2(t))$ and $D(t)$ given by (9.7) and (9.8) in their definitions (Exercise 9.3). For example, the difference in fixed biases at time t is the mean difference $\xi(t) = \mu_2(t) - \mu_1(t)$. Likewise, the agreement at time t is measured by

$$\text{CCC}(t) = \frac{2(\sigma_b^2 + \sigma_{b*}^2)}{\xi^2(t) + 2(\sigma_b^2 + \psi^2 + \sigma_{b*}^2) + \sigma_{e1}^2 + \sigma_{e2}^2} \tag{9.22}$$

and

$$\text{TDI}(t, p) = \left\{ (2\psi^2 + \sigma_{e1}^2 + \sigma_{e2}^2) \chi_{1,p}^2 \left(\frac{\xi^2(t)}{2\psi^2 + \sigma_{e1}^2 + \sigma_{e2}^2} \right) \right\}^{1/2}. \tag{9.23}$$

The precision ratio λ does not depend on t.

The ML estimators of these measures are obtained in the usual way by replacing the unknowns with their estimators. For inference on measures that depend on t, we need their simultaneous confidence bands over the domain $\mathcal{T}$. In particular, we need a two-sided confidence band for the similarity measure $\xi(t)$, and one-sided confidence bands for agreement measures—a lower band for $\text{CCC}(t)$ and an upper band for $\text{TDI}(t, p)$. Section 3.3.5 discusses the construction of a simultaneous confidence band for a parametric function over a finite number of points. That methodology is directly applied here if t is discrete because, in this case, $\mathcal{T} = \{1, \ldots, \tilde{m}\}$ has a finite set of points. We apply it for continuous t as well by discretizing $\mathcal{T}$ into a grid of a moderately large number of points, say, 20–30. As before, the confidence bands are initially obtained for the Fisher's z-transformation of the CCC function and the log transformation of the TDI function. The bands are then transformed back to the original scale (see also Section 9.7). It follows from the distribution of $D(t)$ in (9.8) that the 95% limits of agreement as a function of t are

$$\hat{\xi}(t) \pm 1.96 \, \hat{\tau}. \tag{9.24}$$

If the model (9.2) without the interaction b_{ij} is adopted, the corresponding agreement measures and their estimates are obtained by simply setting $\psi^2 = 0$ or $\hat{\psi}^2 = 0$ in their expressions. From (9.22) and (9.23), we obtain (Exercise 9.5)

$$\text{CCC}(t) = \frac{2(\sigma_b^2 + \sigma_{b*}^2)}{\xi^2(t) + 2(\sigma_b^2 + \sigma_{b*}^2) + \sigma_{e1}^2 + \sigma_{e2}^2}. \tag{9.25}$$

and

$$\text{TDI}(t, p) = \left\{ (\sigma_{e1}^2 + \sigma_{e2}^2) \, \chi_{1,p}^2 \left(\frac{\xi^2(t)}{\sigma_{e1}^2 + \sigma_{e2}^2} \right) \right\}^{1/2}. \tag{9.26}$$

In a similar manner, we get the 95% limits of agreement from (9.24) as

$$\hat{\xi}(t) \pm 1.96 \, \sqrt{\hat{\sigma}_{e1}^2 + \hat{\sigma}_{e2}^2}. \tag{9.27}$$

9.5 CASE STUDY

We now return to the percentage body fat data introduced in Section 9.2.2. Our first task is to find an adequate model of the form (9.2). The observed age range in the data, $(10.7, 17.3)$ years, is taken to be the time interval $\mathcal{T}$. After a preliminary analysis, we decide to model the mean functions as cubic functions of age, that is, use the form (9.10) with $q = 3$. Initially, the model (9.2) is fit with method $\times$ subject interaction and independent within-subject errors for the two methods. These data are not equally spaced in time because not every subject is measured on each measurement occasion. Therefore, to explore models for correlation structure we take age as a continuous time variable and examine the semivariograms for the two methods as functions of age difference, representing the "distance." Figure 9.6 plots the averages of estimated semivariograms (9.16) against the midpoints of various distance intervals. The estimates are computed using standardized residuals of the model with independent errors. The caliper (method 1) semivariogram shows an increasing trend throughout. The DEXA (method 2) semivariogram first shows an increasing trend up to 2 years, and then stabilizes around 0.7. These trends unequivocally suggest that the within-subject errors of the methods should not be regarded as independent. They also indicate that the dependence may be modeled using a continuous AR(1) structure (9.13), which is equivalent to the exponential correlation model (9.17).

Next, we revise the initial model by assuming a continuous AR(1) structure for within-subject errors with ω as the common correlation parameter for both methods. The likelihood ratio test of the correlation hypotheses (9.20) has a p-value under 0.001, confirming the need for incorporating dependence. Further, to assess whether the subject $\times$ method interaction becomes redundant under this correlation model, we perform a likelihood ratio test of (9.21). It has a p-value of 0.18, indicating that the interaction b_{ij} in (9.2) may indeed be dropped. Hence, from now on we focus on this model without the interaction term. However, all key conclusions remain unchanged if the interaction is kept in the model (Exercise 9.8).

Table 9.1 provides ML estimates of model parameters, their standard errors, and 95% confidence intervals. The variance-covariance parameters are reparameterized to have unconstrained parameter spaces. None of the standard errors appears unduly large. The correlation parameter ω is estimated as 0.54 with $(0.48, 0.61)$ as its 95% confidence interval. The adequacy of the assumed continuous AR(1) correlation structure can be checked by examining either the sample autocorrelation functions (9.11) of normalized residuals under the fitted model, or the estimated semivariograms (9.16). The latter are left for Exercise 9.7. The autocorrelation functions are presented in Figure 9.7. As there are nine visits by design, we expect autocorrelations at lags one through eight. However, DEXA's autocorrelations are available only through lag seven because its measurements are missing from the first visit. Also plotted in the figure are the bounds (9.19) with $\alpha = 0.05$. The bounds increase with lag, in absolute value terms, because they are computed using fewer observation pairs

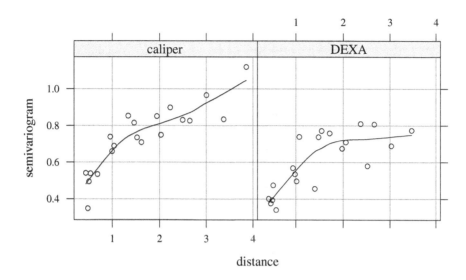

Figure 9.6 Estimated semivariogram functions for caliper and DEXA methods computed using standardized residuals from a model fit to percentage body fat data with independent within-subject errors. A nonparametric smooth curve is added to each plot to show the underlying trend.

as the lag increases. Only one autocorrelation falls outside the bounds, that too barely, suggesting that the assumed correlation structure may be considered adequate. Further model adequacy checking is pursued in Exercise 9.7. It also explores other degrees for the polynomial mean functions. In particular, the model with constant means β_{0j} has a p-value under 0.001, justifying the need for letting the means be functions of age. This exercise additionally explores other spatial correlation models for errors. Overall, the model (9.2) with cubic mean functions and continuous AR(1) errors but without the subject × method interaction appears to provide an adequate fit.

From (9.7), (9.8), and Exercise 9.5, the distributions of $(Y_1(t), Y_2(t))$ and $D(t)$ for $t \in \mathcal{T}$ under the fitted model are

$$\begin{pmatrix} Y_1(t) \\ Y_2(t) \end{pmatrix} \sim \mathcal{N}_2 \left(\begin{pmatrix} \hat{\mu}_1(t) \\ \hat{\mu}_2(t) \end{pmatrix}, \begin{pmatrix} 15.3 & 9.9 \\ 9.9 & 14.1 \end{pmatrix} \right), \quad D(t) \sim \mathcal{N}_1 \left(\hat{\mu}_2(t) - \hat{\mu}_1(t), 9.7 \right). \quad (9.28)$$

Here $\hat{\mu}_1(t)$ and $\hat{\mu}_2(t)$ are the fitted mean functions given by (9.18) using the estimates given in Table 9.1. They and their difference $\hat{\xi}(t)$ were shown as gray curves in Figures 9.1 and 9.2. The mean difference is also plotted in Figure 9.8. The caliper's mean is lower than DEXA's for young women below age 11.5 and it is higher in the age range $(11.5, 14.5)$. Their values are similar beyond age 14.5. With the exception of the left endpoint of $\mathcal{T}$, the mean difference function is less than 3.5 in absolute value. From (9.28), the correlation between the methods is about 0.7. One reason why this correlation is not very high is that the error variations are not very small relative to the between-subject variation. The standard deviation of the difference is about 3.1. This variability is solely attributed to the error variations of the methods. The 95% limits of agreement as functions of age, given by (9.27), are also plotted in Figure 9.8. The lower and the upper limits range between -9.5

Parameter	Estimate	SE	95% Interval
β_{01}	-319.10	62.98	$(-442.54, -195.66)$
β_{11}	74.81	13.75	$(47.87, 101.75)$
β_{21}	-5.40	0.99	$(-7.34, -3.45)$
β_{31}	0.13	0.02	$(0.08, 0.18)$
β_{02}	473.89	82.87	$(311.47, 636.32)$
β_{12}	-95.50	17.67	$(-130.14, -60.86)$
β_{22}	6.64	1.25	$(4.19, 9.09)$
β_{32}	-0.15	0.03	$(-0.21, -0.09)$
$\log(\sigma_b^2)$	2.24	0.16	$(1.92, 2.56)$
$\log(\sigma_{b*}^2)$	-0.75	0.16	$(-1.06, -0.44)$
$\log(\sigma_{e1}^2)$	1.70	0.09	$(1.52, 1.88)$
$\log(\sigma_{e2}^2)$	1.44	0.10	$(1.25, 1.63)$
$\log\{\omega/(1-\omega)\}$	0.17	0.14	$(-0.09, 0.44)$

Table 9.1   Summary of estimates of model parameters for percentage body fat data. Methods 1 and 2 refer to caliper and DEXA, respectively.

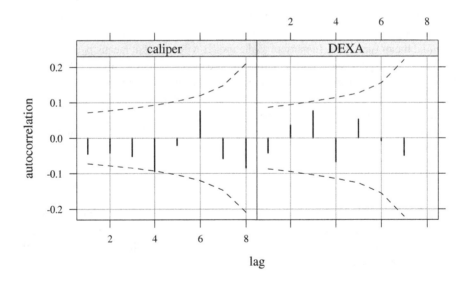

Figure 9.7   Sample autocorrelation functions for normalized residuals of caliper and DEXA methods under a model fit to percentage body fat data with AR(1) errors. The dashed curves represent the 95% bounds (9.19).

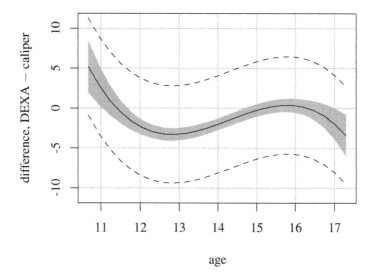

Figure 9.8 Estimate of mean difference in percentage body fat using caliper and DEXA methods (solid curve), its 95% two-sided simultaneous confidence band (shaded region), and the 95% limits of agreement (broken curves).

and -0.9 and 2.7 and 11.3, respectively. They indicate rather weak agreement between the methods on most of $\mathcal{T}$. The limits have a constant width because the standard deviation of the difference does not depend on age.

We proceed next to the evaluation of similarity. Figure 9.8 presents estimate of the mean difference along with its 95% two-sided simultaneous confidence band. This as well as the other simultaneous bands reported here are computed on a grid of 25 equally spaced points in $\mathcal{T}$. The critical point for the band in Figure 9.8 is 2.67. As is often the case in practice, this band is widest near the endpoints because there is not much data near the extremes. The zero line falls within the band except near the endpoints and also when the age is roughly between 11.5 and 14.5, in which case the band is below the line. Thus, the means of the two methods cannot be considered equal over the entire age interval. In particular, the caliper's estimated mean percentage body fat exceeds that of DEXA's by about 2–3 between the ages of 11.5 and 14.5. The precision ratio λ is estimated as 1.30 with $(1.06, 1.58)$ as its 95% confidence interval. Clearly, DEXA appears more precise than caliper. Taken together, these findings suggest that the methods cannot be regarded as similar.

For agreement evaluation, Figure 9.9 displays estimates of CCC and TDI with $p = 0.90$ as functions of age, defined by (9.25) and (9.26), respectively. The estimates near the endpoints cannot be trusted because of their relatively high standard errors. Also presented are their 95% one-sided simultaneous confidence bands over $\mathcal{T}$. The critical points used for CCC and TDI bands are -2.27 and 2.47, respectively. Both measures show essentially the

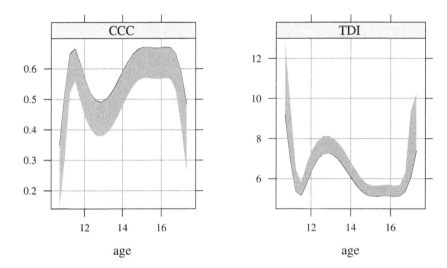

Figure 9.9   Estimates of CCC and TDI functions (solid curves) and their 95% one-sided simultaneous confidence bands (shaded regions) for percentage body fat data.

same pattern of change in the extent of agreement with age: increase from the beginning till about age 11.5, then decrease till about age 13, then increase again till about age 14.5, remain constant near the peak till about age 16.5, and decrease again thereafter. This behavior appears to be driven by the behavior of the estimated mean difference function in Figure 9.8. In particular, the age interval $(11.5, 14.5)$ over which the extent of agreement decreases from its initial peak, attains nadir, and eventually peaks again roughly coincides with the interval over which DEXA's mean is significantly lower than the caliper's mean. The agreement is best around age 11.5 and between the ages of 14.5 and 16.5. It is worst around age 13. There may be a physiological explanation of this phenomenon that is tied to how the two methods measure percentage body fat in adolescent women.

It is evident that even in the best case scenario, the agreement between caliper and DEXA methods is not high enough for interchangeable use. For example, the largest value of CCC lower bound is 0.60, which may only be considered modest. Further, the smallest value of TDI upper bound is 5.5, which is about 23% of the average body fat measurement in the data, a particularly large value. Besides a difference in their means, the lack of agreement is also due to the relatively large error variations of the methods that lead to a somewhat low correlation between them and a high standard deviation for their difference. The latter issues cannot be addressed by a simple recalibration of the methods. DEXA may be preferred because of its higher precision than the skinfold caliper.

9.6 CHAPTER SUMMARY

1. A methodology for analysis of longitudinal method comparison data is presented. It generalizes the one for linked repeated measurements data and allows systematic effects of time on measurements (Chapter 5).

2. Time covariate may be discrete or continuous.

3. Means of the methods are modeled using functions of time of the same form but with method-specific parameters.

4. If time is discrete, each of its levels is given its own intercept.

5. If time is continuous, its effect is modeled as in regression analysis with a continuous predictor.

6. The extent of agreement between the methods may change over time.

7. The model does not require observations from both methods on every measurement occasion.

8. The model allows dependence in the within-subject errors of the same method. The errors of different methods are assumed independent.

9. Time series or spatial correlation models can be used to model dependence in the within-subject errors.

10. By default, the model has a subject × method interaction term. However, it may not be needed when the errors are assumed to be correlated.

11. Simultaneous confidence bands are used for measures that depend on time.

12. The methodology assumes a common scale for the methods and is applicable when the number of subjects is large.

9.7 TECHNICAL DETAILS

First, we focus on the general model (9.2) that includes subject × method interaction.

Let $\mathbf{Y}_{ij} = (Y_{ij1}, \ldots, Y_{ijm_{ij}})^T$ be the $m_{ij} \times 1$ vector of measurements from method j on subject i, and $\mathbf{e}_{ij} = (e_{ij1}, \ldots, e_{ijm_{ij}})^T$ be the corresponding $m_{ij} \times 1$ vector of random errors. Define

$$\mathbf{Y}_i = \begin{pmatrix} \mathbf{Y}_{i1} \\ \mathbf{Y}_{i2} \end{pmatrix}, \quad \mathbf{e}_i = \begin{pmatrix} \mathbf{e}_{i1} \\ \mathbf{e}_{i2} \end{pmatrix}$$

as $M_i \times 1$ vectors of observations and random errors associated with subject i, respectively. Regardless of whether t is discrete or continuous, let β_j be the $(p+1) \times 1$ vector of regression coefficients associated with the mean function of method j and $\mathbf{X}_{ij}$ be the corresponding $m_{ij} \times (p+1)$ design matrix. Define

$$\beta = \begin{pmatrix} \beta_1 \\ \beta_2 \end{pmatrix}, \quad \mathbf{X}_i = \begin{pmatrix} \mathbf{X}_{i1} & \mathbf{0} \\ \mathbf{0} & \mathbf{X}_{i2} \end{pmatrix},$$

respectively, as a $2(p+1) \times 1$ vector and a $M_i \times 2(p+1)$ matrix.

Next, let $\mathbf{u}_i$ be the $(\tilde{m}+3) \times 1$ vector of random effects involving this subject and $\mathbf{Z}_i$ be the $M_i \times (\tilde{m}+3)$ design matrix associated with $\mathbf{u}_i$. These are defined as

$$
\mathbf{u}_i = \begin{pmatrix} u_i \\ b_{i1} \\ b_{i2} \\ b_{i1}^* \\ \vdots \\ b_{i\tilde{m}}^* \end{pmatrix}, \ \mathbf{Z}_i = \begin{pmatrix} 1 & 1 & 0 & I(o_{i11}=1) & \ldots & I(o_{i11}=\tilde{m}) \\ \vdots & \vdots & \vdots & \vdots & \ldots & \vdots \\ 1 & 1 & 0 & I(o_{i1m_{i1}}=1) & \ldots & I(o_{i1m_{i1}}=\tilde{m}) \\ 1 & 0 & 1 & I(o_{i21}=1) & \ldots & I(o_{i21}=\tilde{m}) \\ \vdots & \vdots & \vdots & \vdots & \ldots & \vdots \\ 1 & 0 & 1 & I(o_{i2m_{i2}}=1) & \ldots & I(o_{i2m_{i2}}=\tilde{m}) \end{pmatrix}, \quad (9.29)
$$

where $o_{ijk} \in \{1, \ldots, \tilde{m}\}$ is the measurement occasion of Y_{ijk}. It is assumed that

$$
\mathbf{u}_i \sim \text{independent } \mathcal{N}_{(\tilde{m}+3)}(\mathbf{0}, \mathbf{G}), \ \mathbf{G} = \text{diag}\{\sigma_b^2, \psi^2, \psi^2, \sigma_{b^*}^2, \ldots, \sigma_{b^*}^2\},
$$
$$
\mathbf{e}_i \sim \text{independent } \mathcal{N}_{M_i}(\mathbf{0}, \mathbf{R}_i), \ \mathbf{R}_i = \text{diag}\{\mathbf{R}_{i1}, \mathbf{R}_{i2}\}, \quad (9.30)
$$

where $\mathbf{R}_{ij}$ is an $m_{ij} \times m_{ij}$ covariance matrix whose (k,l)th element is $\sigma_{ej}^2 h(|t_{ijk}-t_{ijl}|, \boldsymbol{\omega})$, with h as the correlation function defined in (9.1). It reduces to a diagonal matrix when the correlation parameter $\boldsymbol{\omega} = \mathbf{0}$. The random vectors $\mathbf{u}_i$ and $\mathbf{e}_i$ are mutually independent.

Now, the model (9.2) can be written in matrix notation as

$$
\mathbf{Y}_i = \mathbf{X}_i \boldsymbol{\beta} + \mathbf{Z}_i \mathbf{u}_i + \mathbf{e}_i, \ i = 1, \ldots, n, \quad (9.31)
$$

where $\mathbf{u}_i$ and $\mathbf{e}_i$ follow the distributions given in (9.30). The vector of transformed model parameters is

$$
\boldsymbol{\theta} = \left(\boldsymbol{\beta}^T, \log(\sigma_b^2), \log(\psi^2), \log(\sigma_{b^*}^2), \log(\sigma_{e1}^2), \log(\sigma_{e2}^2), \boldsymbol{\omega}^T\right)^T.
$$

The fitting of such a mixed-effects model and associated inference based on the large-sample theory of ML estimators have been described in Chapter 3. Of particular interest is the construction of simultaneous confidence bands for measures that depend on t over its domain $\mathcal{T}$. The methodology of Section 3.3.5 is used for this task.

To represent the model (9.2) without the interaction, we simply drop (b_{i1}, b_{i2}) from $\mathbf{u}_i$ in (9.29). Essentially, this amounts to redefining $\mathbf{u}_i$ and $\mathbf{Z}_i$ in (9.29) as

$$
\mathbf{u}_i = \begin{pmatrix} u_i \\ b_{i1}^* \\ \vdots \\ b_{i\tilde{m}}^* \end{pmatrix}, \ \mathbf{Z}_i = \begin{pmatrix} 1 & I(o_{i11}=1) & \ldots & I(o_{i11}=\tilde{m}) \\ \vdots & \vdots & \ldots & \vdots \\ 1 & I(o_{i1m_{i1}}=1) & \ldots & I(o_{i1m_{i1}}=\tilde{m}) \\ 1 & I(o_{i21}=1) & \ldots & I(o_{i21}=\tilde{m}) \\ \vdots & \vdots & \ldots & \vdots \\ 1 & I(o_{i2m_{i2}}=1) & \ldots & I(o_{i2m_{i2}}=\tilde{m}) \end{pmatrix},
$$

redefining $\mathbf{G}$ in (9.30) as $\mathbf{G} = \text{diag}\{\sigma_b^2, \sigma_{b^*}^2, \ldots, \sigma_{b^*}^2\}$, dropping $\log(\psi^2)$ as an unknown parameter from $\boldsymbol{\theta}$, making the corresponding changes in the estimates, and replacing $(\tilde{m}+3)$ with $(\tilde{m}+1)$ (Exercise 9.5).

9.8 BIBLIOGRAPHIC NOTE

The topic of longitudinal data analysis has been covered in a number of books, including Diggle et al. (2002) and Fitzmaurice et al. (2011). However, the analysis of longitudinal method comparison data has been considered by only a handful of authors. Chinchilli et al. (1996), King et al. (2007a), and Hiriote and Chinchilli (2011) generalize the usual CCC to obtain overall summary measures for longitudinal data. Specifically, Chinchilli et al. develop subject-specific CCCs under a random-coefficient growth curve model and combine them into an overall weighted CCC. Both King et al. and Hiriote and Chinchilli assume that each subject contributes two $\tilde{m} \times 1$ vectors, consisting of paired measurements by the two methods on each measurement occasion. King et al. develop a "repeated measures" CCC that characterizes how close the two vectors are through a single index. They also incorporate an $\tilde{m} \times \tilde{m}$ weight matrix into the index to allow differential emphasis on within- and between-occasion agreement between the methods. Hiriote and Chinchilli develop a "matrix-based" CCC by first constructing an $\tilde{m} \times \tilde{m}$ matrix that measures agreement between the two vectors. Then they transform the matrix into a scalar quantity by taking its Frobenius norm and scaling it to lie between -1 and 1. The inference procedures proposed by both King et al. and Hiriote and Chinchilli do not make any assumptions about the correlation structure between the measurements. However, they require measurements from both methods on each measurement occasion. Carrasco et al. (2009) focus on a special case of the repeated measures CCC developed by King et al. but consider likelihood-based inference on the measure by assuming a mixed-effects model for the data. Their model allows missing observations and is a special case of the model we consider here. See Carrasco et al. (2009) and Hiriote and Chinchilli (2011) for comparisons of the various approaches.

The above articles summarize the extent of agreement in a single CCC-type index. None is concerned with examining how the agreement changes over time, which is a goal of Choudhary (2007). It works with differences in paired longitudinal measurements, models them semiparametrically as a function of time via penalized splines, and measures agreement using TDI as a function of time. It uses a Bayesian approach for inference. Our approach in this chapter is to directly model the paired longitudinal data instead of modeling their differences. This has two advantages. Firstly, we can use all data, whereas working with differences necessitates discarding observations whose paired counterparts are missing—a common occurrence in longitudinal studies. Secondly, we have the additional flexibility of using any measure of agreement we like because it can be expressed in terms of parameters of the model for the entire data.

Our discussion of correlation models for errors is kept quite brief and is primarily based on Pinheiro and Bates (2000). The books by Brockwell and Davis (2002) on time series analysis and Cressie (1993) on spatial statistics detail a variety of correlation models. More focussed discussions in the specific contexts of longitudinal data and mixed-effects models can be found in Pinheiro and Bates (2000), Diggle et al. (2002), and Fitzmaurice et al. (2011). These books also explain diagnostics for checking the adequacy of the fitted correlation models. Quite a few correlation models are implemented in the `nlme` package of Pinheiro and Bates for fitting mixed-effects models in R. The conservative nature of the likelihood ratio test of zero variance of a random effect is described in Pinheiro and Bates (2000, Section 2.4).

Data Source

The percentage body fat data are from Chinchilli et al. (1996). They have also been analyzed by a number of authors, including Choudhary (2007), King et al. (2007a), and Hiriote and Chinchilli (2011). They can be obtained from the book's website.

EXERCISES

9.1 Consider random variables $Y_1, \ldots, Y_m$ with a common mean. They are said to follow a *compound symmetric* correlation structure if they have a common variance σ^2 and a common correlation ρ, that is,

$$\text{var}(Y_k) = \sigma^2, \quad \text{cor}(Y_k, Y_l) = \rho, \quad k \neq l = 1, \ldots, m.$$

Show that this correlation structure is valid only if $-1/(m-1) \leq \rho \leq 1$. [Hint: Examine the variance of the average $\overline{Y}$.]

9.2 Consider the model (9.2) with errors following independent $\mathcal{N}_1(0, \sigma_{ej}^2)$ distributions for $k = 1, \ldots, m_{ij}, j = 1, 2, i = 1, \ldots, n$.

    (a) Define $e_{ijk}^* = b_{ij} + e_{ijk}$, and write the model as $Y_{ijk} = \mu_j(t_{ijk}) + u_i + b_{io_{ijk}}^* + e_{ijk}^*$. Show that for a given (i, j), the new errors $e_{ij1}^*, \ldots, e_{ijm_{ij}}^*$ have a compound symmetric correlation structure with $\psi^2 + \sigma_{ej}^2$ as the common variance and $\psi^2/(\psi^2 + \sigma_{ej}^2)$ as the common correlation. (This correlation is an intraclass correlation.)

    (b) Write the model in (a) by replacing e_{ijk}^* with $\tilde{e}_{ijk}$ that follow normal distributions with mean zero and a compound symmetric correlation structure with σ_{ej}^2 as the common variance and ω as the common correlation. Are the two models equivalent? Justify your answer.

9.3   (a) Verify that the distributions of $(Y_1(t), Y_2(t))$ and $D(t)$ for $t \in \mathcal{T}$ under the model (9.6) are given by (9.7) and (9.8), respectively.

    (b) Use (a) to verify that the longitudinal version of the similarity measure β_0 is $\xi(t) = \mu_2(t) - \mu_1(t)$ and the longitudinal versions of CCC and TDI are given by (9.22) and (9.23), respectively.

9.4 Consider the model (9.2). Replace the assumption of a common correlation function (9.1) for within-subject errors of the two methods with

$$\text{cor}(e_{ijk}, e_{ijl}) = h_j(|t_{ijk} - t_{ijl}|, \boldsymbol{\omega}_j), \quad j = 1, 2.$$

This allows each method to have its own correlation function as well as correlation parameters. Derive the measures of similarity and agreement under this model.

9.5 Consider the model (9.2) without the subject $\times$ method interaction b_{ij}, that is,

$$Y_{ijk} = \mu_j(t_{ijk}) + u_i + b_{io_{ijk}}^* + e_{ijk}, \quad k = 1, \ldots, m_{ij}, j = 1, 2, i = 1, \ldots, n.$$

    (a) Express this model in the matrix notation.

(b) Argue that the analogs of the moments in (9.3) to (9.5) and the distributions in (9.7) and (9.8) under the new model can be obtained by simply setting $\psi^2 = 0$ in these expressions.

(c) Verify the expressions in (9.25)–(9.27).

9.6 Consider the longitudinal data model (9.2). Derive expressions for CCC and TDI under this model for measuring agreement between an observation from method 1 at time t and an observation from method 2 at time $t + \Delta$, where $|\Delta| > 0$. How do these expressions compare with the case when $\Delta = 0$? (See also King et al., 2007a.)

9.7 Consider the percentage body fat data from Section 9.5.

(a) Fit the model (9.2) with cubic mean functions and continuous AR(1) within-subject errors and without the method × subject interaction. Verify the estimates in Table 9.1. Perform diagnostics to check the various model assumptions.

(b) Refit the model in (a) with polynomial mean functions of degree $q = 1, 2, 4$. Perform model comparison to determine which degree should be used. Would you still recommend $q = 3$?

(c) Refit the model in (a) with compound symmetric correlation structure for the errors. Does this correlation model provide a better fit than the continuous AR(1) structure?

9.8 Reanalyze the body fat data by modeling them using (9.2) with subject × method interaction, and compare conclusions with those obtained in Section 9.5.

CHAPTER 10

A NONPARAMETRIC APPROACH

10.1 PREVIEW

Here we present a nonparametric approach for analysis of continuous method comparison data. Attention is restricted to the evaluation of similarity and agreement. The methodology makes no assumption about either the shape of the data distribution or how the observed measurements are related to the underlying true values. It is an alternative to the normality-based parametric approaches of previous chapters, and is especially attractive for data with marked deviations from normality. It works for unreplicated as well as unlinked repeated measurements data. It takes a statistical functional approach that treats the population quantities, including the measures of similarity and agreement, as features of a population distribution and estimates them using the same features of an empirical distribution. Under certain assumptions, the resulting estimators are approximately normal for large samples. This result is used to develop nonparametric analogs of the procedures in Chapter 7 involving multiple methods. Its application is illustrated using two case studies.

10.2 INTRODUCTION

Consider the setup of Chapter 7. We have measurements from $J \, (\geq 2)$ methods on n subjects. It is assumed that n is large. The measurements may be unreplicated or repeated. The latter are assumed to be unlinked. The unreplicated measurements are denoted by Y_{ij}, $j = 1, \ldots, J$, $i = 1, \ldots, n$. The repeated measurements are denoted by

Measuring Agreement: Models, Methods, and Applications. By P. K. Choudhary and H. N. Nagaraja
Copyright © 2017 John Wiley & Sons, Inc.

Y_{ijk}, $k = 1, \ldots, m_{ij}$, $j = 1 \ldots, J$, $i = 1, \ldots, n$. In the balanced case when all m_{ij} are equal, m denotes the common value. To present a unified framework encompassing both data types, we treat unreplicated data as a special case of repeated measurements data with all $m_{ij} = 1$. Thus, Y_{ij} is essentially an alias for Y_{ij1}, and $m = 1$ refers to the unreplicated case. As before, $(Y_1, \ldots, Y_J)$ denotes the population vector of single measurements from the J methods on the same subject. Let $F(y_1, \ldots, y_J)$ be its joint cdf. A cdf is also used to refer to the distribution it characterizes.

The methods used in previous chapters are *parametric* in that the data are assumed to follow a probability distribution of a known form, specifically a normal distribution, characterized in terms of model parameters. The parameters are estimated by the ML method. Under certain assumptions, the ML estimators are *efficient*, essentially meaning that, if the assumed model is correct and n is large, one cannot find more accurate estimators than them. This optimality property breaks down if the assumed model is wrong, in which case the ML estimators may be a poor choice. In contrast, the methodology of this chapter is *nonparametric* or *distribution-free* in that no particular form is assumed for the data distribution, thereby allowing the methodology to be broadly applicable. However, there is a trade-off. Although a nonparametric estimator may be more accurate than the ML estimator if the assumed model is wrong, the converse is true if the assumed model is correct because of the latter's efficiency. This motivates the common practice of initially attempting a parametric analysis wherein a normality-based model is first fit, followed by model diagnostics to verify the normality assumption. If no serious violations are seen, one proceeds with the parametric analysis, otherwise a nonparametric analysis is pursued. The violations include skewness and outliers in the data. Often, however, the two analyses produce similar inferences regardless of how serious the violations are.

The nonparametric approach also has limitations brought upon by its assumptions or lack thereof, including the following two that are relevant here. First, it does not decompose the observed values into true values and errors. As a result, the usual characteristics of measurement methods such as biases and precisions considered in Section 1.7, and hence the associated measures of similarity are left undefined. Thus, there is a need for alternative measures. Second, the approach does not generalize well to data with features such as heteroscedasticity and covariate effects that call for explicit modeling. It is easier to analyze such data within a parametric framework.

Notwithstanding its limitations, a nonparametric approach remains useful for analysis of basic types of method comparison data. To describe it, we let

$$c_i = \prod_{j=1}^{J} m_{ij},$$

and assume that the distribution of $(Y_1, \ldots, Y_J)$ is continuous; the measurements on different subjects are independent; and for each $i = 1, \ldots, n$, the c_i possible J-tuples formed by selecting one measurement per method from the available measurements on the ith subject, that is,

$$\{(Y_{i1k_1}, \ldots, Y_{iJk_J}), k_j = 1, \ldots, m_{ij}, j = 1, \ldots, J\},$$

are identically distributed as $(Y_1, \ldots, Y_J)$.

For unreplicated data, there is only one J-tuple per subject. The assumptions imply they are i.i.d. draws from the distribution of $(Y_1, \ldots, Y_J)$. For repeated measurements data, there are c_i J-tuples from the ith subject, resulting in a total of $\sum_{i=1}^{n} c_i$ tuples. These tuples are also identically distributed draws from the distribution of $(Y_1, \ldots, Y_J)$, but independence holds only for the tuples from different subjects. Those from the same subject are dependent. This also means that a subject's multiple tuples are treated the same way in that they carry the same amount of information.

The population moments and functions thereof, viz., means, variances, and correlations, play a key role in the analysis of method comparison data. These quantities are fine for normal data, but one may question their value for non-normal data. Their usage may be considered particularly problematic if the data have outliers because the nonparametric estimators of population moments are sample moments, which are not robust to outliers. However, a discussion of robust alternatives to moments and measures based on them is beyond the scope of this book (see Bibliographic Note for a reference). Instead, if outliers are seen in the data, then as in a parametric approach, we perform the analysis twice— with and without the outliers—and compare the conclusions. The analysis also involves inference on percentiles. But their nonparametric estimators are relatively more robust to outliers than those of moments.

10.3 THE STATISTICAL FUNCTIONAL APPROACH

This approach is a general method for constructing nonparametric estimators. It treats the population quantities as *statistical functionals*, that is, functions of the form $h(F)$, where h is a known function and F is the population cdf. Writing a population quantity in this way highlights it as a feature h of the population distribution F. The cdf F is estimated nonparametrically by the empirical cdf $\hat{F}$. Thereafter, F in $h(F)$ is replaced by $\hat{F}$ to get the *plug-in estimator* $h(\hat{F})$—the same feature h of the sample distribution $\hat{F}$. This estimator may be considered a "natural" estimator for $h(F)$. Parameters such as population moments and percentiles and functions thereof are readily written as statistical functionals (Exercise 10.1), and their sample analogs can be thought of as plug-in estimators (Exercise 10.2).

For a concrete example, consider the population mean μ_j of the jth measurement method. The feature h here is the mean of the jth component of the distribution F of $(Y_1, \ldots, Y_J)$. From unreplicated data, F can be estimated by the empirical cdf,

$$\hat{F}(y_1, \ldots, y_J) = \frac{1}{n} \sum_{i=1}^{n} I(Y_{i1} \leq y_1, \ldots, Y_{iJ} \leq y_J), \qquad (10.1)$$

where $I(A)$ is the indicator function of an event A, defined as

$$I(A) = \begin{cases} 1, & \text{if event } A \text{ occurs,} \\ 0, & \text{otherwise.} \end{cases}$$

It is readily seen that the mean of the jth component of the distribution $\hat{F}$ is the sample mean $\overline{Y}_{\cdot j} = \sum_{i=1}^{n} Y_{ij}/n$ (Exercise 10.2). Thus, we have the anticipated result that the sample mean is a plug-in estimator of the population mean.

10.3.1 A Weighted Empirical CDF

It is clear that we need a nonparametric estimator $\hat{F}$ of F to construct plug-in estimators of population quantities. For unreplicated data, the empirical cdf (10.1) is a natural choice. But no such candidate is apparent for repeated measurements data in general. Here we focus on a weighted generalization of (10.1) of the form:

$$\hat{F}(y_1, \ldots, y_J) = \sum_{i=1}^{n} w(n, \mathbf{m}_i) \left\{ \sum_{k_1=1}^{m_{i1}} \cdots \sum_{k_J=1}^{m_{iJ}} I(Y_{i1k_1} \leq y_1, \ldots, Y_{iJk_J} \leq y_J) \right\},$$
(10.2)

where w is a weight function; $\mathbf{m}_i = (m_{i1}, \ldots, m_{iJ})^T$; and $\{(Y_{i1k_1}, \ldots, Y_{iJk_J}), k_j = 1, \ldots, m_{ij}, j = 1, \ldots, J\}$ are the c_i J-tuples formed by the measurements on the ith subject. The J-tuples from a subject receive the same weight. The weight depends on the number of replications on the subject and not on $(y_1, \ldots, y_J)$. The weight function is non-negative and is assumed to satisfy an unbiasedness condition,

$$\sum_{i=1}^{n} c_i\, w(n, \mathbf{m}_i) = 1,$$
(10.3)

so that $\hat{F}$ is an unbiased estimator of F.

When the design is balanced with all $m_{ij} = m$, the weight function in (10.2) does not depend on the subject index. In fact, in this case c_i is a constant and the unique weight function satisfying (10.3) is the constant function

$$w(n, \mathbf{m}_i) = \frac{1}{nm^J}.$$
(10.4)

It gives equal weight to all J-tuples in the data. Due to its uniqueness, the resulting $\hat{F}$ may be considered a "standard" empirical cdf for balanced designs. Besides, when $m = 1$, it reduces to the cdf (10.1) for unreplicated data. Therefore, hereafter we use (10.4) as the weight function for unreplicated as well as balanced repeated measurements data.

For unbalanced data, we focus on two candidate weight functions. They are

$$w_1(n, \mathbf{m}_i) = \frac{1}{nc_i}, \quad w_2(n, \mathbf{m}_i) = \frac{1}{\sum_{i=1}^{n} c_i}.$$
(10.5)

The first gives equal weight to each subject i in the data and distributes that weight equally over all its c_i J-tuples. The second gives equal weight to all the J-tuples in the entire dataset. These two are extreme but useful special cases of an optimal weight function (Exercise 10.6). All these weight functions reduce to (10.4) for balanced designs. Thus, choosing between w_1 and w_2 is an issue only for unbalanced designs. In this case, we suggest analyzing data using both of them and comparing the conclusions because neither is a uniformly better choice than the other (see Bibliographic Note).

10.3.2 Distributions Induced by Empirical CDF

The cdf $\hat{F}$ in (10.2) induces a discrete multivariate empirical distribution for $(Y_1, \ldots, Y_J)$, whose possible values are the observed $\sum_{i=1}^{n} c_i$ J-tuples in the dataset. Despite the fact that the underlying population distribution is continuous, there may be ties among a method's measurements and hence among the J-tuples. Allowing for the possibility of ties, the joint probability mass function (pmf) of $(Y_1, \ldots, Y_J)$ under $\hat{F}$ is

$$p_{\hat{F}}(y_1, \ldots, y_J) = \sum_{i=1}^{n} w(n, \mathbf{m}_i) \left\{ \sum_{k_1=1}^{m_{i1}} \cdots \sum_{k_J=1}^{m_{iJ}} I(Y_{i1k_1} = y_1, \ldots, Y_{iJk_J} = y_J) \right\}.$$
(10.6)

The notation $p_{\hat{F}}$ emphasizes that the pmf is associated with the distribution $\hat{F}$. The inner sum on the right in (10.6) essentially counts the frequency of $(y_1, \ldots, y_J)$ among each subject's tuples. A weighted sum of these frequencies is the probability of observing $(y_1, \ldots, y_J)$. Upon summing (10.6) over the remaining components, we get the joint pmf of (Y_j, Y_l), $j \neq l$ as

$$p_{\hat{F}}(y_j, y_l) = \sum_{i=1}^{n} w(n, \mathbf{m}_i) \left(\frac{c_i}{m_{ij} m_{il}} \right) \left\{ \sum_{k_j=1}^{m_{ij}} \sum_{k_l=1}^{m_{il}} I(Y_{ijk_j} = y_j, Y_{ilk_l} = y_l) \right\}, \quad (10.7)$$

and the marginal pmf of Y_j as

$$p_{\hat{F}}(y_j) = \sum_{i=1}^{n} w(n, \mathbf{m}_i) \left(\frac{c_i}{m_{ij}} \right) \left\{ \sum_{k_j=1}^{m_{ij}} I(Y_{ijk_j} = y_j) \right\}. \quad (10.8)$$

The expressions for these pmfs are verified in Exercise 10.3. Their special cases when there are no within-method ties are derived in Exercise 10.4 for unbalanced designs and in Exercise 10.5 for balanced designs.

Now that we have the pmfs (10.7) and (10.8) under $\hat{F}$, we can compute certain moments and percentiles involving (Y_j, Y_l) by simply invoking their definitions. They serve as plug-in estimators of their population analogs under F. In particular, the estimators of first- and second-order moments are

$$E_{\hat{F}}(Y_j^r) = \sum_{y_j} y_j^r \, p_{\hat{F}}(y_j), \quad E_{\hat{F}}(Y_l^r) = \sum_{y_l} y_l^r \, p_{\hat{F}}(y_l), \quad r = 1, 2,$$

$$E_{\hat{F}}(Y_j Y_l) = \sum_{y_j} \sum_{y_l} y_j y_l \, p_{\hat{F}}(y_j, y_l). \quad (10.9)$$

As before, the notation $E_{\hat{F}}$ emphasizes that the expectation is associated with the distribution $\hat{F}$. It follows that the corresponding estimators of means and variances of Y_j and Y_l and their correlation are

$$\hat{\mu}_j = E_{\hat{F}}(Y_j), \quad \hat{\mu}_l = E_{\hat{F}}(Y_l),$$

$$\hat{\sigma}_j^2 = E_{\hat{F}}(Y_j^2) - \hat{\mu}_j^2, \quad \hat{\sigma}_l^2 = E_{\hat{F}}(Y_l^2) - \hat{\mu}_l^2, \quad \hat{\rho}_{jl} = \frac{E_{\hat{F}}(Y_j Y_l) - \hat{\mu}_j \hat{\mu}_l}{\hat{\sigma}_j \hat{\sigma}_l}. \quad (10.10)$$

These estimators can also be used in the usual manner to get the corresponding estimators of mean and variance of the difference $D_{jl} = Y_l - Y_j$.

Next, let G_{jl} be the cdf of $|D_{jl}|$. It can be written as an expectation as

$$G_{jl}(x) = P_F(|Y_l - Y_j| \leq x) = E_F\{I(|Y_l - Y_j| \leq x)\}, \quad x > 0.$$

Hence its plug-in estimator is

$$\hat{G}_{jl}(x) = P_{\hat{F}}(|Y_l - Y_j| \le x) = \sum_{y_j}\sum_{y_l} I(|y_l - y_j| \le x)\, p_{\hat{F}}(y_j, y_l), \quad x > 0. \quad (10.11)$$

Exercise 10.8 gives alternative expressions for the estimators in (10.9) and (10.11); those may be simpler to evaluate. The 100γth percentile of $|D_{jl}|$ is defined as the inverse cdf $G_{jl}^{-1}(\gamma)$, where

$$G_{jl}^{-1}(\gamma) = \min\{x : G_{jl}(x) \ge \gamma\}, \quad 0 < \gamma < 1.$$

Its sample counterpart $\hat{G}_{jl}^{-1}$ is also similarly defined, that is,

$$\hat{G}_{jl}^{-1}(\gamma) = \min\{x : \hat{G}_{jl}(x) \ge \gamma\}, \quad 0 < \gamma < 1. \quad (10.12)$$

10.4   EVALUATION OF SIMILARITY AND AGREEMENT

The nonparametric approach of this chapter does not make any assumptions about: (a) the shape of the data distribution, and (b) how the observed measurements are related to the true values. Although this does not pose any difficulty with measures of agreement such as CCC and TDI, the limits of agreement discussed earlier are not meaningful anymore because their definition is tied to normality of data. In addition, (b) precludes us from defining measures of similarity such as the difference in fixed biases and ratio of precisions. A similar situation occurred in Chapter 4 for paired measurements data when we switched from the mixed-effects model (4.1) to the bivariate normal model (4.6). However, as in that chapter, the similarity of two methods can be examined by directly comparing their means and variances using mean difference and variance ratio, respectively.

Just like Chapter 7, suppose there are Q specified pairwise comparisons of interest involving the J methods in the study. The population vector of their measurements is $(Y_1, \ldots, Y_J)$. Its cdf F is estimated by the weighted empirical cdf $\hat{F}$ given in (10.2) with weights given by (10.4) for balanced designs and by (10.5) for unbalanced designs. For a method pair (j, l), $j < l = 1, \ldots, J$ of interest, the measures of similarity are the mean difference $\mu_l - \mu_j$ and the variance ratio σ_l^2/σ_j^2. Moreover, the measures of agreement are CCC_{jl} and $\mathrm{TDI}_{jl}(p)$. These measures are statistical functionals of the distribution F (Exercise 10.7). The plug-in estimators of the similarity measures are $\hat{\mu}_l - \hat{\mu}_j$ and $\hat{\sigma}_l^2/\hat{\sigma}_j^2$, and those of the agreement measures are

$$\widehat{\mathrm{CCC}}_{jl} = \frac{2\hat{\rho}_{jl}\hat{\sigma}_j\hat{\sigma}_l}{(\hat{\mu}_j - \hat{\mu}_l)^2 + \hat{\sigma}_j^2 + \hat{\sigma}_l^2}, \quad \widehat{\mathrm{TDI}}_{jl}(p) = \hat{G}_{jl}^{-1}(p), \quad (10.13)$$

where the quantities involved are given by (10.9) and (10.12).

Thus, we have nonparametric estimators of measures of similarity and agreement for each of the Q pairs of interest. Under certain assumptions, these plug-in estimators are approximately normal from the large-sample theory of statistical functionals, and their SEs can be approximated using estimated moments of *influence functions* (see Section 10.7). As in Chapter 7, we examine Q two-sided simultaneous confidence intervals for a similarity measure, and Q one-sided simultaneous confidence bounds for an agreement measure. These are of the usual form

$$\text{estimate} \pm \text{critical point} \times \text{SE(estimate)}, \quad (10.14)$$

possibly on a transformed scale. Specifically, a log transformation is applied for the variance ratios and a Fisher's z-transformation is applied for the CCCs. One exception to (10.14) is TDI for which upper confidence bounds of the following from is suggested (Section 10.7):

$$\hat{G}_{jl}^{-1}\left[p - \text{critical point} \times \text{SE}\{\hat{G}_{jl}(\widehat{\text{TDI}}_{jl}(p))\}\right]. \tag{10.15}$$

These bounds avoid the estimation of the pdf of $|D_{jl}|$ in the tails, which is needed for the bounds in (10.14). Such density estimates are generally not stable unless n is quite large. The critical points are $\mathcal{N}_1(0, 1)$ percentiles when $Q = 1$. For $Q > 1$, they are computed numerically as described in Section 3.3 (see also Section 10.7).

Two observations are now in order about the nonparametric estimators of means, variances, and correlation of Y_j and Y_l given by (10.10). First, in the case of unreplicated data with $J = 2$, these estimators are identical to the ML estimators given by (4.8) under the bivariate normal model (4.6) (Exercise 10.2). Second, in the case of balanced repeated measurements data, the estimators in (10.10) often tend to be close to the ML estimators under the mixed-effects model (7.4). Consequently, the nonparametric and the ML estimators of the moment-based measures, $\mu_l - \mu_j$, σ_l^2/σ_j^2 and CCC_{jl}, coincide in the first case and tend to be close in the second case.

10.5 CASE STUDIES

In this section, we illustrate the nonparametric methodology by using it to analyze two datasets. Both consist of measurements of systolic blood pressure (mm Hg), but the first has unreplicated observations from two methods, whereas the second has replicated observations from three methods. For convenience, we refer to the first as "unreplicated blood pressure data" and the second as "replicated blood pressure data."

10.5.1 Unreplicated Blood Pressure Data

This dataset has paired blood pressure measurements of 200 subjects taken by a standard method using arm pressure (method 1) and a test method using finger pressure (method 2). There is a total of $200 \times 2 = 400$ observations in the data. They range between 60 and 228 mm Hg. Figure 10.1 shows their trellis plot. The measurements from the two methods do not have much overlap. The finger's measurements exceed their arm counterparts for most subjects. The former also exhibit somewhat larger variability than the latter. A handful of subjects have relatively large differences, suggesting that the differences have a skewed distribution. However, there are no clear outliers. There is considerable within-subject variation in the measurements, but this variation is small in relation to the between-subject variation. The data can be considered homoscedastic. The scatterplot in Figure 10.2 shows modest correlation in the methods. The Bland-Altman plot in the same figure shows a mild upward trend, corroborating the somewhat unequal variances of the methods. This trend may also be indicative of unequal scales of the methods but we cannot be sure due to lack of replications. The boxplots in Figure 10.3 confirm the difference in their marginal distributions. They also show right-skewness in the data. The non-normality is confirmed by model diagnostics in Exercise 10.14.

To perform the nonparametric analysis, we first need the empirical cdf $\hat{F}$. Since these are unreplicated data, $\hat{F}$ is the bivariate cdf that gives $1/n$ weight to each observed pair.

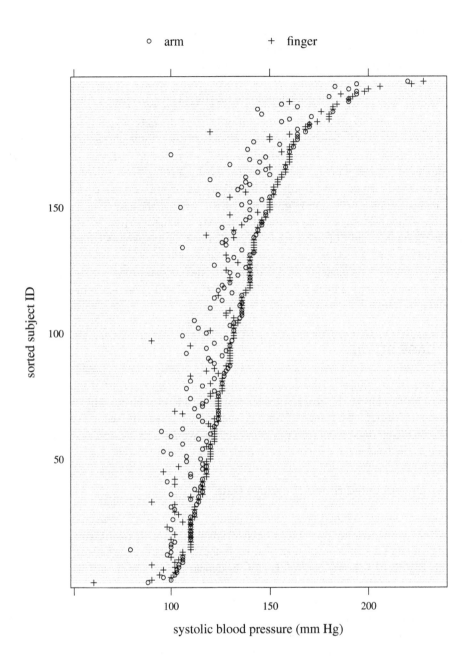

Figure 10.1 Trellis plot of unreplicated blood pressure data.

Under this $\hat{F}$, the sample means, variances (with divisor n), and correlation of (Y_1, Y_2) are plug-in estimators of their population counterparts (Exercise 10.2). The estimates are

$$(\hat{\mu}_1, \hat{\mu}_2) = (128.5, 132.8), \ (\hat{\sigma}_1, \hat{\sigma}_2) = (23.2, 25.6), \ \hat{\rho} = 0.83.$$

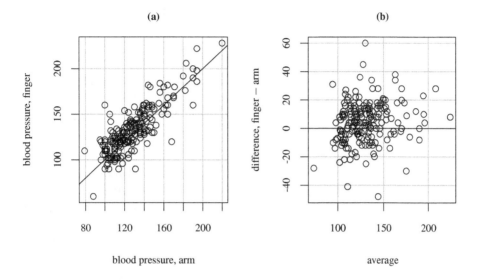

Figure 10.2   A scatterplot with line of equality (left panel) and a Bland-Altman plot with zero line (right panel) for unreplicated blood pressure data.

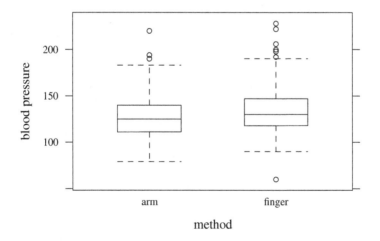

Figure 10.3   Side-by-side boxplots for unreplicated blood pressure data.

	Nonparametric		Parametric	
		95% Interval		95% Interval
Measure	Estimate	or Bound	Estimate	or Bound
$\mu_2 - \mu_1$	4.30	$(2.28, 6.31)$	4.30	$(2.28, 6.31)$
σ_2^2/σ_1^2	1.21	$(1.04, 1.42)$	1.21	$(1.04, 1.42)$
CCC	0.81	0.75	0.81	0.77
TDI(0.90)	23.00	28.00	25.00	27.10

Table 10.1   Nonparametric and parametric estimates for measures of similarity and agreement for unreplicated blood pressure data. The parametric estimates are based on the bivariate normal model (4.6). Lower bounds for CCC and upper bounds for TDI are presented. Methods 1 and 2 refer to arm and finger methods, respectively.

They are consistent with what we expect from the exploratory analysis. They also lead to an estimated mean of 4.3 and standard deviation of 14.5 for the difference $D = Y_2 - Y_1$. The standard deviation is rather large mainly due to the modest correlation between the methods.

Table 10.1 presents plug-in estimates of the similarity measures $\mu_2 - \mu_1$ and σ_2^2/σ_1^2, and the agreement measures CCC and TDI(0.90). Also presented are two-sided 95% intervals for the similarity measures and one-sided 95% bounds for the agreement measures. These use percentiles of a standard normal distribution as critical points because only two methods are compared. The critical points are 1.96 for the mean difference and log of variance ratio, 1.645 for the Fisher's z-transformation of CCC, and -1.645 for the TDI bound, which is computed using (10.15). The interval for $\mu_2 - \mu_1$ ranges from 2.3 to 6.3, implying a larger mean for the finger method compared to the arm method. The interval for σ_2^2/σ_1^2 is barely to the right of one, providing borderline evidence for higher variability of the finger method. Thus, on the whole, the methods do not have similar characteristics.

The CCC lower bound of 0.75 suggests a weak agreement in the methods. The TDI upper bound of 28 also suggests this conclusion by clearly showing that the methods cannot be considered to have acceptable agreement because doing so would amount to treating a 28 mm Hg difference in blood pressure as clinically acceptable. It is also apparent from the similarity evaluation that no simple recalibration can bring the two methods into acceptable agreement. Although subtracting 4.3 from the finger's measurements makes its mean match that of the arm's, the resulting improvement in CCC and TDI bounds, now at 0.77 and 26.3, respectively, is not large enough for the conclusion to change. For further improvement, the correlation between the methods needs to increase, for example, by increasing the precisions of the methods, thereby reducing the size of the differences.

Even though the normality assumption does not hold for these data, it is of interest to analyze them anyway using a normality-based approach and compare conclusions. The relevant methodology is the one in Chapter 4 that assumes the bivariate normal model (4.6) for the data. Table 10.1 also presents the resulting parametric inferences. We see that the two estimates of every moment-based measure are identical. This is expected because the ML estimators of the first- and second-order moments under (4.6) are also the nonparametric plug-in estimators (Exercise 10.2). But even the confidence intervals and bounds for these measures are identical to the number of decimal places reported. In addition, although the two estimates and bounds for TDI are not identical, there is little practical difference between them. Overall, this seems to suggest that the skewness of these data is not severe enough to invalidate the parametric analysis. Note also that the number of subjects here ($n = 200$) is relatively large.

10.5.2 Replicated Blood Pressure Data

This dataset, introduced in Exercise 7.12, has three replicate measurements of systolic blood pressure (mm Hg) taken in quick succession on 85 subjects by each of two experienced observers named "J" (method 1) and "R" (method 2) using a sphygmomanometer, and by a semi-automatic blood pressure monitor (method 3). We treat these as unlinked repeated measurements data. The design is balanced with a total of $85 \times 3 \times 3 = 765$ observations ranging from 74 to 228 mm Hg. We are interested in all-pairwise comparisons involving the three methods.

A trellis plot of the data is displayed in Figure 10.4. The measurements of the two observers largely overlap, but those of the monitor tend be larger than theirs. It also has a higher within-subject variation than the observers. This variation does not seem to depend on the measurement's magnitude in a consistent manner. Also, as in the previous dataset, some subjects have large differences between monitor's and observers' measurements, suggesting skewness in the distributions of their differences. But none of the observations is a clear outlier. Figure 10.5 displays a matrix of scatterplots and the corresponding Bland-Altman plots for a subset of data consisting of one measurement per method selected randomly for every subject. The scatterplots show a very high correlation between the observers but only modest correlations between the observers and the monitor. The Bland-Altman plots do not have any trend, implying a common scale for the methods. These plots also corroborate the monitor's tendency to produce larger measurements than the observers'. The side-by-side boxplots of all measurements from the three methods are displayed in Figure 10.6. Besides confirming the foregoing observation, they also show that the two observers have remarkably similar marginal distributions. In addition, there is clear right-skewness in all three marginal distributions, invalidating the normality assumption for the data (Exercise 7.12).

To get the empirical cdf $\hat{F}$, $3^3 = 27$ triplets (or 3-tuples) are formed for each subject using the repeated measurements of the three methods. This results in a total of $85 \times 27 = 2295$ triplets in the data. Therefore, from (10.4), $\hat{F}$ is a trivariate cdf that gives a weight of $1/2295$ to each triplet. From Exercise 10.15, the plug-in estimates of (mean, standard deviation) of measurements from methods 1, 2, and 3 are $(127.4, 31.0)$, $(127.3, 30.7)$, and $(143.0, 32.5)$, respectively. In addition, the estimated correlation between the methods in the pairs $(1, 2)$, $(1, 3)$, and $(2, 3)$ are 0.97, 0.79, and 0.79, respectively. Thus, the two observers have practically the same estimated means and variances, and their correlation is very high. On the other hand, the monitor produces higher readings than the observers by about 16 mm Hg on average and correlates less with their measurements. It also has a somewhat higher variability than the observers. The standard deviation of the difference between two observers is about 7 and it is three times as much for the difference between the monitor and an observer.

For similarity evaluation, Table 10.2 presents estimates and 95% simultaneous confidence intervals for the three all-pairwise mean differences and variance ratios. The critical point for the former is 2.24 and it is 2.25 for the latter on the log scale. The first interval for mean difference is tight around zero, implying no difference in the means of the two

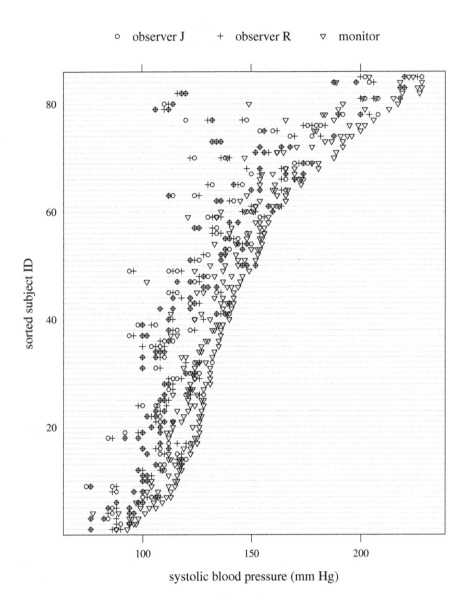

Figure 10.4   Trellis plot of replicated blood pressure data.

observers. The other two intervals are essentially identical and confirm that the monitor has a higher mean than the observers. The first interval for variance ratio, although barely covering one, is quite tight around 1.02. The value of 1 is deep inside the remaining two intervals, which are also essentially identical. This suggests that all methods can be taken to have the same variance. Overall, the two observers have very similar characteristics, but the same is not true for the monitor-observer pairs due to the larger mean of the monitor.

For agreement evaluation, Table 10.3 presents estimates and 95% simultaneous one-sided confidence bounds for the three all-pairwise CCCs and TDIs with $p = 0.90$. The

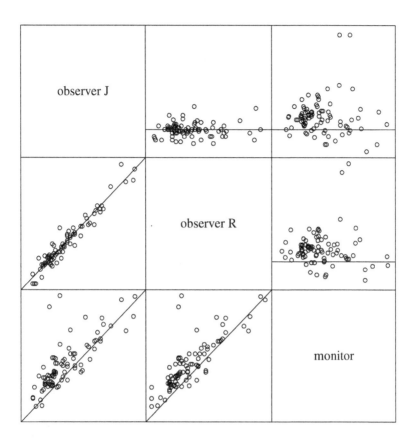

Figure 10.5 A matrix of scatterplots of systolic blood pressures with line of equality (below the diagonal) and Bland-Altman plots with zero line (above the diagonal) for replicated blood pressure data. One measurement per method from each of the 85 subjects is randomly selected for this plot. The measurements range from 76 to 227 mm Hg and their differences range from −25 to 111 mm Hg.

critical point is 1.92 for CCC after applying the Fisher's z-transformation. The TDI critical point, for use in (10.15), is 1.99. The TDI bounds imply that for 90% of subjects the measurement differences between method pairs (1, 2), (1, 3), and (2, 3) are estimated to lie between ±14, ±54, and ±53, respectively. The value of 14 is about 11% of the average value for the observers. This extent of agreement can be considered acceptable. However, this is clearly not the case for the two monitor-observer pairs that have quite similar extent of agreement. The same conclusion is reached on the basis of CCC bounds. It is also evident that the monitor's unacceptable agreement with the observers is caused by a large mean difference and a relatively low correlation that itself is a consequence of the monitor's relatively high within-subject variation (see the trellis plot in Figure 10.4). The first cause can be fixed by subtracting 15.6 from the monitor's measurements. But this recalibration

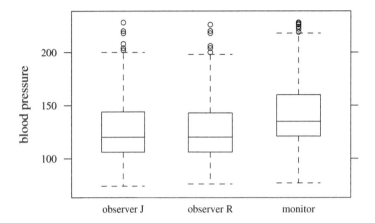

Figure 10.6   Side-by-side boxplots for all measurements of replicated blood pressure data.

Pair	$\mu_l - \mu_j$		σ_l^2/σ_j^2	
(j, l)	Estimate	95% Interval	Estimate	95% Interval
$(1, 2)$	-0.1	$(-0.4, 0.2)$	1.02	$(1.00, 1.04)$
$(1, 3)$	15.6	$(11.0, 20.2)$	0.91	$(0.69, 1.21)$
$(2, 3)$	15.7	$(11.2, 20.3)$	0.90	$(0.68, 1.18)$

Table 10.2   Estimates and two-sided 95% simultaneous confidence intervals for all-pairwise mean differences and variance ratios for replicated blood pressure data. Methods 1, 2, and 3 refer to observers J and R and the monitor, respectively.

Pair	CCC_{jl}		TDI_{jl}	
(j, l)	Estimate	95% Lower Bound	Estimate	95% Upper Bound
$(1, 2)$	0.97	0.96	12	14
$(1, 3)$	0.70	0.52	34	54
$(2, 3)$	0.70	0.52	35	53

Table 10.3   Estimates and one-sided 95% simultaneous confidence bounds for all-pairwise CCCs and TDIs (with $p = 0.90$) for replicated blood pressure data. Methods 1, 2, and 3 refer to observers J and R and the monitor, respectively.

helps only to a limited extent as the new TDI bounds for (1, 3) and (2, 3) pairs are still high at 40 and 38, respectively, and both the new CCC bounds are still relatively low at 0.78. Further improvement requires reducing the monitor's error variation, which cannot be achieved by a simple recalibration.

For these data also, it may be of interest to compare these results with a normality-based parametric analysis even though the normality assumption does not hold here. However, the standard mixed-effects model (7.4) for unlinked repeated measurements data does not provide a reliable fit and an alternative model is fit in Exercise 7.12. Comparison of results under this model is left to Exercise 10.15.

10.6 CHAPTER SUMMARY

1. The methodology presented here is a nonparametric analog of the normality-based approach developed in Chapters 4, 5 and 7 for J (≥ 2) methods for unreplicated and unlinked repeated measurements data.

2. It makes no assumption about the shape of the data distribution.

3. No assumption is needed about scales for the measurement methods. But the data are assumed to be homoscedastic.

4. It allows for simultaneous inference on pairwise measures when more than two methods are compared.

5. It takes a statistical functional approach where population quantities are considered features of the population distribution and are estimated using the same features of the empirical distribution.

6. Weights are used to get the empirical distribution for repeated measurements data.

7. The design for repeated measurements data may be balanced or unbalanced.

8. For balanced designs and large number of subjects, the nonparametric inferences on moment-based measures are often similar to their normality-based counterparts.

9. The observed measurements are not decomposed into true values and errors, precluding the use of similarity measures such as bias difference and precision ratio. Instead, mean difference and variance ratio are used.

10. The methodology is valid for large number of subjects.

10.7 TECHNICAL DETAILS

Let $\mathcal{Y}$ be the support of the population vector $\mathbf{Y} = (Y_1, \ldots, Y_J)^T$ with cdf $F(\mathbf{y})$ and pdf or pmf $p_F(\mathbf{y})$. Let $\mathcal{S}$ denote the index set of Q pairs of the form (j, l), $j < l = 1, \ldots, J$ indicating the specific method pairs of interest. For a $(j, l) \in \mathcal{S}$, a measure of similarity or agreement can be written as a statistical functional $\phi_{jl} = h_{jl}(F)$, where h_{jl} is a known real-valued function defined over a class $\mathcal{F}$ of J-variate cdfs on $\mathcal{Y}$ for which ϕ_{jl} is well-defined. The measures of interest in this chapter are represented as statistical functionals and these are defined in terms of expectations that are assumed to exist. An expectation can be explicitly written as a statistical functional in the following manner:

$$E_F\{a(\mathbf{Y})\} = \int_{\mathcal{Y}} a(\mathbf{y})dF(\mathbf{y}), \tag{10.16}$$

where

$$\int_{\mathcal{Y}} a(\mathbf{y})dF(\mathbf{y}) = \begin{cases} \int_{\mathcal{Y}} a(\mathbf{y})p_F(\mathbf{y})dy, & \text{if } \mathbf{Y} \text{ is continuous,} \\ \sum_{\mathbf{y} \in \mathcal{Y}} a(\mathbf{y})p_F(\mathbf{y}), & \text{if } \mathbf{Y} \text{ is discrete.} \end{cases}$$

Let ϕ denote the $Q \times 1$ vector of values of a measure for the method pairs of interest. Its components are ϕ_{jl}, $(j, l) \in \mathcal{S}$, and it is also a statistical functional $\phi = \mathbf{h}(F)$, where the function $\mathbf{h} : \mathcal{F} \mapsto \mathbb{R}^Q$ essentially stacks the h_{jl} in a $Q \times 1$ vector. The plug-in estimator of ϕ is $\hat{\phi} = \mathbf{h}(\hat{F})$, a $Q \times 1$ vector with components $\hat{\phi}_{jl} = h_{jl}(\hat{F})$. Under certain assumptions, $\hat{\phi}$ approximately follows a $\mathcal{N}_Q(\phi, n^{-1}\hat{\Omega})$ distribution when n is large. Assuming that we know how to compute the $Q \times Q$ estimated covariance matrix $\hat{\Omega}$, this result can be used just as in Chapter 7 to obtain appropriate simultaneous confidence bounds and intervals for the Q values of a measure of interest.

10.7.1 The Ω Matrix

To compute $\hat{\Omega}$, we first need its population counterpart, the $Q \times Q$ covariance matrix Ω. It is defined in terms of variances and covariances of the *influence function* of the measure. The influence function of a scalar functional $h(F)$ measures the rate at which the functional changes when F is contaminated by a small probability of contamination $\mathbf{y}$. It plays a key role in the theory of nonparametric and robust estimators. To define it, let $\delta_{\mathbf{y}}$ be the cdf of a J-variate distribution that assigns probability 1 to the point $\mathbf{y}$. Then, the influence function of $h(F)$ is

$$L(\mathbf{y}, F) = \frac{d}{d\epsilon} h\{(1 - \epsilon)F + \epsilon\delta_{\mathbf{y}}\}|_{\epsilon=0}. \tag{10.17}$$

Here $(1-\epsilon)F + \epsilon\delta_{\mathbf{y}}$ is the cdf of a contaminated distribution under which the random vector follows the distribution F with probability $1 - \epsilon$ and the distribution $\delta_{\mathbf{y}}$ with probability ϵ. Being a function of $\mathbf{Y} = \mathbf{y}$, the influence function is a random quantity. Its expectation is taken to be zero by definition. For example, consider the expectation functional $E_F\{a(\mathbf{Y})\}$ given by (10.16). Its influence function is (Exercise 10.9)

$$L(\mathbf{y}, F) = a(\mathbf{y}) - E_F\{a(\mathbf{Y})\}, \tag{10.18}$$

which obviously has expectation zero.

Let $L_{jl}(y_j, y_l) \equiv L_{jl}(\mathbf{y}, F)$ denote the influence function of the measure ϕ_{jl}, $(j, l) \in \mathcal{S}$. Next, let ω_{jl}^2 and $\omega_{jl,st}$, $(j, l) \neq (s, t) \in \mathcal{S}$, respectively, denote the diagonal and the off-diagonal elements of Ω. Also let Y_j^* be a replication of Y_j, $j = 1, \ldots, J$ from the same subject. The elements of Ω can be written in terms of the influence functions as:

$$\omega_{jl}^2 = n \sum_{i=1}^{n} w^2(n, \mathbf{m}_i) \left(\frac{c_i^2}{m_{ij}m_{il}} \right) [E\{L_{jl}^2(Y_j, Y_l)\}$$
$$+ (m_{ij} - 1)E\{L_{jl}(Y_j, Y_l)L_{jl}(Y_j^*, Y_l)\} + (m_{il} - 1)E\{L_{jl}(Y_j, Y_l)L_{jl}(Y_j, Y_l^*)\}$$
$$+ (m_{ij} - 1)(m_{il} - 1)E\{L_{jl}(Y_j, Y_l)L_{jl}(Y_j^*, Y_l^*)\}],$$
$$\omega_{jl,st} = n \sum_{i=1}^{n} w^2(n, \mathbf{m}_i) c_i^2 \times$$

$$\begin{cases} \frac{1}{m_{ij}}\left[E\{L_{jl}(Y_j,Y_l)L_{jt}(Y_j,Y_t)\}+(m_{ij}-1)E\{L_{jl}(Y_j,Y_l)L_{jt}(Y_j^*,Y_t)\}\right], & s=j, t\neq l,\\ \frac{1}{m_{il}}\left[E\{L_{jl}(Y_j,Y_l)L_{lt}(Y_l,Y_t)\}+(m_{il}-1)E\{L_{jl}(Y_j,Y_l)L_{lt}(Y_l^*,Y_t)\}\right], & s=l, t\neq j,\\ \frac{1}{m_{il}}\left[E\{L_{jl}(Y_j,Y_l)L_{sl}(Y_s,Y_l)\}+(m_{il}-1)E\{L_{jl}(Y_j,Y_l)L_{sl}(Y_s,Y_l^*)\}\right], & s\neq j, t=l,\\ \frac{1}{m_{ij}}\left[E\{L_{jl}(Y_j,Y_l)L_{sj}(Y_s,Y_j)\}+(m_{ij}-1)E\{L_{jl}(Y_j,Y_l)L_{sj}(Y_s,Y_j^*)\}\right], & s\neq l, t=j,\\ E\{L_{jl}(Y_j,Y_l)L_{st}(Y_s,Y_t)\}. & s\neq j, t\neq l. \end{cases}$$
$$(10.19)$$

The expectations here are with respect to the distribution F; it has been dropped from the notation to reduce clutter. The expressions simplify when the design is balanced (Exercise 10.10). In particular, $\boldsymbol{\Omega}$ does not depend on n anymore. Further simplification occurs for unreplicated measurements. Taking $m_{ij}=1$ for all i,j in (10.19) yields

$$\omega_{jl}^2 = E\{L_{jl}^2(Y_j,Y_l)\}, \quad \omega_{jl,st} = E\{L_{jl}(Y_j,Y_l)L_{st}(Y_s,Y_t)\}. \qquad (10.20)$$

Thus, in the unreplicated case, ω_{jl}^2 is the variance of the influence function of ϕ_{jl}, and $\omega_{jl,st}$ is the covariance between the influence functions of ϕ_{jl} and ϕ_{st}, regardless of whether the method pairs (j,l) and (s,t) contain any common methods. In addition, if $J=2$, we have $Q=1$, and the matrix $\boldsymbol{\Omega}$ simply represents the scalar quantity ω_{12}^2.

10.7.2 Estimation of Ω

Let $\hat{L}_{jl}(y_j,y_l) \equiv L_{jl}(\mathbf{y},\hat{F})$ denote the empirical counterpart of the influence function $L_{jl}(y_j,y_l) \equiv L_{jl}(\mathbf{y},F)$, $(j,l) \in \mathcal{S}$. The estimator $\hat{\boldsymbol{\Omega}}$ of $\boldsymbol{\Omega}$ can be obtained by replacing the population moments of $L_{jl}(Y_j,Y_l)$ in (10.19) with their sample analogs based on $\hat{L}_{jl}(Y_j,Y_l)$. Essentially the latter can be obtained by first computing the corresponding sample moments for each subject separately and then averaging them to come up with overall estimates. Specifically, the four moments needed for estimating ω_{jl}^2 can be estimated in the following manner:

$$E\{L_{jl}^2(Y_j,Y_l)\}: \quad \frac{1}{n}\sum_{i=1}^{n}\frac{1}{m_{ij}m_{il}}\sum_{k_j=1}^{m_{ij}}\sum_{k_l=1}^{m_{il}}\hat{L}_{jl}^2(Y_{ijk_j},Y_{ilk_l}),$$

$$E\{L_{jl}(Y_j,Y_l)L_{jl}(Y_j^*,Y_l)\}: \quad \frac{1}{\#\{i:m_{ij}>1\}}\sum_{i=1}^{\#\{i:m_{ij}>1\}}\frac{1}{m_{ij}m_{il}(m_{ij}-1)}$$
$$\times \sum_{k_j=1}^{m_{ij}}\sum_{k_l=1}^{m_{il}}\sum_{r_j\neq k_j=1}^{m_{ij}}\hat{L}_{jl}(Y_{ijk_j},Y_{ilk_l})\hat{L}_{jl}(Y_{ijr_j},Y_{ilk_l}),$$

$$E\{L_{jl}(Y_j,Y_l)L_{jl}(Y_j,Y_l^*)\}: \quad \frac{1}{\#\{i:m_{il}>1\}}\sum_{i=1}^{\#\{i:m_{il}>1\}}\frac{1}{m_{ij}m_{il}(m_{il}-1)}$$
$$\times \sum_{k_j=1}^{m_{ij}}\sum_{k_l=1}^{m_{il}}\sum_{r_l\neq k_l=1}^{m_{il}}\hat{L}_{jl}(Y_{ijk_j},Y_{ilk_l})\hat{L}_{jl}(Y_{ijk_j},Y_{ilr_l}),$$

$$E\{L_{jl}(Y_j,Y_l)L_{jl}(Y_j^*,Y_l^*)\}: \quad \frac{1}{\#\{i:m_{ij}>1,m_{il}>1\}}$$
$$\times \sum_{i=1}^{\#\{i:m_{ij}>1,m_{il}>1\}}\frac{1}{m_{ij}m_{il}(m_{ij}-1)(m_{il}-1)}$$

$$\times \sum_{k_j=1}^{m_{ij}} \sum_{k_l=1}^{m_{il}} \sum_{r_j \neq k_j=1}^{m_{ij}} \sum_{r_l \neq k_l=1}^{m_{il}} \hat{L}_{jl}(Y_{ijk_j}, Y_{ilk_l}) \hat{L}_{jl}(Y_{ijr_j}, Y_{ilr_l}).$$

Next, consider the moments needed for $\omega_{jl,st}$. We can estimate the moment of the form $E\{L_{jl}(Y_j, Y_l) L_{st}(Y_s, Y_t)\}$ by

$$\frac{1}{n} \sum_{i=1}^{n} \frac{1}{m_{ij} m_{il} m_{is} m_{it}} \sum_{k_j=1}^{m_{ij}} \sum_{k_l=1}^{m_{il}} \sum_{k_s=1}^{m_{is}} \sum_{k_t=1}^{m_{it}} \hat{L}_{jl}(Y_{ijk_j}, Y_{ilk_l}) \hat{L}_{st}(Y_{isk_s}, Y_{itk_t}),$$

where if $s = j$ (or $s = l$), m_{is} is removed from the denominator and the sum over k_s is restricted to $k_s = k_j$ (or $k_s = k_l$); and a similar modification is made if $t = j$ or $t = l$. Further, $E\{L_{jl}(Y_j, Y_l) L_{jt}(Y_j^*, Y_t)\}$ can be estimated as

$$\frac{1}{\#\{i : m_{ij} > 1\}} \sum_{i=1}^{\#\{i : m_{ij} > 1\}} \frac{1}{m_{ij} m_{il}(m_{ij} - 1) m_{it}}$$

$$\times \sum_{k_j=1}^{m_{ij}} \sum_{k_l=1}^{m_{il}} \sum_{r_j \neq k_j=1}^{m_{ij}} \sum_{k_t=1}^{m_{it}} \hat{L}_{jl}(Y_{ijk_j}, Y_{ilk_l}) \hat{L}_{jt}(Y_{ijr_j}, Y_{itk_t}).$$

One can proceed in a similar manner to estimate the remaining three moments, namely, $E\{L_{jl}(Y_j, Y_l) L_{lt}(Y_l^*, Y_t)\}$, $E\{L_{jl}(Y_j, Y_l) L_{sl}(Y_s, Y_l^*)\}$, and $E\{L_{jl}(Y_j, Y_l) L_{sj}(Y_s, Y_j^*)\}$. See Exercises 10.11 and 10.12 for compact expressions for the inner multiple sums involved in these estimates.

10.7.3   Influence Functions for the Measures

The influence functions $L_{jl}(y_j, y_l)$ for the measures ϕ_{jl} of similarity and agreement considered in Section 10.4 are as follows (Exercise 10.13):

$$\mu_l - \mu_j : (y_l - y_j) - (\mu_l - \mu_j),$$

$$\sigma_l^2 / \sigma_j^2 : \frac{\sigma_j^2 \{(y_l - \mu_l)^2 - \sigma_l^2\} - \sigma_l^2 \{(y_j - \mu_j)^2 - \sigma_j^2\}}{\sigma_j^4},$$

$$\mathrm{CCC}_{jl} : \frac{2(y_j - \mu_j)(y_l - \mu_l) - \mathrm{CCC}_{jl}(y_j^2 + y_l^2 - 2y_j \mu_l - 2y_l \mu_j + 2\mu_j \mu_l)}{\sigma_j^2 + \sigma_l^2 + (\mu_l - \mu_j)^2},$$

$$\mathrm{TDI}_{jl}(p) : \frac{-I\{|y_l - y_j| \leq \mathrm{TDI}_{jl}(p)\} + p}{g_{jl}\{\mathrm{TDI}(p)\}}, \tag{10.21}$$

where g_{jl} is the pdf of $|Y_l - Y_j|$ with cdf G_{jl}. The empirical counterparts of these influences are used as in Section 10.7.2 to estimate the covariance matrix for the estimated measures.

10.7.4   TDI Confidence Bounds

From the TDI's influence function in (10.21), it is clear that an estimate of the pdf g_{jl} at an estimated TDI—typically a relatively large percentile—is needed to compute SEs and confidence bounds. However, as mentioned previously, density estimates in the tails are generally not stable unless n is quite large. If one is willing to forgo the SEs, the density estimation can be avoided by using the confidence bounds (10.15). For this, one works with the cdf G_{jl} instead of its inverse. To be precise, $\phi_{jl} = G_{jl}(x)$ for an appropriate x is taken as the agreement measure. (Recall from Chapter 2 that this measure is in fact the index *coverage probability* defined by (2.24).) It is estimated as $\hat{\phi}_{jl} = \hat{G}_{jl}(x)$. Being an expectation functional, its influence function from Exercise 10.9 is

$$L_{jl}(y_j, y_l) = I(|y_l - y_j| \leq x) - G_{jl}(x). \tag{10.22}$$

With $\widehat{\text{TDI}}_{jl}(p)$ as x, one proceeds in the same way as for other measures to compute simultaneous upper confidence bounds for ϕ_{jl}, $(j, l) \in \mathcal{S}$. These have the form

$$\hat{G}_{jl}\big(\widehat{\text{TDI}}_{jl}(p)\big) - \text{critical point} \times \text{SE}\big\{\hat{G}_{jl}\big(\widehat{\text{TDI}}_{jl}(p)\big)\big\}.$$

Thereupon, the estimate $\hat{G}_{jl}\big(\widehat{\text{TDI}}_{jl}(p)\big)$ in the first term in the expression above is replaced by p, the quantity it actually estimates, and G_{jl}^{-1} is evaluated at the resulting value, yielding the bounds given in (10.15).

10.7.5 Summary of Steps

To summarize, the steps involved in constructing nonparametric simultaneous confidence intervals for ϕ_{jl}, $(j, l) \in \mathcal{S}$ are as follows:

1. Estimate the cdf F by the empirical cdf $\hat{F}$ using (10.2).

2. Compute the plug-in estimate $\hat{\phi}_{jl} = h_{jl}(\hat{F})$ using the joint pmf (10.7) of (Y_j, Y_l) under $\hat{F}$.

3. Compute the empirical influences $\hat{L}_{jl}(y_j, y_l)$ for each observed pair (Y_{ijk_j}, Y_{ilk_l}), $k_j = 1, \ldots, m_{ij}$, $k_l = 1, \ldots, m_{il}$ using (10.21) or (10.22).

4. Repeat steps 2 and 3 for each $(j, l) \in \mathcal{S}$ to get the estimate $\hat{\phi}$ of the vector ϕ and compute its estimated covariance matrix $n^{-1}\hat{\Omega}$.

5. Apply the methodology of Section 3.3 to compute appropriate critical points for simultaneous bounds and intervals and use them in (10.14) and (10.15).

10.8 BIBLIOGRAPHIC NOTE

The nonparametric methodology of this chapter is largely based on Choudhary (2010). The article provides the underlying technical details, including a derivation of the asymptotic normality of plug-in estimators under a specified set of assumptions. The use of weights to compute empirical cdf from repeated measurements data is motivated by Olsson and Rootzén (1996), who focus on nonparametric estimation of quantiles of a single variable. Both articles also present a comparison of estimators obtained using different weight functions in the case of unbalanced designs. Lehmann (1998) provides a gentle introduction to nonparametric estimation, statistical functionals, and influence functions. More rigorous and complete accounts are given by Fernholz (1983) and van der Vaart (1998).

A key attraction of the statistical functional approach is that it provides a unified nonparametric framework for inference on various measures of similarity and agreement. In the method comparison literature, it was first used by Guo and Manatunga (2007), although only for inference on CCC with unreplicated data under univariate censoring. For CCC, an alternative approach based on U-statistics has been developed by King and Chinchilli and their coauthors in a number of articles, including King and Chinchilli (2001a, b) and King et al. (2007a, b). The two nonparametric approaches for CCC differ in assumptions, but are expected to lead to similar inferences when n is large. For TDI, an alternative approach based on order statistics is proposed in Perez-Jaume and Carrasco (2015). This article also compares the two nonparametric approaches for TDI.

The normality-based methodologies may lead to inaccurate inferences for non-normal method comparison data. This has been demonstrated by Carrasco et al. (2007) for CCC and by Perez-Jaume and Carrasco (2015) for TDI. We have illustrated a nonparametric approach for handling non-normal data. An alternative is to use a parametric mixed-effects model approach based on distributions other than the normal, for example, a lognormal distribution for random effects (Carrasco et al., 2007), or more general skewed and heavy-tailed distributions for random effects or errors that include the normal as a special case (Sengupta et al., 2015). These model-based approaches work for both CCC and TDI. Yet another alternative, though only for moment-based measures such as CCC, is to use GEE to directly model the moments rather than modeling the entire data distribution. Such a semiparametric approach has been taken by a number of authors, including Barnhart and Williamson (2001), Barnhart et al. (2002, 2005), and Lin et al. (2007). The moment-based measures may be unduly affected by outliers in the data. King and Chinchilli (2001b) address this issue for CCC in the case of paired measurements data by developing its robust versions. Their approach is to replace the squared-error distance function built into the definition of CCC by alternate functions that are less susceptible to outliers, for example, absolute error distance functions and their Winsorized versions. A similar approach can be adopted for the other measures.

Data Sources

The unreplicated and the replicated blood pressure data are from Bland and Altman (1995b) and Bland and Altman (1999), respectively. They can be obtained from the book's website.

EXERCISES

10.1 Suppose a scalar random variable X follows a probability distribution with cdf $G(x)$. Let $g(x)$ denote the pdf if X is continuous and the pmf if it is discrete. Define the notation,

$$\int_{\mathcal{X}} a(x)dG(x) = \begin{cases} \int_{\mathcal{X}} a(x)g(x)dx, & \text{if } X \text{ is continuous,} \\ \sum_{x \in \mathcal{X}} a(x)g(x), & \text{if } X \text{ is discrete,} \end{cases}$$

where $\mathcal{X}$ is the support of X. Also, define the inverse cdf $G(x)$ as $G^{-1}(u) = \min\{x : G(x) \geq u\}$.

(a) Write the mean and variance of X as statistical functionals.

(b) Write the $100p$th percentile of X as a statistical functional.

10.2 Consider the empirical cdf $\hat{F}$ given by (10.1) for estimating F from unreplicated data. There may be ties among observations from a given method.

(a) Show that the joint pmf of $(Y_1, \ldots, Y_J)$ under $\hat{F}$ is

$$p_{\hat{F}}(y_1, \ldots, y_J) = \frac{1}{n} \sum_{i=1}^{n} I(Y_{i1} = y_1, \ldots, Y_{iJ} = y_J).$$

(b) Show that the joint pmf of (Y_j, Y_l) under $\hat{F}$ is

$$p_{\hat{F}}(y_j, y_l) = \frac{1}{n} \sum_{i=1}^{n} I(Y_{ij} = y_j, Y_{il} = y_l), \ j \neq l = 1, \ldots, J.$$

(c) Show that the marginal pmf of Y_j under $\hat{F}$ is

$$p_{\hat{F}}(y_j) = \frac{1}{n} \sum_{i=1}^{n} I(Y_{ij} = y_j), \ j = 1, \ldots, J.$$

(d) Let $h(F)$ be the population mean of Y_j. Show that the plug-in estimator $h(\hat{F})$ is the sample mean $\overline{Y}_{\cdot j}$.

(e) Let $h(F)$ be the population variance of Y_j. Show that the plug-in estimator $h(\hat{F})$ is the sample variance $\sum_{i=1}^{n} (Y_{ij} - \overline{Y}_{\cdot j})^2 / n$ with divisor n.

(f) Let $h(F)$ be the population covariance between Y_j and Y_l. Show that the plug-in estimator is the sample covariance $h(\hat{F}) = \sum_{i=1}^{n} (Y_{ij} - \overline{Y}_{\cdot j})(Y_{il} - \overline{Y}_{\cdot l})/n$ with divisor n.

(g) Let $h(F)$ be the population correlation between Y_j and Y_l. Show that the plug-in estimator $h(\hat{F})$ is the sample correlation between Y_j and Y_l.

(h) Let $h(F)$ be the $100p$th population percentile of Y_j. Show that the plug-in estimator $h(\hat{F}) = \min\{y : \hat{F}_j(y) \geq p\}$, where $\hat{F}_j$ is the cdf associated with the pmf given in part (c).

(i) Show that the plug-in estimators of means, variances, and correlation of Y_j and Y_l obtained in previous parts are identical to the ones in (10.10). (When $J = 2$, they are also identical to the ML estimators given by (4.8) under the bivariate normal model (4.6).)

10.3 Verify the expressions for the pmfs given in (10.6)–(10.8) under the empirical distribution (10.2) for $(Y_1, \ldots, Y_J)$.

10.4 (Continuation of Exercise 10.3) Assume now that there are no within-method ties in the data. Establish the following:

(a) The joint pmf of $(Y_1, \ldots, Y_J)$ in (10.6) can be written as

$$p_{\hat{F}}(y_{i1k_1}, \ldots, y_{iJk_J}) = w(n, \mathbf{m}_i).$$

(b) The joint pmf of (Y_j, Y_l) in (10.7) can be written as

$$p_{\hat{F}}(y_{ijk_j}, y_{ilk_l}) = w(n, \mathbf{m}_i) \left(\frac{c_i}{m_{ij} m_{il}} \right).$$

(c) The marginal pmf of Y_j in (10.8) can be written as

$$p_{\hat{F}}(y_{ijk_j}) = w(n, \mathbf{m}_i) \left(\frac{c_i}{m_{ij}} \right).$$

Here $k_j = 1, \ldots, m_{ij}, j \neq l = 1, \ldots, J, i = 1, \ldots, n$.

10.5 (Continuation of Exercise 10.4) Assume further that the design is balanced with all $m_{ij} = m$. Show that the pmfs in Exercise 10.4 simplify to the following expressions:

$$p_{\hat{F}}(y_{i1k_1}, \ldots, y_{iJk_J}) = \frac{1}{nm^J},$$

$$p_{\hat{F}}(y_{ijk_j}, y_{ilk_l}) = \frac{1}{nm^2},$$

$$p_{\hat{F}}(y_{ijk_j}) = \frac{1}{nm},$$

for $k_j = 1, \ldots, m, j \neq l = 1, \ldots, J, i = 1, \ldots, n$.

10.6 Consider the cdf $\hat{F}$ defined in (10.2) with weight function w satisfying the unbiasedness condition (10.3). Assume that the indicator functions I involved in $\hat{F}$ have a common correlation $\rho(\mathbf{y})$, with $\mathbf{y} = (y_1, \ldots, y_J)^T$.

(a) Show that the optimal weight function that makes $\hat{F}(\mathbf{y})$ the minimum variance unbiased estimator of $F(\mathbf{y})$ in the family of estimators satisfying (10.2) and (10.3) is

$$w(n, \mathbf{m}_i) = \frac{\{1 + (c_i - 1)\rho(\mathbf{y})\}^{-1}}{\sum_{l=1}^{n} c_l \{1 + (c_l - 1)\rho(\mathbf{y})\}^{-1}}.$$

(b) The optimal weight function depends on $\mathbf{y}$ through $\rho(\mathbf{y})$. Discuss its impact on the properties of $\hat{F}$. In particular, does it guarantee $\hat{F}(\mathbf{y})$ to be non-decreasing in $\mathbf{y}$—a property necessary for $\hat{F}$ to be a valid cdf?

(c) For a balanced design, show that the optimal function reduces to (10.4).

(d) For an unbalanced design, show that the optimal function reduces to w_1 and w_2 given in (10.5) when $\rho(\mathbf{y}) = 1$ and $\rho(\mathbf{y}) = 0$, respectively.

(This exercise offers a straightforward generalization of a similar result in Olsson and Rootzén (1996) for univariate distribution.)

10.7 Show that the measures of similarity and agreement considered in Section 10.4 can be written as statistical functionals in the following manner:

$$\mu_l - \mu_j = E_F(Y_l - Y_j),$$

$$\frac{\sigma_l^2}{\sigma_j^2} = \frac{E_F(Y_l^2) - \{E_F(Y_l)\}^2}{E_F(Y_j^2) - \{E_F(Y_j)\}^2},$$

$$\text{CCC}_{jl} = \frac{2\{E_F(Y_j Y_l) - E_F(Y_j)E_F(Y_l)\}}{E_F(Y_j^2) + E_F(Y_l^2) - 2E_F(Y_j)E_F(Y_l)},$$

$$\text{TDI}_{jl}(p) = G_{jl}^{-1}(p),$$

where $G_{jl}(x) = E_F\{I(|Y_l - Y_j| \le x)\}$, $x > 0$ is the cdf of $|Y_l - Y_j|$.

10.8 (a) Show that the estimated cdf in (10.11) can be written as

$$\hat{G}_{jl}(x) = \sum_{i=1}^{n} w(n, \mathbf{m}_i) \left(\frac{c_i}{m_{ij}m_{il}} \right) \sum_{k_j=1}^{m_{ij}} \sum_{k_l=1}^{m_{il}} I(|Y_{ijk_j} - Y_{ilk_l}| \le x), \quad x > 0.$$

(b) Show that the estimated moments in (10.9) can be written as

$$E_{\hat{F}}(Y_j^r) = \sum_{i=1}^{n} w(n, \mathbf{m}_i) \left(\frac{c_i}{m_{ij}} \right) \sum_{k_j=1}^{m_{ij}} Y_{ijk_j}^r, \quad r = 1, 2,$$

$$E_{\hat{F}}(Y_j Y_l) = \sum_{i=1}^{n} w(n, \mathbf{m}_i) \left(\frac{c_i}{m_{ij}m_{il}} \right) \sum_{k_j=1}^{m_{ij}} \sum_{k_l=1}^{m_{il}} Y_{ijk_j} Y_{ilk_l}.$$

10.9 Consider the expectation functional $E_F\{a(\mathbf{Y})\}$ given by (10.16). Show that its influence function is $L(\mathbf{y}, F) = a(\mathbf{y}) - E_F\{a(\mathbf{Y})\}$.

10.10 When the design is balanced with all $m_{ij} = m$, show that the elements of $\boldsymbol{\Omega}$ given in (10.19) have the following simplified expressions:

$$\omega_{jl}^2 = \frac{1}{m^2} \big[E\{L_{jl}^2(Y_j, Y_l)\} + (m-1)E\{L_{jl}(Y_j, Y_l)L_{jl}(Y_j^*, Y_l)\}$$
$$+ (m-1)E\{L_{jl}(Y_j, Y_l)L_{jl}(Y_j, Y_l^*)\} + (m-1)^2 E\{L_{jl}(Y_j, Y_l)L_{jl}(Y_j^*, Y_l^*)\} \big],$$

$$\omega_{jl,st} = \frac{1}{m} \times$$

$$\begin{cases} \big[E\{L_{jl}(Y_j, Y_l)L_{jt}(Y_j, Y_t)\} + (m-1)E\{L_{jl}(Y_j, Y_l)L_{jt}(Y_j^*, Y_t)\} \big], & s = j, t \ne l, \\ \big[E\{L_{jl}(Y_j, Y_l)L_{lt}(Y_l, Y_t)\} + (m-1)E\{L_{jl}(Y_j, Y_l)L_{lt}(Y_l^*, Y_t)\} \big], & s = l, t \ne j, \\ \big[E\{L_{jl}(Y_j, Y_l)L_{sl}(Y_s, Y_l)\} + (m-1)E\{L_{jl}(Y_j, Y_l)L_{sl}(Y_s, Y_l^*)\} \big], & s \ne j, t = l, \\ \big[E\{L_{jl}(Y_j, Y_l)L_{sj}(Y_s, Y_j)\} + (m-1)E\{L_{jl}(Y_j, Y_l)L_{sj}(Y_s, Y_j^*)\} \big], & s \ne l, t = j, \\ mE\{L_{jl}(Y_j, Y_l)L_{st}(Y_s, Y_t)\}, & s \ne j, t \ne l. \end{cases}$$

10.11 Let $\mathbf{A}$ denote an $m_{ij} \times m_{il}$ matrix with (p, q)th element $a_{pq} = \hat{L}_{jl}(Y_{ijp}, Y_{ilq})$. Define the column sum $a_{p\cdot} = \sum_q a_{pq}$, the row sum $a_{\cdot q} = \sum_p a_{pq}$ and the overall sum $a_{\cdot\cdot} = \sum_p \sum_q a_{pq}$. Also define the sums of squares: $a_1 = \sum_p \sum_q a_{pq}^2$, $a_2 = \sum_q a_{\cdot q}^2$, $a_3 = \sum_p a_{p\cdot}^2$, and $a_4 = a_{\cdot\cdot}^2$. Verify the following compact expressions for the multiple sums involved in estimation of ω_{jl}^2 in Section 10.7.2:

$$\sum_{k_j=1}^{m_{ij}} \sum_{k_l=1}^{m_{il}} \hat{L}_{jl}^2(Y_{ijk_j}, Y_{ilk_l}) = a_1,$$

$$\sum_{k_j=1}^{m_{ij}} \sum_{k_l=1}^{m_{il}} \sum_{r_j \ne k_j=1}^{m_{ij}} \hat{L}_{jl}(Y_{ijk_j}, Y_{ilk_l}) \hat{L}_{jl}(Y_{ijr_j}, Y_{ilk_l}) = a_2 - a_1,$$

$$\sum_{k_j=1}^{m_{ij}} \sum_{k_l=1}^{m_{il}} \sum_{r_l \ne k_l=1}^{m_{il}} \hat{L}_{jl}(Y_{ijk_j}, Y_{ilk_l}) \hat{L}_{jl}(Y_{ijk_j}, Y_{ilr_l}) = a_3 - a_1,$$

$$\sum_{k_j=1}^{m_{ij}}\sum_{k_l=1}^{m_{il}}\sum_{r_j\neq k_j=1}^{m_{ij}}\sum_{r_l\neq k_l=1}^{m_{il}}\hat{L}_{jl}(Y_{ijk_j},Y_{ilk_l})\hat{L}_{jl}(Y_{ijr_j},Y_{ilr_l})=a_4-a_3-a_2+a_1.$$

10.12 (Continuation of Exercise 10.11) Let $\mathbf{B}$ denote an $m_{is}\times m_{it}$ matrix with (u,v)th element $b_{uv}=\hat{L}_{st}(Y_{isu},Y_{itv})$. Define the column sum $b_{u\cdot}=\sum_v b_{uv}$, the row sum $b_{\cdot v}=\sum_u b_{uv}$ and the overall sum $b_{\cdot\cdot}=\sum_u\sum_v b_{uv}$. Verify the following expressions for the multiple sums involved in estimation of $\omega_{jl,st}$ in Section 10.7.2:

$$\sum_{k_j=1}^{m_{ij}}\sum_{k_l=1}^{m_{il}}\sum_{k_s=1}^{m_{is}}\sum_{k_t=1}^{m_{it}}\hat{L}_{jl}(Y_{ijk_j},Y_{ilk_l})\hat{L}_{st}(Y_{isk_s},Y_{itk_t})=a_{\cdot\cdot}b_{\cdot\cdot},$$

$$\sum_{k_j=1}^{m_{ij}}\sum_{k_l=1}^{m_{il}}\sum_{k_t=1}^{m_{it}}\hat{L}_{jl}(Y_{ijk_j},Y_{ilk_l})\hat{L}_{jt}(Y_{ijk_j},Y_{itk_t})=\sum_p a_{p\cdot}b_{p\cdot},$$

$$\sum_{k_j=1}^{m_{ij}}\sum_{k_l=1}^{m_{il}}\sum_{r_j\neq k_j=1}^{m_{ij}}\sum_{k_t=1}^{m_{it}}\hat{L}_{jl}(Y_{ijk_j},Y_{ilk_l})\hat{L}_{jt}(Y_{ijr_j},Y_{itk_t})=a_{\cdot\cdot}b_{\cdot\cdot}-\sum_p a_{p\cdot}b_{p\cdot}.$$

10.13 Use the definition (10.17) of an influence function to verify the forms for influence functions given in (10.21) for the measures of similarity and agreement considered. [*Hint*: For the first three, use Exercise 10.9 and apply the chain rule if needed. For the last, use implicit differentiation.]

10.14 Consider the unreplicated blood pressure data from Section 10.5.1.

   (a) Perform model diagnostics to verify that the bivariate normal model (4.6) does not fit these data well.

   (b) Verify the results of the nonparametric and parametric analyses in Table 10.1.

10.15 (Continuation of Exercise 7.12) Consider the replicated blood pressure data from Exercise 7.12 and Section 10.5.2.

   (a) Determine the nonparametric estimates of means, variances, and correlations for the three methods.

   (b) Determine the nonparametric estimates of means and standard deviations of $D_{ij}, j=1,2,3$.

   (c) Verify the results of the nonparametric analysis in Tables 10.2 and 10.3.

   (d) Compare conclusions with those of the parametric analysis carried out in Exercise 7.12.

   (e) Which analysis, nonparametric or parametric, would you recommend? Why?

10.16 Table 10.4 presents lengths (in mm) of 25 fiddler crab claws measured by an observer using two Mitutoyo vernier calipers. There are three unlinked replications of each measurement. These data are a subset of the data analyzed in Choudhary et al. (2014) and focus only on observer 1.

   (a) Perform an exploratory analysis of the data.

Claw	Caliper 1	Caliper 2
1	37.9, 37.8, 38.8	37.5, 37.9, 37.8
2	40.8, 40.9, 40.8	41.0, 41.0, 40.9
3	31.0, 31.1, 31.1	31.2, 31.2, 31.1
4	26.9, 26.9, 26.9	27.0, 27.0, 26.8
5	25.3, 25.3, 25.3	25.3, 25.4, 25.2
6	38.9, 39.7, 38.8	38.5, 38.8, 38.7
7	40.1, 40.1, 40.1	40.1, 40.2, 40.0
8	20.4, 20.5, 20.4	20.6, 20.4, 20.5
9	43.7, 43.7, 43.8	43.8, 43.7, 43.7
10	33.4, 33.4, 33.4	33.6, 33.6, 33.5
11	24.3, 24.3, 24.3	24.4, 24.3, 24.3
12	35.2, 35.2, 35.1	35.3, 35.2, 35.2
13	29.6, 29.6, 29.6	29.7, 29.7, 29.6
14	34.8, 34.7, 34.5	35.0, 34.6, 34.8
15	23.3, 23.2, 23.3	23.3, 23.3, 23.3
16	46.7, 46.7, 46.7	46.9, 46.8, 46.7
17	42.6, 42.4, 42.5	42.7, 42.6, 42.5
18	37.7, 37.5, 37.6	37.7, 37.7, 37.0
19	38.4, 38.1, 38.4	38.6, 38.5, 38.4
20	31.7, 31.6, 31.7	31.3, 31.7, 31.7
21	27.0, 26.9, 27.1	27.1, 27.7, 27.1
22	30.6, 30.7, 30.7	30.8, 30.7, 31.8
23	27.0, 27.1, 27.1	27.0, 27.2, 27.2
24	40.1, 40.2, 40.1	40.2, 40.5, 40.2
25	37.1, 37.0, 37.1	37.7, 37.2, 37.2

Table 10.4 Crab claws data consisting of lengths of crab claws (in mm) for Exercise 10.16. They are provided by P. Cassey.

(b) Fit model (7.4) and perform model diagnostics. Does the normality assumption for residuals appear reasonable? Proceed with the normality-based parametric analysis regardless of your finding.

(c) Analyze the data using an appropriate nonparametric approach.

(d) Compare conclusions of the parametric and nonparametric analyses. Which analysis would you prefer? Why?

CHAPTER 11

SAMPLE SIZE DETERMINATION

11.1 PREVIEW

This chapter presents a simulation-based methodology to determine sample sizes for planing method comparison studies involving two methods. The focus is on two designs that are most common in practice, namely, the paired measurements design and the repeated measurements designs for unlinked data. For a paired design, we determine the number of subjects that ensure a specified level of precision for estimate of a measure of inter-method agreement. For a repeated measurements design, we determine the number of subjects as well as the number of replications of a measurement that ensure a specified level of precision for estimates of both inter- and intra-method versions of an agreement measure. The methodology is illustrated through an example.

11.2 INTRODUCTION

So far in this book we have focussed on analysis of method comparison data. This chapter considers sample size determination for planning a method comparison study involving two measurement methods. Generally, by "sample size" we mean n—the number of independent subjects in the study. A study with too small a sample size may not be conclusive. On the other extreme, a study with too large a sample size is wasteful. Therefore, statistical considerations are needed to determine a sample size that may be considered adequate.

Measuring Agreement: Models, Methods, and Applications. By P. K. Choudhary and H. N. Nagaraja
Copyright © 2017 John Wiley & Sons, Inc.

Two approaches for sample size determination are common. One is designed for the situation when testing hypotheses is the inference of primary interest. In this case, the sample size is determined to ensure that the test with a specified level of significance has a desirable power at a given point in the alternative (research) hypothesis region. The other is designed for the situation when a two-sided confidence interval for a parameter is the inference of primary interest. In this case, the sample size is determined to achieve a specified value for either the width or the expected width of the confidence interval. The former is used if the width is a fixed quantity and the latter is used if the width is a random quantity.

In this book, we have primarily relied on confidence intervals for inference instead of hypotheses testing. Therefore, it is natural for us to adopt a sample size approach based on the confidence intervals. To consider this approach in more detail, note that the width of a two-sided confidence interval is often a constant multiple of the estimated standard error of the estimator used. This is certainly the case here because the $100(1 - \alpha)\%$ confidence interval for a parameter or a parametric function ϕ is based on a large-sample normal approximation for its estimator $\hat{\phi}$ and has the form

$$\hat{\phi} \pm z_{1-\alpha/2}\mathrm{SE}(\hat{\phi}).$$

The standard error used above is estimated from the data. It depends on n, albeit this dependence is suppressed in the notation. From the large sample theory, both the true standard error that $\mathrm{SE}(\hat{\phi})$ estimates and the expectation $E\{\mathrm{SE}(\hat{\phi})\}$ of this estimator tend to zero as $n \to \infty$. This implies that we can achieve a specified value for the expected width of the interval, $2z_{1-\alpha/2}E\{\mathrm{SE}(\hat{\phi})\}$, by taking a sufficiently large sample size.

As this sample size approach for a two-sided confidence interval focuses on the width of the interval, it cannot be directly used for the situation when a one-sided confidence interval of the form

$$\left(-\infty, \hat{\phi} - z_{1-\alpha}\mathrm{SE}(\hat{\phi})\right) \ \text{ or } \ \left(\hat{\phi} + z_{1-\alpha}\mathrm{SE}(\hat{\phi}), \infty\right)$$

is of primary interest. This is because such intervals have infinite width. However, by turning the focus away from the width of the interval to the standard error of the estimator, the approach can be easily generalized to handle one-sided intervals as well. The general approach determines the sample size that provides a specified value for $E\{\mathrm{SE}(\hat{\phi})\}$. In the case of two-sided intervals, it is equivalent to the one based on the width because the expected width equals the expected standard error times a known constant.

We now consider some issues that come up while adopting this approach for method comparison studies. First, the analysis of method comparison data involves performing inference on a number of measures of similarity and agreement. In this situation, we may determine the sample size required for each measure and take the maximum of the resulting sample sizes. This maximum simultaneously satisfies the requirements for all the measures. However, given that agreement evaluation is the inference of primary interest, it seems appropriate for sample size determination to target only the agreement measures.

Second, herein we use one-sided confidence bounds for two agreement measures, TDI and CCC. The bounds are obtained by first computing them on transformed scales—$\log(\mathrm{TDI})$ and $z(\mathrm{CCC})$—and then applying the corresponding inverse transformations to the results. This means we need to consider standard errors for estimators on the transformed scale and not on the original scale.

Third, the practitioner may choose one of the agreement measures and base sample size computation on that measure. Alternatively, the computation may be done for both the measures and the larger of the two sample sizes may be taken.

Fourth, the expected standard errors do not have closed-form expressions. Therefore, they need to be computed using Monte Carlo simulation.

Finally, sample size determination necessarily depends on the data design and the model assumed for the data. Therefore, these as well as a *ballpark* value θ_0 for the model parameter vector θ also needs to be specified.

We describe the sample size methodology for paired and repeated measurements designs in terms of a general agreement measure ϕ. These are the two of the most common designs used in method comparison studies. The methodology is illustrated using a case study. Robustness of the methodology with respect to the choice of θ_0 is also discussed.

11.3 THE SAMPLE SIZE METHODOLOGY

11.3.1 Paired Measurements Design

Suppose that the data are to be collected using a paired measurements design and they will be modeled using the bivariate normal model (4.6). We need to determine the number of subjects n that would provide an acceptably small value for $E\{SE(\hat{\phi})\}$. For a given value of n and the ballpark value θ_0, the expected standard error is computed as follows:

Step 1. Simulate the observations Y_{ij}, $j = 1, 2$, $i = 1, \ldots, n$ from the assumed bivariate normal model (4.6) by taking $\theta = \theta_0$.

Step 2. Fit this model to the simulated data by the ML method and follow the prescribed estimation algorithm based on large-sample theory (see Section 4.6) to compute the estimated measure $\hat{\phi}$ and the associated $SE(\hat{\phi})$.

Step 3. Repeat Steps 1 and 2 a large number of times, say L. Let SE_l denote the value of $SE(\hat{\phi})$ in the lth repetition. Approximate $E\{SE(\hat{\phi})\}$ as the average,

$$E\{SE(\hat{\phi})\} \approx \frac{1}{L} \sum_{l=1}^{L} SE_l.$$

This algorithm is used to compute $E\{SE(\hat{\phi})\}$ on a grid of realistic values of n. We can take $L = 500$ for this computation. The results can be summarized graphically by plotting $E\{SE(\hat{\phi})\}$ against n. The practitioner can examine this graph to come up with a level of standard error that is acceptable and take the corresponding n as the desired sample size.

11.3.2 Repeated Measurements Design

Suppose now that unlinked repeated measurements data are to be collected and they will be modeled using the mixed-effects model (5.1). At the planning stage, it is reasonable to assume that the design is balanced with m replications from each method on every subject. In addition to the number of subjects n, we also need to determine m because it also affects precision of the estimates. For this, however, we restrict attention to $m = 2$ and 3 because more than 3 replications is rare in practice and is generally not needed (see Section 11.4).

Unlike the paired data, which only allow the evaluation of inter-method agreement, the repeated measurements data additionally allow the evaluation of intra-method agreement—a key objective of method comparison studies (Section 5.6). Therefore, the sample size determination should be targeted towards both the inferences. To this end, let ϕ_j denote the intra-method version of ϕ for jth method, $j = 1, 2$. We need to determine the number of subjects n and the number of replications m that would provide an acceptably small value for $\max\{E\{\text{SE}(\hat{\phi})\}, E\{\text{SE}(\hat{\phi}_1)\}, E\{\text{SE}(\hat{\phi}_2)\}\}$. This would imply that all the three standard errors exceed the desired level of accuracy. Presumably, the expected standard errors involved in this criterion are decreasing functions of n. They are also assumed to decrease as m increases from 2 to 3. This assumption needs to be verified.

Just like the paired design case, the expected standard errors for a given (n, m) combination and the ballpark value $\boldsymbol{\theta}_0$ can be computed in the following manner:

Step 1. Simulate the observations $Y_{ijk}, k = 1, \ldots, m; j = 1, 2; i = 1, \ldots, n$ from the assumed mixed-effects model (5.1) by taking $\boldsymbol{\theta} = \boldsymbol{\theta}_0$.

Step 2. Fit this model to the simulated data by the ML method, and follow the prescribed estimation algorithm based on large-sample theory (see Section 5.9) to compute the estimated measures $\hat{\phi}$, $\hat{\phi}_1$, and $\hat{\phi}_2$, as well as the associated $\text{SE}(\hat{\phi})$, $\text{SE}(\hat{\phi}_1)$, and $\text{SE}(\hat{\phi}_2)$.

Step 3. Repeat Steps 1 and 2 a large number of times, say L. Let SE_l, $\text{SE}_{1,l}$, and $\text{SE}_{2,l}$ denote the respective values of $\text{SE}(\hat{\phi})$, $\text{SE}(\hat{\phi}_1)$, and $\text{SE}(\hat{\phi}_2)$ in the lth repetition. Approximate the expected standard errors as the averages,

$$E\{\text{SE}(\hat{\phi})\} \approx \frac{1}{L} \sum_{l=1}^{L} \text{SE}_l, \quad E\{\text{SE}(\hat{\phi}_j)\} \approx \frac{1}{L} \sum_{l=1}^{L} \text{SE}_{j,l}, \; j = 1, 2.$$

This algorithm is used to compute the three expected standard errors on a grid of realistic values of n for both $m = 2$ and 3. We can take $L = 500$ for this computation. The results can be summarized graphically by plotting them against n separately for $m = 2$ and 3, possibly on the same graph. The practitioners can examine these results to come up with a level of $\max\{E\{\text{SE}(\hat{\phi})\}, E\{\text{SE}(\hat{\phi}_1)\}, E\{\text{SE}(\hat{\phi}_2)\}\}$ that is acceptable and get the corresponding two combinations of (n, m) values. Thereafter, they can calculate the total cost of sampling associated with the options and choose the cheaper one.

11.4 CASE STUDY

To illustrate the sample size methodology, we need $\boldsymbol{\theta}_0$—the ballpark value for the relevant parameter vector $\boldsymbol{\theta}$. For the paired design, this $\boldsymbol{\theta}$ represents

$$(\mu_1, \mu_2, \log(\sigma_1^2), \log(\sigma_2^2), z(\rho))^T,$$

the vector of parameters of the bivariate normal model (4.6). For the repeated measurements design, the relevant $\boldsymbol{\theta}$ is the vector

$$(\beta_0, \mu_b, \log(\sigma_b^2), \log(\psi^2), \log(\sigma_{e1}^2), \log(\sigma_{e2}^2))^T$$

of parameters of the mixed-effects model (5.1).

We use estimates obtained from the kiwi data analyzed in Section 5.7.1 to get the θ_0. Since these data are unlinked repeated measurements data and are modeled using (5.1), we can directly use the estimates in Table 5.1. This means

$$\theta_0 = (11.3, 311.8, 7.6, 4.6, 4.5, 4.4)^T. \tag{11.1}$$

Further, the corresponding values of inter- and intra-method versions of log transformation of TDI(0.90) are

$$(\log\{\mathrm{TDI}(0.90)\}, \log\{\mathrm{TDI}_1(0.90)\}, \log\{\mathrm{TDI}_2(0.90)\}) = (3.59, 3.07, 3.03),$$

and those of Fisher's z-transformation of CCC are

$$(z(\mathrm{CCC}), z(\mathrm{CCC}_1), z(\mathrm{CCC}_2)) = (1.4, 2.0, 2.0).$$

For the paired design, we take

$$\theta_0 = (311.8, 323.2, 7.7, 7.7, 1.6)^T. \tag{11.2}$$

These are parameters of the fitted bivariate normal distribution (5.35) for kiwi data implied by (11.1). It also follows that the underlying values of TDI and CCC and hence their transformations are the same under the two models.

For the illustration, we target sample size determination on the agreement measure TDI. This is primarily because TDI is easier to interpret and, unlike CCC, is not influenced by the between-subject variation in the data. Nevertheless, we also examine the precision of the estimated $z(\mathrm{CCC})$ for the TDI-based sample size.

We begin with sample size determination for a paired design with θ_0 given by (11.2). The simulation algorithm from Section 11.3.1 is used with $L = 500$ to compute the expected standard errors of $\log\{\mathrm{TDI}(0.90)\}$ and $z(\mathrm{CCC})$ on a grid of values of n between 30 and 200. The results are presented in Figure 11.1. As anticipated, the expected standard error curves for both measures are decreasing in n. Specifically, the standard error decreases from 0.12 to 0.05 in the case of $\log\{\mathrm{TDI}\}$ and from 0.17 to 0.05 in the case of $z(\mathrm{CCC})$.

Suppose the target standard error for $\log\{\mathrm{TDI}(0.90)\}$ is 0.06. If we would like to use a 95% upper confidence bound for $\log\{\mathrm{TDI}(0.90)\}$, the standard error of 0.06 implies that the true TDI(0.90) is no more than $\exp(1.645 \times 0.06) = 1.1$ times its estimate with 95% confidence (Exercise 11.1). Thus, for example, if the estimated TDI is $\exp(3.59) = 36.2$, the 95% upper confidence bound for the true TDI would be $1.1 \times 36.2 = 39.8$. Figure 11.1 shows that the target 0.06 for the expected standard error is achieved by $n = 125$. Therefore, we may take $n = 125$ as the required sample size. This figure also shows that $n = 125$ yields 0.085 as the expected standard error for $z(\mathrm{CCC})$. Thus, for example, if the estimated CCC is $\tanh(1.4) = 0.89$, then with this standard error the 95% lower confidence bound for the true CCC would be

$$\tanh(1.4 - 1.645 \times 0.085) = 0.85.$$

Next, we consider sample size determination for a repeated measurements design with θ_0 given by (11.1). The simulation algorithm from Section 11.3.2 is used to compute expected standard errors of estimators of inter- and intra-method versions of $\log\{\mathrm{TDI}(0.90)\}$ and $z(\mathrm{CCC})$ on the same grid for n as before, separately for $m = 2$ and 3. Figure 11.2 presents

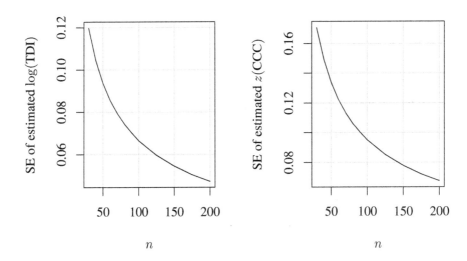

Figure 11.1   Expected standard errors for estimators of $\log\{\text{TDI}(0.90)\}$ (left panel) and $z(\text{CCC})$ (right panel) as functions of n for a paired measurements design.

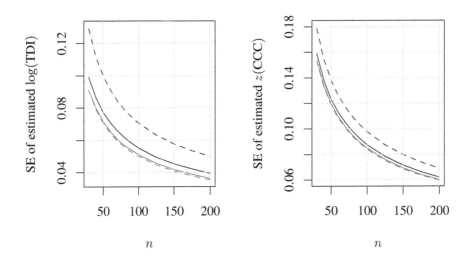

Figure 11.2   Expected standard errors for estimators of inter- and intra-method versions of $\log\{\text{TDI}(0.90)\}$ (left panel) and $z(\text{CCC})$ (right panel) as functions of n for a repeated measurements design with $m = 2$ and 3 replications. In both figures, solid curves are for the inter-method version, with black color for $m = 2$ and gray for $m = 3$. The broken curves are for intra-method version for method 1. (Method 2 results are similar and are not shown.)

(n, m)	$\log\{\text{TDI}(0.90)\}$	$\log\{\text{TDI}_1(0.90)\}$	$z(\text{CCC})$	$z(\text{CCC}_1)$
$(140, 2)$	0.05	0.06	0.07	0.08
$(73, 3)$	0.06	0.06	0.10	0.10
$(73, 4)$	0.06	0.05	0.10	0.09

Table 11.1 Expected standard errors for estimators of various measures.

the results. The results for the two intra-method versions of a measure are virtually indistinguishable. Therefore, only those for method 1 are shown. We see that all the expected standard error curves are decreasing in n for a fixed m, and also in m for a fixed n. Further, for both measures, the curve for the intra-method version remains above its counterpart for the inter-method version when $m = 2$. There is indication that the converse may be true for $m = 3$; nevertheless, the two curves in this case are quite similar.

The target of 0.06 for the maximum of the expected standard errors for estimators of inter- and intra-method versions of $\log\{\text{TDI}(0.90)\}$ can be achieved by two (n, m) combinations—$(140, 2)$ and $(73, 3)$. Although a practitioner can now distinguish between the two options by bringing in sampling cost considerations, it seems rather obvious that $(73, 3)$ is likely to be the cheaper option. This is because the cost of taking an additional replication on an existing subject is usually a small fraction of the cost of recruiting an entirely new subject. The maximum over the expected standard errors for the estimated $z(\text{CCC})$ is approximately 0.08 for the $(140, 2)$ combination of (n, m) and is 0.10 for the $(73, 3)$ combination.

These results indicate that there is much gain in increasing m from 2 to 3. It is then natural to wonder whether the same holds when m is increased from 3 to 4. Exercise 11.2 shows that for $(n, m) = (73, 4)$, the expected standard errors, rounded to two decimal places, in the case of inter- and intra-method versions of $\log\{\text{TDI}(0.90)\}$ are 0.06 and 0.05, respectively. The corresponding values in the case of $z(\text{CCC})$ are 0.10 and 0.09, respectively. Thus, it is clear that there is little gain in increasing m from 3 to 4 because both $(73, 3)$ and $(73, 4)$ combinations of (n, m) lead to the same value for the maximum expected standard error for the estimators of interest. The actual expected standard errors for these (n, m) combinations are given in Table 11.1.

To examine the robustness of the sample sizes determined above, we repeat the calculation for both paired and repeated measurements designs by making a number of changes to θ_0. For the paired design, we set

$$\mu_1 = \mu_2 = 0, \ \rho = 0.9, \ \sigma_1^2 = \sigma_2^2 = \sigma^2, \ \sigma^2 = 2208c, \tag{11.3}$$

where $2208 = \exp(7.7)$ represents the common approximate value for the variances σ_1^2 and σ_2^2 reported in (11.2), and take $c \in \{0.1, 0.5, 2, 4\}$. For the repeated measurements design, we set

$$\beta_0 = \mu_b = 0, \ \sigma_b^2 = (9/10)\sigma^2, \ \psi^2 = \sigma_{e1}^2 = \sigma_{e2}^2 = (1/20)\sigma^2, \tag{11.4}$$

where σ^2 is as defined in (11.3) and varies with $c \in \{0.1, 0.5, 2, 4\}$. From (5.7) and (5.24), these choices imply that the methods have mean zero, their overall variances equal σ^2, their correlation equals 0.9, and two measurements from the same method have a correlation of 0.95. Thus, for both paired and repeated measurements designs, we consider 4 parameter settings, with widely different values for σ^2, that also differ substantially from the original θ_0. It turns out that the results in all cases are practically the same as the ones presented for the original θ_0 (Exercise 11.2). This shows that the sample sizes are quite robust to the choice of θ_0. Essentially, all one needs is a ballpark figure for σ^2, the variance of the measurements. As then the sample size determination can proceed by taking the θ_0 implied by either (11.3) for the paired measurements design or (11.4) for the repeated measurements design.

Finally, in this book, we have advocated the virtues of replicating measurements by arguing that it allows reliable estimation of error variances, which makes the evaluation of intra-method agreement possible. The above results also show that, even for estimation of measures of inter-method agreement, replicated data require fewer subjects than unreplicated data to achieve the same expected standard error. The reduction may be especially substantial in the case of $m = 3$. For example, to achieve the target of 0.06 in the case of $\log\{\mathrm{TDI}(0.90)\}$, we need $n = 125$ for a paired measurements design, whereas only $n = 73$ is needed for a repeated measurements design with $m = 3$. Moreover, we have seen that $n = 125$ for a paired measurements design leads to 0.085 as the expected standard error in the case of $z(\mathrm{CCC})$. The same target is achieved by $n = 100$ for a repeated measurements design with $m = 3$. This is another advantage of a repeated measurements design over a paired measurements design.

11.5 CHAPTER SUMMARY

1. Sample size can be determined by requiring a desirable precision for the estimate of an agreement measure.

2. For a paired measurements design, sample size determination involves computing the number of subjects.

3. For a repeated measurements design, sample size determination involves computing the number of subjects as well as the number of replications per subject.

4. Generally, more than three replications are not necessary.

5. A repeated measurements design may require fewer subjects than a paired measurements design to provide the same precision for estimated measure of inter-method agreement.

6. The sample size methodology is quite robust to the choice of the ballpark values for the model parameters under the assumption of bivariate normality.

11.6 BIBLIOGRAPHIC NOTE

Sample size determination for method comparison studies based on power of a hypothesis test involving an agreement measure has been discussed by a number of authors. They include Lin (1992) using CCC, Lin et al. (2002) and Choudhary and Nagaraja (2007) using TDI and CP measures, and Lin et al. (1998) using limits of agreement. See Exercise 12.20 in Chapter 12 for an example of sample size calculation through power analysis. Liao (2009) provides an approach based on notions of discordance rate and tolerance probability. Yin et al. (2008) present a Bayesian approach for sample size determination. Giraudeau and Mary (2001) present a method for computing number of subjects and number of replicates per subject to get a specified expected width of a two-sided confidence interval for an intraclass correlation coefficient.

EXERCISES

11.1 Let $\log\{\widehat{\text{TDI}}(p_0)\} + z_{1-\alpha}\,\text{SE}[\log\{\widehat{\text{TDI}}(p_0)\}]$ denote a $100(1-\alpha)\%$ upper confidence bound for $\log\{\text{TDI}(p_0)\}$. For a given value s_0 for the standard error, deduce that

$$P\{\text{TDI}(p_0) \leq \widehat{\text{TDI}}(p_0)\exp(z_{1-\alpha}s_0)\} = 1 - \alpha.$$

Thus, the true $\text{TDI}(p_0)$ is no more than $\exp(z_{1-\alpha}s_0)$ times its estimated value with $100(1-\alpha)\%$ confidence.

11.2 Verify the various expected standard error estimates reported in Section 11.4 for sample size determination using estimates from the kiwi data given in Table 5.1 on page 129.

11.3 Proceed as in Section 11.4 to perform sample size determination for paired and repeated measurements designs with $m = 2$ and 3 using estimates obtained from the knee joint angle data presented in Exercise 5.8 on page 138. Assess robustness of the sample sizes to the choice of the ballpark parameter value θ_0. How do these sample sizes compare to those reported in Section 11.4?

CHAPTER 12

CATEGORICAL DATA

12.1 PREVIEW

Throughout this book our attention thus far was focussed on the problem of measuring agreement when data were observed on a continuous scale. This concluding chapter discusses the agreement problem when different raters or methods assign categories and presents basic models and measures for examining agreement. The categories could be on a nominal or an ordinal scale and there could be two or more. We discuss in detail a popular measure called *kappa* (κ) and examine its properties under a variety of setups including multiple raters and categories. We also illustrate the methods introduced with case studies.

12.2 INTRODUCTION

There are numerous instances of measuring agreement between two or more raters or methods or devices where the response variable is nominal or ordinal. A recent Google search of the phrase "agreement kappa" produced over 15 million hits; in the medical field alone, the search engine on the PubMed website provided links to more than 22,000 research papers. This problem is also frequent in the fields of psychology, education, and social sciences. In this chapter, we provide a basic introduction to the agreement problem with categorical ratings. The phrase "Cohen's kappa" itself produced nearly 400,000 links on Google and about 3,200 papers on PubMed. Consequently, the kappa coefficient is the focus of our exploration, in spite of its shortcomings and perceived paradoxes.

Measuring Agreement: Models, Methods, and Applications. By P. K. Choudhary and H. N. Nagaraja
Copyright © 2017 John Wiley & Sons, Inc. **289**

First, we introduce typical categorical datasets that arise in measuring agreement with two raters and a not so widely known graph that is useful in visualizing the strength of agreement for ordinal data. We carry out an in-depth study of the properties of the kappa coefficient under a variety of settings when there are two raters and only two categories. We provide explicit expressions for the relevant parameters and their estimates, and describe associated inferential procedures, including the sample size determination. We explain the perceived paradoxes in the properties of the kappa coefficient using its mathematical properties.

Next, we investigate the problem of measuring agreement when there are two or more raters and there are more than two rating categories. We will consider both nominal and ordinal scales and the data on ordinal scale leads us to the exploration of weighted kappa coefficients and ANOVA models. We briefly touch upon the prominent modeling approaches to study agreement as well as disagreement. They include conditional logistic regression models and a generalized linear mixed-effects model approach for the dichotomous case, and log-linear models for multi-category ratings. This chapter also contains detailed case studies and a discussion on appropriate interpretation of the kappa statistic.

12.3   EXPERIMENTAL SETUPS AND EXAMPLES

12.3.1   Types of Data

While measuring agreement between two or more raters with categorical ratings, the ratings could be nominal or ordinal. With nominal ratings, a good measure of agreement treats all the disagreements between two raters equally and the entire focus is on the cases where the raters agree. In contrast, when the ratings are ordinal in nature, it becomes necessary to quantify the degree of disagreement and incorporate it into the measure of agreement. Whatever be the scale used for ratings, it also matters whether the raters involved can be treated as fixed raters or can be assumed to be randomly chosen raters. In the former case, there are two possible scenarios. The raters could be two specific raters using their own internal mechanism or two mechanisms or protocols that are followed by arbitrary rating personnel; the basic assumption is that ratings are done across randomly chosen subjects. In both these cases, there is a possibility of rater bias, in that the marginal probability that the first rater assigns a rating category of say 1 is not the same for the second rater and this bias (either due to a specific rater or due to the protocol used) affects the common measures of agreement. This leads to the fixed rater setup with a potential for rater bias and the classical Cohen's κ. Our most basic model assumes this possibility a priori; we also consider the case where the marginal probabilities of categories are taken to be identical across raters. This second scenario can arise when randomly chosen raters are doing the rating, and this leads to the intraclass version of the κ measure. Such a situation arises when each subject is rated by two randomly chosen raters who are similarly professionally trained; for example, two radiologists interpreting the same X-ray using a similar methodology.

12.3.2   Illustrative Examples

12.3.2.1   *Agreement Between Meta Analyses and Subsequent Randomized Clinical Trials*   A study investigated the agreement or lack thereof between meta analyses and subsequent large randomized clinical trials (involving 1000 or more subjects) published

in four of the most prominent medical journals. The researchers examined altogether 40 compatible hypotheses on primary or secondary outcomes coming out of 12 large trials and 19 meta analyses. Table 12.1 provides the distribution of "Positive" or "Negative" conclusions drawn from paired cases. Here the method of using meta analysis and the method of doing a large randomized clinical trial are treated as two fixed raters.

Result of	Result of Randomized Clinical Trial	
Meta Analysis	Positive	Negative
Positive	13	6
Negative	7	14

Table 12.1   Observed conclusions of randomized clinical trials and preceding meta analyses.

In this simple example, $27 (= 13 + 14)$ out of the 40 or 67.5% of conclusions of preceding meta analyses agree with the large-scale randomized clinical trials that were carried out later. Given that the well-conducted meta analyses as well as the randomized trials were based on large sample sizes, we would have anticipated a higher level of agreement between them. Another perspective on this agreement statistic is obtained by asking the question: if occurred by chance alone, what would we expect in those cells that corresponded to agreement? We would have anticipated the two conclusions to agree $\{(20 \times 19)/40\} + \{(20 \times 21)/40\} = 20$ or 50% of the time. That is, agreement was only 17.5% beyond anticipated by chance.

12.3.2.2 *Agreement Between Physicians and Nurses*   A study examined the agreement between the assessments of physicians (rater 1) and nurses (rater 2) using a retrospective chart review of 1025 Medicare beneficiaries aged 65 years or older. It compared samples of cases that were flagged by the Complications Screening Program (CSP, a computer program that screens hospital discharge abstracts for potentially substandard care) for one of 15 surgical complications and five medical complications. We consider the agreement problem for the totals of surgical and medical complications. This can be viewed as a two fixed raters problem, since physicians and nurses are trained differently.

Table 12.2 provides the distribution of the confirmation of CSP-flagged cases by the physicians and nurses on two types of complications.

Physician	Nurse Response			
Response	Surgical Complications		Medical Complications	
	Yes	No	Yes	No
Yes	349	36	51	14
No	89	63	20	90

Table 12.2   Summary of observed responses of physicians and nurses on medical and surgical cases flagged by the CSP system.

12.3.2.3 *Multi-Category Agreement Data: Agreement in Multiple Sclerosis Assessment*   Multiple sclerosis (MS) is an autoimmune disorder affecting the central

nervous system in adults with debilitating effects on the activities of their daily life. Two neurologists (one from Winnipeg, Canada, labeled 1; and the other from New Orleans, USA, labeled 2) classified two groups of patients on the certainty of MS using the following ordinal scale labeled 1 through 4 for certain (=1), probable (=2), possible (=3, with odds 1 : 1), and doubtful, unlikely, or definitely not (=4) categories. The data from the individual groups have been separately studied extensively. In Table 12.3, we pool the data and study the problem of agreement using basic models introduced in this chapter. These are two fixed raters using multi-category ratings scheme using an ordinal scale.

Neurologist 1	Neurologist 2 Rating				Total
Rating	1	2	3	4	
1	43	8	0	1	52
2	36	22	7	0	65
3	12	27	8	10	57
4	4	9	7	24	44
Total	95	66	22	35	218

Table 12.3 Diagnosis by two neurologists of patients on the likelihood of multiple sclerosis.

An example of random raters and multiple nominal categories is discussed in Exercise 12.17.

12.3.3 A Graphical Approach

Bangdiwala introduced a chart that illuminates the inter-rater bias as well as the strength of agreement between two raters. It provides a simple, powerful visual assessment of both inter-rater bias and agreement within ordinal categories.

Suppose two raters are classifying n subjects on an ordinal scale into one of c categories labeled $1, \ldots, c$, and the data are arranged in the form of a $c \times c$ contingency table. Let n_{ij}, frequency of the (i, j)th cell, represent the number of subjects who were classified into category i by rater 1 and j by rater 2. Denote by $n_i.$ and $n._j$ the total frequency of the ith row and jth column, respectively, for $i, j = 1, \ldots, c$. Further, define $n_{0.} = n_{.0} = 0$, and partial sums $s_i. = \sum_{j=1}^{i} n_j., s._i = \sum_{j=1}^{i} n._j, i = 0, \ldots, c$.

The agreement chart is constructed using the following steps:

1. Draw an $n \times n$ square and a 45° reference line.

2. Draw c rectangles $R_i, i = 1, \ldots, c$, inside the square such that R_i has dimension $n_i. \times n._i$. These rectangles are placed sequentially inside the $n \times n$ square such that rectangle R_i has lower left vertex at $(s_{i-1.}, s._{i-1})$, and upper right vertex at $(s_i., s._i)$, for $i = 1, \ldots, c$. Note that if either $n_i.$ or $n._i$ is zero, then R_i reduces to a vertical or horizontal line.

3. Divide R_i into a $c \times c$ grid where the embedded $n_{ij} \times n_{ki}$ rectangle $r(j, k)$ corresponding to the (j, k)th grid has lower left vertex at $(s_{i-1.} + \sum_{t=1}^{j-1} n_{it}, s._{i-1} + \sum_{t=1}^{k-1} n_{ti})$ and upper right vertex at $(s_{i-1.} + \sum_{t=1}^{j} n_{it}, s._{i-1} + \sum_{t=1}^{k} n_{ti})$ for $j, k = 1, \ldots c$.

4. Within R_i shade the region $r(j, k)$ based on the values of $l = \max\{|j - i|, |k - i|\}$ where the intensity of the shade is a strictly decreasing function of l. The $n_{ii} \times n_{ii}$ square region $r(i, i)$ corresponding to the (i, i)th grid (and $l = 0$) is the region of perfect agreement and will have the darkest shade.

5. Repeat Steps 3 and 4 for $i = 1, \ldots, c$ with the same choice of shading levels.

If there is very limited inter-rater bias, the $n_{i\cdot}$ and $n_{\cdot i}$ remain close and hence the rectangle R_i comes close to being a square. When this happens for most of the i, the rectangles come close to the reference line in the original $n \times n$ square. As the inter-rater bias becomes more pronounced, the rectangles move farther away from the diagonal and can move either below or above it. The shading pattern within the ith rectangle provides an insight into the level of agreement as well as of disagreement when at least one of the raters has classified a subject into category i. The agreement chart can be drawn with multi-category nominal data, but then the shading pattern would not correlate with the magnitude of disagreement and hence becomes less informative.

Figure 12.1 provides the agreement chart for the multi-category ordinal MS data introduced in Section 12.3. The numbers along the top and right edges of the outer square represent, respectively, the total frequencies corresponding to the four ratings of Neurologists 1 and 2. Discrepancies in the marginal frequencies of the two neurologists for categories 1, 3, and 4 lead to non-square shapes. For category 2, we obtain nearly a square due to the closeness of the marginal frequencies, but even then, the full agreement is limited there as shown by the small black square within it.

12.4 COHEN'S KAPPA COEFFICIENT FOR DICHOTOMOUS DATA

Consider a sample of n subjects or specimens that are classified into one of two categories labeled $1, 2$ by J raters. Let Y_{ij} denote the rating of the ith subject by the jth rater; $j = 1, \ldots, J$. We assume that $(Y_{i1}, \ldots, Y_{iJ})$, $i = 1, \ldots, n$ form a random sample from the joint distribution of $(Y_1, \ldots, Y_J)$ over the J-dimensional cube $\{1, 2\}^J$. The interest is to assess the agreement of two raters taken in pairs and to obtain a summary measure of agreement that provides an overall measure for the group of J raters. Cohen's *kappa* coefficients, introduced in 1960 for two raters classifying into two categories and generalized to several raters and multiple categories in later years, provide commonly used measures for this purpose. We introduce these measures, and study their properties under suitable models with the goal of providing measures for intra-rater as well as inter-rater agreement. We take up the two raters case first; that is, take $J = 2$.

12.4.1 Definition and Basic Properties: Two Raters

Let (Y_1, Y_2) have the joint pmf and marginal pmfs of Y_1 and Y_2 given, respectively, by

$$p_{ij} = P(Y_1 = i, Y_2 = j), \ p_{i\cdot} = P(Y_1 = i), \text{ and } p_{\cdot j} = P(Y_2 = j); \ i, j = 1, 2. \quad (12.1)$$

The parameter space for this multinomial trial is

$$\{(p_{11}, p_{12}, p_{21}, p_{22}) : p_{ij} \geq 0; \sum_{i,j} p_{ij} = 1\}.$$

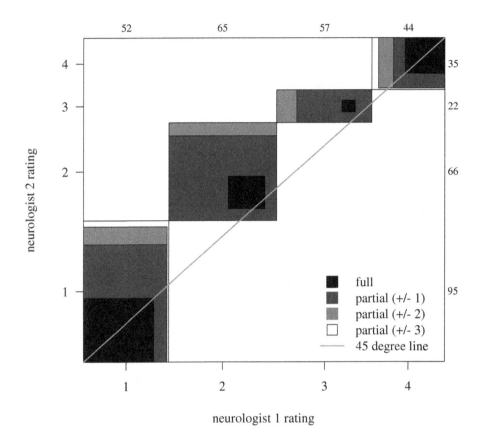

Figure 12.1   Bangdiwala agreement chart for the MS data in Table 12.3.

Then a simple metric for measuring agreement is the probability

$$\theta = P(Y_1 = Y_2) = \sum_{i=1}^{2} p_{ii}. \tag{12.2}$$

Note that $0 \leq \theta \leq 1$, and θ is 0 when $p_{11} = p_{22} = 0$ leading to perfect disagreement, and is 1 when $p_{12} = p_{21} = 0$ leading to perfect agreement. In both these extreme cases, the joint distribution has at most two points in its support.

There can be an agreement between the two raters even if they were choosing categories randomly. To adjust for this, Cohen proposed a measure that is *corrected for chance* by introducing the probability of such an event due to random causes,

$$\begin{aligned} \theta_0 &= P(Y_1 = Y_2 | \text{independence}) = \sum_{i=1}^{2} p_{i\cdot} p_{\cdot i} \\ &= (p_{11} + p_{12})(p_{11} + p_{21}) + (p_{22} + p_{21})(p_{12} + p_{22}). \end{aligned} \tag{12.3}$$

The parameter θ_0 is also between 0 and 1, and θ_0 is 0 when p_{12} or p_{21} is 1 (with perfect disagreement), and it is 1 when p_{11} or p_{22} is 1 with perfect agreement. In both the extreme cases, however, the joint distribution is degenerate.

Cohen's *kappa* measure is then given by

$$\kappa = \frac{\theta - \theta_0}{1 - \theta_0}, \tag{12.4}$$

where we assume that $\theta_0 < 1$. Clearly, $\kappa \leq \theta \leq 1$ and when θ_0 is specified, $\kappa \geq -(1 - \theta_0)^{-1} \geq -1$. Further, $\kappa = 0$ only when $\theta = \theta_0$ or when $P(Y_1 = Y_2)$ remains the same as due to chance. Upon substituting for θ and θ_0 in terms of the p_{ij} and simplifying the right-hand side of (12.4) we obtain

$$\kappa = \frac{2(p_{11}p_{22} - p_{12}p_{21})}{p_{12} + p_{21} + 2(p_{11}p_{22} - p_{12}p_{21})}. \tag{12.5}$$

This form suggests that $\kappa = 0$ if and only if the odds ratio $OR = p_{11}p_{22}/p_{12}p_{21} = 1$. Further, it expresses κ as an explicit function of the multinomial probabilities. Hence $\hat{\kappa}$, the ML estimator of κ, can be computed from the ML estimators of the p_{ij} and an expression for the standard error of $\hat{\kappa}$ can be given using the well-known asymptotic properties of the ML estimators. Details are given in the next section.

There are numerous investigations in the psychology and medical literature that discuss different scenarios where the raw agreement metric θ is high, but κ is very low and even negative. To explain this phenomenon with mathematical clarity, we will reparameterize the space of the p_{ij} by writing

$$p_{11} = \frac{\theta - \delta_1}{2}, \; p_{22} = \frac{\theta + \delta_1}{2}, \; p_{12} = \frac{1 - \theta - \delta_2}{2}, \; p_{21} = \frac{1 - \theta + \delta_2}{2}, \tag{12.6}$$

where δ_1 represents the magnitude of asymmetry when there is agreement and δ_2 represents a similar discrepancy measure when there is a disagreement between the two raters. The corresponding parameter space is

$$\{(\theta, \delta_1, \delta_2) : 0 \leq \theta \leq 1, -\theta \leq \delta_1 \leq \theta, -(1 - \theta) \leq \delta_2 \leq (1 - \theta)\}.$$

In terms of these parameters, it follows that

$$\kappa = \frac{2\theta - 1 + (\delta_2^2 - \delta_1^2)}{1 + (\delta_2^2 - \delta_1^2)}. \tag{12.7}$$

With $x = \delta_2^2 - \delta_1^2$, $x \in [-\theta^2, (1 - \theta)^2]$. For a fixed θ, $\kappa(x)$ is increasing in x (Exercise 12.3). Consequently,

$$\kappa_{\min} = \kappa(-\theta^2) = -\frac{1 - \theta}{1 + \theta} \quad \text{and} \quad \kappa_{\max} = \kappa((1 - \theta)^2) = \frac{\theta^2}{1 + (1 - \theta)^2} \tag{12.8}$$

provide lower and upper limits for the possible values of κ for a given probability of agreement θ. Figure 12.2 provides these bounds as θ moves in $(0, 1)$. It shows that even in the best case scenario, κ remains small for θ under 0.80. Further, even when θ is close to 1, it is possible to have κ being negative, and it happens when $p_{21} = p_{12}$ while either p_{11} or p_{22} remains close to θ.

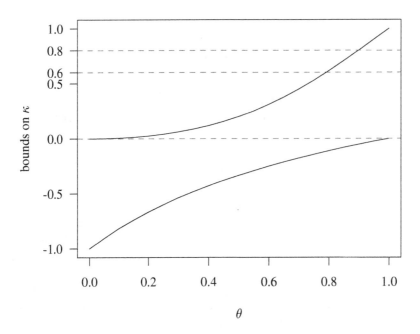

Figure 12.2   Range of κ values for a given probability of agreement θ. Given $\theta = 0.8$, κ cannot exceed 0.6; even when θ is as high as 0.90, κ cannot exceed 0.8, and can be negative.

Another useful parameterization of the parameter space with κ as a component exists. It can be used to further explore bounds on κ. With $\theta_1 = p_{11} + p_{12} \equiv p_{1.}$, $\theta_2 = p_{11} + p_{21} \equiv p_{.1}$, the p_{ij} can be expressed in terms of θ_1, θ_2, and κ as:

$$
\begin{aligned}
p_{11} &= \frac{1}{2}\{\kappa(\theta_1 + \theta_2) + 2(1 - \kappa)\theta_1\theta_2\}, \\
p_{12} &= \frac{1}{2}\{\kappa(\theta_1 - \theta_2) + 2(1 - \kappa)\theta_1(1 - \theta_2)\}, \\
p_{21} &= \frac{1}{2}\{2\theta_2 - \kappa(\theta_1 + \theta_2) + 2(1 - \kappa)\theta_1\theta_2\}, \\
p_{22} &= \frac{1}{2}\{2(1 - \theta_1 - \theta_2) + \kappa(\theta_1 + \theta_2) + 2(1 - \kappa)\theta_1\theta_2\}.
\end{aligned}
\tag{12.9}
$$

Non-negativity of the p_{ij} leads to further bounds on κ in terms of θ_1 and θ_2. The parameter space $\{(p_{11}, p_{12}, p_{21}, p_{22}) : p_{ij} \geq 0; \sum_{i,j} p_{ij} = 1\}$ is equivalent to the space

$$\{(\theta_1, \theta_2, \kappa) : 0 \leq \theta_1, \theta_2 \leq 1; \kappa_{\min}(\theta_1, \theta_2) \leq \kappa \leq \kappa_{\max}(\theta_1, \theta_2)\},$$

where (Exercise 12.4)

$$\kappa_{\min}(\theta_1, \theta_2) = \frac{2\{\max(0, \theta_1 + \theta_2 - 1) - \theta_1\theta_2\}}{\theta_1 + \theta_2 - 2\theta_1\theta_2};$$

$$\kappa_{\max}(\theta_1, \theta_2) = \frac{2\{\min(\theta_1, \theta_2) - \theta_1\theta_2\}}{\theta_1 + \theta_2 - 2\theta_1\theta_2}. \tag{12.10}$$

There are two other forms for κ defined in (12.4). To develop them, first consider

$$
\begin{aligned}
\text{cov}(Y_1, Y_2) &= \text{cov}(Y_1 - 1, Y_2 - 1) = p_{22} - p_{2\cdot}p_{\cdot 2} \\
&= p_{22} - (p_{21} + p_{22})(p_{12} + p_{22}) = p_{11}p_{22} - p_{12}p_{21} \\
&= \frac{1}{2}(\theta - \theta_0).
\end{aligned}
$$

Let $\mu_j = E(Y_j)$ and $\sigma_j^2 = \text{var}(Y_j)$, $j = 1, 2$. Then

$$
\begin{aligned}
\sigma_1^2 + \sigma_2^2 + (\mu_1 - \mu_2)^2 &= (1 - p_{2\cdot})p_{2\cdot} + (1 - p_{\cdot 2})p_{\cdot 2} + (p_{2\cdot} - p_{\cdot 2})^2 \\
&= p_{2\cdot} + p_{\cdot 2} - 2p_{2\cdot}p_{\cdot 2} \\
&= 1 - p_{1\cdot} + p_{\cdot 2} - p_{2\cdot}p_{\cdot 2} - p_{2\cdot}p_{\cdot 2} \\
&= (1 - \theta_0),
\end{aligned}
$$

upon simplification. This leads to another important form for the κ coefficient given by

$$\kappa = \frac{2\text{cov}(Y_1, Y_2)}{\sigma_1^2 + \sigma_2^2 + (\mu_1 - \mu_2)^2} = \frac{2\rho\sigma_1\sigma_2}{\sigma_1^2 + \sigma_2^2 + (\mu_1 - \mu_2)^2}, \tag{12.11}$$

where ρ is the Pearson correlation of Y_1 and Y_2. In this form, Cohen's kappa can be seen as the concordance correlation coefficient (CCC) introduced in (2.6) of Section 2.4. The form in (12.11) also shows that when $p_{\cdot 2} = p_{2\cdot}$ or equivalently when $p_{12} = p_{21}$ or when Y_1 and Y_2 are identically distributed, $\kappa = \rho$; in other cases it is smaller than ρ.

There is another easily interpretable representation for $1 - \theta_0$ that can be used to give yet another expression for κ; see Exercise 12.5.

12.4.2 Sample Kappa Coefficient

The original multinomial parameterization with expression for κ given in (12.5) leads us to simple forms for the ML estimator $\hat{\kappa}$. Suppose we have n subjects being classified by raters 1 and 2. As in Section 12.3.3, let n_{ij} denote the number of subjects being classified into category i by rater 1 and j by rater 2, $i, j = 1, 2$. Let $n_{i\cdot} = \sum_{j=1}^{2} n_{ij}$, $n_{\cdot j} = \sum_{i=1}^{2} n_{ij}$ and $n_{\cdot\cdot} = \sum_{i=1}^{2} \sum_{j=1}^{2} n_{ij} = n$. The data are usually tabulated as in Table 12.4. We assume that the n subjects being rated form a random sample from the multinomial population. Thus, the log-likelihood function is given by

$$\log\{L(p_{11}, p_{12}, p_{21}, p_{22})\} = \sum_{i=1}^{2} \sum_{j=1}^{2} n_{ij} \log(p_{ij}) + \text{constant},$$

and consequently the ML estimator of p_{ij} is $\hat{p}_{ij} = n_{ij}/n$. By the invariance property of the ML estimators, the ML estimator of κ represented by (12.5) is given by

$$\hat{\kappa} = \frac{2(n_{11}n_{22} - n_{12}n_{21})}{n(n_{12} + n_{21}) + 2(n_{11}n_{22} - n_{12}n_{21})}. \tag{12.12}$$

Rater 1	Rater 2 Response (Y_2)		
Response (Y_1)	1	2	Total
1	n_{11}	n_{12}	$n_{1.}$
2	n_{21}	n_{22}	$n_{2.}$
Total	$n_{.1}$	$n_{.2}$	$n_{..} = n$

Table 12.4   Summary of observed responses of raters 1 and 2.

We can use the other forms of κ given above and write down the corresponding equivalent forms for $\hat{\kappa}$. A large-sample estimate of $\text{var}(\hat{\kappa})$ is given by

$$\widehat{\text{var}}(\hat{\kappa}) = \frac{1}{n(1 - \hat{\theta}_0)^2} \left\{ \sum_{i=1}^{2} \hat{p}_{ii} \left[1 - (\hat{p}_{i.} + \hat{p}_{.i})(1 - \hat{\kappa}) \right]^2 + (1 - \hat{\kappa})^2 \left[\hat{p}_{12}(\hat{p}_{1.} + \hat{p}_{.2})^2 \right. \right.$$
$$\left. \left. + \hat{p}_{21}(\hat{p}_{2.} + \hat{p}_{.1})^2 \right] - \left[\hat{\kappa} - \hat{\theta}_0(1 - \hat{\kappa}) \right]^2 \right\}, \tag{12.13}$$

where $\hat{\theta}_0$ is the ML estimator of θ_0 defined in (12.3), and $\hat{\kappa}$ is given by (12.12). This estimate along with the assumption of normal approximation to the distribution of $\hat{\kappa}$ can be used to find large-sample confidence bounds and intervals for κ as well as to test the agreement hypotheses (of common interest) of the form (1.13), $H_0 : \kappa \le \kappa_0$ versus $H_1 : \kappa > \kappa_0$. For example, the fact that

$$\frac{\hat{\kappa} - \kappa}{\sqrt{\widehat{\text{var}}(\hat{\kappa})}} \sim \mathcal{N}_1(0, 1)$$

approximately, can be used to suggest $\hat{\kappa} - z_{1-\alpha}\sqrt{\widehat{\text{var}}(\hat{\kappa})}$ as a $100(1 - \alpha)\%$ lower confidence bound for κ.

For the meta analysis and randomized clinical trial agreement example in Section 12.3.2.1, the cell frequencies are $n_{11} = 13$, $n_{12} = 6$, $n_{21} = 7$, and $n_{22} = 14$. Consequently, the sample kappa coefficient $\hat{\kappa}$ given in (12.12) turns out to be 0.35 with an estimated standard error of 0.1479 upon using the formula in (12.13). The associated lower confidence bound of 0.1067 has an approximate confidence level of 95%.

But the coverage level for the above confidence bound can vary from the nominal level $100(1 - \alpha)\%$ even for $n = 100$ for some combinations of $\kappa, p_{i.}$, and $p_{.i}$. Hence we recommend confidence bounds and intervals based on bootstrapping for small sample sizes.

12.4.3 Agreement with a Gold Standard

Now suppose rater 1 is the gold standard. Then there are measures of agreement other than κ that are relevant and readily interpretable. By taking response category of 1 as *positive*, the commonly used measures are the conditional probabilities *sensitivity* η_1 and *specificity* η_2, given, respectively, by

$$\eta_1 = \frac{p_{11}}{p_{1.}} \text{ and } \eta_2 = \frac{p_{22}}{1 - p_{1.}}, \tag{12.14}$$

where $\theta_1 \equiv p_1.$ is the *prevalence* parameter. Then κ can be expressed in terms of these parameters as (Exercise 12.6)

$$\kappa = \frac{2\theta_1(1-\theta_1)(\eta_1 + \eta_2 - 1)}{\theta_1^2 + (1-\theta_1)^2 + (1 - 2\theta_1)\{\theta_1\eta_1 - (1-\theta_1)\eta_2\}}. \tag{12.15}$$

When η_1 and η_2 are known, κ will be a function of prevalence θ_1, and its maximum possible value is given by

$$\kappa_{\max}(\eta_1, \eta_2) = \frac{2(\eta_1 + \eta_2 - 1)}{\eta_1 + \eta_2 + 2\sqrt{(1-\eta_1)(1-\eta_2)}}. \tag{12.16}$$

12.4.4 Unbiased Raters: Intraclass Kappa

In the kappa coefficient introduced above, there was no constraint on the propensity of the two raters to classify the same proportion of subjects into any specific category; that is, we assumed that inter-rater bias may exist. In certain situations, an assumption of no inter-rater bias appears reasonable. One is where the same rater rates a subject twice, as in a repeatability study, and the other is the case where we can draw a random sample of two raters from the available raters and use their ratings of the same subject. In both these cases, we can assume unbiasedness of two raters. In the first case, the agreement problem corresponds to intra-rater reliability, and in the second, the concern is about inter-rater reliability. Thus, with unbiased raters, we are lead to a situation where the parameter space is restricted by the condition $p._1 = p_1.$ or, equivalently, $p_{12} = p_{21}$, or the case where $\delta_2 = 0$, or the assumption that Y_1 and Y_2 are identically distributed. Further, the expression for κ simplifies to

$$\kappa = \frac{p_{11} - p_{1.}^2}{p_{1.}(1 - p_{1.})} \equiv \kappa_I \tag{12.17}$$

which is nothing but the correlation between Y_1 and Y_2 where the two random variables are now exchangeable. This conclusion also follows from the CCC form for κ given in (12.11). Thus, κ can be identified as the intraclass correlation coefficient when the raters are unbiased. This interpretation is particularly helpful in the case of randomly chosen multiple raters.

It is convenient to use the parameters θ, δ_1, and δ_2 introduced in (12.6) and take $\delta_2 = 0$ to describe κ_I using (12.7), and also to express the likelihood for the observed data. For a random sample of n subjects, the log-likelihood is given by

$$\log\{L(\theta, \delta_1)\} = n_{11}\log(\theta - \delta_1) + n_{22}\log(\theta + \delta_1) + (n_{12} + n_{21})\log(1 - \theta) + \text{constant}.$$

Consequently, the ML estimators under the restricted parameter space are

$$\hat{\theta} = \frac{n_{11} + n_{22}}{n} \quad \text{and} \quad \hat{\delta}_1 = \frac{n_{22} - n_{11}}{n}.$$

Hence we conclude that, for the unbiased raters model, the population κ coefficient is

$$\kappa_I = \frac{2\theta - 1 - \delta_1^2}{1 - \delta_1^2} \quad \text{and} \quad \hat{\kappa}_I = \frac{4n_{11}n_{22} - (n_{12} + n_{21})^2}{(2n_{11} + n_{12} + n_{21})(2n_{22} + n_{12} + n_{21})} \tag{12.18}$$

is its ML estimator. An approximation to the variance of the sample intraclass κ is given by

$$\widehat{\text{var}}(\hat{\kappa}_I) = \frac{1 - \hat{\kappa}_I}{n}\left\{(1 - \hat{\kappa}_I)(1 - 2\hat{\kappa}_I) + \frac{\hat{\kappa}_I(2 - \hat{\kappa}_I)}{2\hat{p}_{1.}(1 - \hat{p}_{1.})}\right\}, \tag{12.19}$$

where $\hat{\kappa}_I$ is given in (12.18), and

$$\hat{p}_{1\cdot} = (1 - \hat{\delta}_1)/2 = \frac{2n_{11} + n_{12} + n_{21}}{2n}.$$

These ML estimators assume the exchangeability of Y_1 and Y_2.

12.4.5 Multiple Raters

Suppose there are J (≥ 2) raters that classify each of the n subjects into one of two categories labeled 1 and 2. Let Y_{ij} be the rating of the ith subject by the jth rater, $j = 1, \ldots, J; i = 1, \ldots, n$. Define Bernoulli random variables Y_{ij}^* as

$$Y_{ij}^* = \begin{cases} 1, & \text{if } Y_{ij} = 1, \\ 0, & \text{if } Y_{ij} = 2. \end{cases}$$

We assume the sample of n subjects is randomly chosen. The agreement question for two raters can be generalized to this setup and we consider two models for this purpose. They are, respectively, the fixed rater and random rater models.

If the goal is measuring agreement between the specified J raters, one can find sample κ for each of the $\binom{J}{2} = J(J-1)/2$ pairs using (12.12) and take the average κ as the estimate of the assumed common κ value. One can simplify this task by grouping the subjects based on the number of positive classifications. In addition, we can use the jackknife procedure to reduce bias in the estimate. We can find the confidence intervals and bounds using bootstrapping by resampling the n subjects, and carry out hypothesis testing using this approach.

When there are multiple raters, one can also test for the rater bias using Cochran's Q test. It is implemented as follows. First define

$$Y_{i\cdot}^* = \sum_{j=1}^{J} Y_{ij}^* \equiv J\overline{Y}_{i\cdot}^*; \quad Y_{\cdot j}^* = \sum_{i=1}^{n} Y_{ij}^* \equiv n\overline{Y}_{\cdot j}^*; \quad Y_{\cdot\cdot}^* = \sum_{i=1}^{n}\sum_{j=1}^{J} Y_{ij}^* \equiv nJ\overline{Y}_{\cdot\cdot}^*. \quad (12.20)$$

The absence of rater bias corresponds to the null hypothesis that $E(\overline{Y}_{\cdot j}^*)$ are the same for $j = 1 \ldots, J$. The test statistic used is

$$Q = \frac{2n^2 \sum_{j=1}^{J}(\overline{Y}_{\cdot j}^* - \overline{Y}_{\cdot\cdot}^*)^2}{\sum_{i=1}^{n} Y_{i\cdot}^*(J - Y_{i\cdot}^*)/\binom{J}{2}} = (J-1)\frac{J\sum_{j=1}^{J} Y_{\cdot j}^{*2} - Y_{\cdot\cdot}^{*2}}{JY_{\cdot\cdot}^* - \sum_{i=1}^{n} Y_{i\cdot}^{*2}}, \quad (12.21)$$

where it is assumed that there is at least one pair of disagreement in the dataset so that the denominator is nonzero. Under the null hypothesis of no bias across raters, Q has an approximate χ^2 distribution with $(J-1)$ degrees of freedom. When $J = 2$, the resulting test reduces to the McNemar's test. Conclusions drawn from this test for homogeneity of the raters can be incorporated into the overall estimate of κ.

When $E(\overline{Y}_{\cdot j}^*)$ are assumed to be the same for $j = 1 \ldots, J$, one can consider the intra-class correlation interpretation for κ under a random effects model (that makes additional assumptions) to obtain an estimate for it. We will discuss that model next.

The one-way random effect model that assumes an exchangeable dependence structure for the ratings on a subject is natural when we have J randomly drawn raters. Let us assume that the Bernoulli variables Y_{ij}^* can be expressed as

$$Y_{ij}^* = \mu + s_i + e_{ij}, \quad j = 1, \ldots, J; \ i = 1, \ldots, n, \quad (12.22)$$

where the independent random variables s_i and e_{ij} have zero means and variances σ_s^2 and σ_e^2, respectively. Then the intraclass correlation, that is, the correlation between any two measurements on subject i is $\sigma_s^2/(\sigma_s^2 + \sigma_e^2)$. Upon recalling (12.17), we note that this is another representation for κ under the assumptions of the model in (12.22). Following the familiar approach used in the normality-based ANOVA models we can use moment estimators of the variance components to obtain another estimator for the intraclass kappa, κ_I. The unbiasedness of the moment estimators of the variance components do not depend on normality. Define the between subject mean square (BMS) and within subject mean square (WMS) as follows:

$$BMS = \frac{J}{n-1}\sum_{i=1}^{n}(\overline{Y}_{i\cdot}^* - \overline{Y}_{\cdot\cdot}^*)^2; \; WMS = \frac{1}{nJ(J-1)}\sum_{i=1}^{n}Y_{i\cdot}^*(J - Y_{i\cdot}^*), \quad (12.23)$$

where $Y_{i\cdot}^*, \overline{Y}_{i\cdot}^*$, and $\overline{Y}_{\cdot\cdot}^*$ are defined in (12.20). Then it can be shown that (Exercise 12.10)

$$E(BMS) = \sigma_e^2 + J\sigma_s^2; \; E(WMS) = \sigma_e^2. \quad (12.24)$$

Thus, $\kappa_I = \sigma_s^2/(\sigma_s^2 + \sigma_e^2)$ can be estimated by

$$\hat{\kappa}_I = \frac{BMS - WMS}{BMS + (J-1)WMS}. \quad (12.25)$$

The above approach has assumed that raters' classifications of different subjects are independent. Thus, it can be used even when the subjects are evaluated by varying number of raters that are possibly different as long as our assumption that the model given in (12.22) holds.

There are other approaches to estimating κ_I, such as jackknifing, that avoid the ANOVA approach. One can also use the bootstrap estimate of κ_I and find the lower confidence limit from the resampled distribution. We recommend this approach to find the confidence limit as the convergence to large-sample properties is very slow.

12.4.6 Combining and Comparing Kappa Coefficients

Suppose there are m experiments comparing two raters (or two methods of classification), each classifying the subjects into one of two categories, and the experiments produce independent estimates of κ. This is a typical scenario in a meta analysis context. Another scenario is when we have the marginal probabilities of classification that may depend on confounding variables and they vary across the experiments.

Let κ_j be the population parameter corresponding to the jth experiment and let $\hat{\kappa}_j$ be the associated sample κ coefficient based on a sample of size $n_j, j = 1, \ldots, m$. Under the assumption that the κ_j are all the same and their common value is κ^*, its estimate is given as a weighted sum by the following formula,

$$\hat{\kappa}^* = \frac{\sum_{j=1}^{m} C_j \hat{\kappa}_j}{\sum_{j=1}^{m} C_j}, \quad (12.26)$$

where $\hat{\kappa}_j$ is computed using the formula for $\hat{\kappa}$ given in (12.12). One can consider two choices for the weights C_j. One is $C_j = n_j$, and another is $C_j = 1/\widehat{var}(\hat{\kappa}_j)$ where $\widehat{var}(\hat{\kappa}_j)$ is computed using the formula in (12.13). The motivation for considering the second set of weights comes from the optimal estimation of the common mean using independent estimators with different variances. One can also consider pooling the data (if available) and then computing the sample kappa coefficient for the combined sample of size $\sum_{j=1}^{m} n_j$. Simulation has shown that weighting by the sample sizes (i.e., taking $C_j = n_j$) produces estimates of κ^* that have smaller bias and mean square error under a variety of settings, including when sample sizes are small.

A test of the null hypothesis that the κ_j are all the same can be constructed using the test statistic T given by

$$T = \sum_{j=1}^{m} \frac{(\hat{\kappa}_j - \hat{\kappa}^*)^2}{C_j}, \tag{12.27}$$

where, $\hat{\kappa}^*$ is computed from (12.26) with $C_j = 1/\widehat{\text{var}}(\hat{\kappa}_j)$. Under the null hypothesis T has approximately a χ^2 distribution with $(m-1)$ degrees of freedom, and the hypothesis is rejected for large values of T. This works well when the sample sizes are large (> 100).

When one can assume that the raters are unbiased in each of the m experiments, we can use the intraclass kappa coefficient κ_I as the measure of agreement. Under this model, using $\hat{\kappa}_I$ in place of $\hat{\kappa}$ and taking $C_j = 1/\widehat{\text{var}}(\hat{\kappa}_{I,j})$, where the variance estimate is given by (12.19) in the statistic T defined in (12.27), leads to a χ^2 test statistic that has better power properties for smaller sample sizes. One can also consider the problem of testing the equality of two dependent κ coefficients with two raters and two categories under this intraclass kappa model. With additional modeling assumptions, one can present a test that is similar in spirit to the test statistic T presented for the comparison of independent κ coefficients, but modified to account for the dependence between the two kappa estimates.

12.4.7 Sample Size Calculations

Consider the problem of measuring agreement between two raters or methods that categorize a given subject into one of two categories. Suppose one wants to test the null hypothesis $H_0 : \kappa = \kappa_0$ versus the one-sided alternative $H_1 : \kappa > \kappa_0$ at level of significance α, and wants a power of $100(1-\beta)\%$ at $\kappa = \kappa_1 (> \kappa_0)$. Typically, one would use the large-sample normal approximation to obtain the sample size

$$n = \hat{\sigma}^2 \frac{(z_{1-\alpha} + z_{1-\beta})^2}{(\kappa_0 - \kappa_1)^2}, \tag{12.28}$$

where $\hat{\sigma}^2/n$ is an estimate of $\text{var}(\hat{\kappa})$ with $\hat{\kappa}$ being the sample κ given in (12.12). Further, $z_{1-\alpha}$ and $z_{1-\beta}$ are the $100(1-\alpha)$th and $100(1-\beta)$th percentile of the standard normal distribution. From the large-sample approximation to $\widehat{\text{var}}(\hat{\kappa})$, given in (12.13), it is clear that the variance estimate depends on estimates of several parameters including κ. With the reparameterization of the cell probabilities in terms of κ, and marginal probabilities $p_1.$ and $p._1$, given in (12.9), it follows that the expression for $\hat{\sigma}^2$ depends on estimates for these three parameters of which κ is the parameter of interest. So, one could use preliminary estimates of $p_1.$ and $p._1$ from a pilot sample or prior prevalence studies in the formula for $\hat{\sigma}^2$ and substitute κ_0 and κ_1 to choose the larger of the two estimates as $\hat{\sigma}^2$. Then the use of (12.28) yields the desired sample size. As we have seen before in (12.10), the choices for $p_1.$ and $p._1$ restrict the range for κ and one needs to choose them so that both κ_0 and κ_1 are feasible under these constraints. If it is appropriate to assume unbiasedness of raters (say when raters are randomly chosen), we use $\hat{\kappa}_I$ defined in (12.18) to carry out the test and take $\hat{\sigma}^2$ from the variance approximation given in (12.19) to compute n using (12.28). With appropriate modifications, the sample size formula in (12.28) can be used for tests involving agreement measures for continuous measurements. See Exercise 12.20.

We recommend the use of simulation studies for sample size calculations, especially for more complex setups.

12.5 KAPPA TYPE MEASURES FOR MORE THAN TWO CATEGORIES

12.5.1 Two Fixed Raters with Nominal Categories

When there are c (≥ 3) categories and $J = 2$ raters, the joint pmf of their ratings of a subject is given by (12.1), where now the possible ratings i, j by the two raters belong to the set $\{1, 2, \ldots, c\}$. Then, the κ coefficient, introduced in (12.4) takes on the form

$$\kappa = \frac{\sum_{i=1}^{c} p_{ii} - \theta_0}{1 - \theta_0}, \tag{12.29}$$

where now θ_0, the probability of agreement due to chance, is $\sum_{i=1}^{c} p_i.p_{.i}$. The ML estimation methodology here follows the description given in Section 12.4.2 and will not be presented.

While the above approach directly generalized the definition of κ in the dichotomous case as a chance adjusted measure of agreement, the available data also provides an opportunity to examine the agreement measure for individual categories. Let κ_t be the kappa coefficient obtained by dichotomizing the categories as t versus non-t, for $t = 1, \ldots, c$. The estimates of κ_t will provide an idea about the variation in the agreement between the two raters in terms of the choice of a particular category. In fact, the overall κ defined above in (12.29) is a weighted sum of these κ_t. It can be shown that $\kappa = \sum_{t=1}^{c} w_t \kappa_t$, where the weight

$$w_t = \frac{1 - p_t.p_{.t} - (1 - p_t.)(1 - p_{.t})}{2\left(1 - \sum_{i=1}^{c} p_i.p_{.i}\right)} \tag{12.30}$$

is non-negative and $\sum_{t=1}^{c} w_t = 1$. See Exercise 12.11.

When there are multiple categories, the kappa coefficient just discussed treats all disagreements equally and in fact ignores them completely. But when categories are ordered, the magnitudes of disagreement can be quantified in some cases using a suitably chosen weight function. In such situations a *weighted* κ, introduced below, provides a more meaningful measure of agreement.

12.5.2 Two Raters with Ordinal Categories: Weighted Kappa

Suppose there are c ordered categories labeled $1, \ldots, c$ and let w_{ij} denote the agreement weight associated with the classification i by rater 1 and j by rater 2; $i, j = 1, \ldots, c$. Take $w_{ii} = 1$ for perfect agreement, and for $j \neq i$, $0 \leq w_{ij} < 1$ for imperfect agreement; further assume $w_{ij} = w_{ji}$. Then the weighted κ is defined by

$$\kappa^w = \frac{\sum_{i=1}^{c} \sum_{j=1}^{c} w_{ij}(p_{ij} - p_i.p_{.j})}{1 - \sum_{i=1}^{c} \sum_{j=1}^{c} w_{ij} p_i.p_{.j}} = 1 - \frac{\sum_{i=1}^{c} \sum_{j=1}^{c}(1 - w_{ij})p_{ij}}{\sum_{i=1}^{c} \sum_{j=1}^{c}(1 - w_{ij})p_i.p_{.j}}. \tag{12.31}$$

Since the w_{ij} are bounded by 1, both the weighted sums in the second form are positive, and consequently κ^w does not exceed 1. The last form also shows that a scale change in $(1 - w_{ij})$ will not alter the value of κ^w.

The ML estimators for the parameters in (12.31) are $\hat{p}_{ij} = n_{ij}/n$, $\hat{p}_{i\cdot} = n_{i\cdot}/n$, and $\hat{p}_{\cdot j} = n_{\cdot j}/n$. Using these, the ML estimator of κ^w, $\hat{\kappa}^w$, can be computed. A close large-sample approximation to its variance estimate is given by

$$\widehat{\mathrm{var}}(\hat{\kappa}^w) = \frac{1}{n(1 - \hat{p}_e)^2}$$

$$\times \left\{ \sum_{i=1}^{c} \sum_{j=1}^{c} \hat{p}_{ij} \left(w_{ij} - (\overline{w}_{i\cdot} + \overline{w}_{j\cdot})(1 - \hat{\kappa}^w) \right)^2 - (\hat{\kappa}^w - \hat{p}_e(1 - \hat{\kappa}^w))^2 \right\},$$

$$(12.32)$$

where $\overline{w}_{i\cdot}$ is the average weight given to category i (recall that $\overline{w}_{i\cdot} = \overline{w}_{\cdot i}$ due to the symmetry of the weight function) and

$$\hat{p}_e = \sum_{i=1}^{c} \sum_{j=1}^{c} w_{ij} \hat{p}_{i\cdot} \hat{p}_{\cdot j}.$$

Two weight functions based on squared distance and absolute distance are generally used. As expressed in the form of disagreement weights, they are given by

$$1 - w_{ij} = \frac{(i - j)^2}{(c - 1)^2}; \ 1 - w_{ij} = \frac{|i - j|}{|c - 1|}. \tag{12.33}$$

When $p_{i\cdot} = p_{\cdot i}$ for all i and $1 - w_{ij} \propto (i - j)^2$, κ^w is identical to the Pearson correlation between the ratings of the two raters (Exercise 12.12).

When $1 - w_{ij} \propto (i - j)^2$, the sample estimate $\hat{\kappa}^w$ is very close (at the order of $1/n$) to the moment estimate of the intraclass correlation coefficient in a two-way random effects model where the two raters as well as the subjects are treated as random effects and the observations are the numerical ratings with support $\{1, \ldots, c\}$. Note that the random effects model assumption here causes the two rating distributions to be exchangeable. Thus, the standard techniques associated with the ANOVA table applicable to two-way ANOVA can be employed to get quick estimates of κ^w. This approach is further discussed in Section 12.5.3 below.

When $w_{ij} = 1$ for $i = j$ and 0 otherwise, the weighted kappa reduces to κ, given in (12.29).

12.5.3 Multiple Raters

When there are $c \ (\geq 3)$ categories and $J \ (\geq 3)$ raters, extensions of the kappa coefficient discussed so far do exist. There are several variance components models that make numerous assumptions. But the interpretation of the estimates of agreement coefficients becomes less clear in most cases. These generally involve the intraclass correlation interpretation of κ and make the assumption of random raters.

Suppose the J raters are distinct across subjects being rated and there are c categories. We suggest the use of pairwise κ^w defined in (12.31) across the J raters, and their average as an overall measure of agreement. Lower confidence bounds can be obtained using the recommended bootstrapping approach.

When the raters can be taken to be random effects, a two-way random effects model given by

$$Y_{ij} = \mu + s_i + r_j + e_{ij}, \; i = 1, \ldots, n; \; j = 1, \ldots, J(\geq 2), \qquad (12.34)$$

can be fit where Y_{ij} is the rating given by rater j for subject i and takes on values $1, \ldots, c\, (\geq 2)$. This is a generalization of the model proposed in (12.22) and assumes that the raters are unbiased and r_j has a constant variance σ_r^2. The intraclass correlation that corresponds to the inter-rater agreement is then given by

$$\rho_C = \sigma_s^2 / (\sigma_s^2 + \sigma_r^2 + \sigma_e^2). \qquad (12.35)$$

This reduces to the weighted κ coefficient introduced above in Section 12.5.2 when $J = 2$, the raters are exchangeable, and the weight function chosen is $w_{ij} = 1 - \{(j-i)/(c-1)\}^2$. The intraclass correlation ρ_C can be estimated using standard ANOVA methods that involve variance component estimates and let $\hat{\rho}_C$ be its estimate obtained by plugging in the moment estimates of these variance components. Then the variance of $\hat{\rho}_C$ can be approximated by

$$\frac{1}{n(\sigma_s^2 + \sigma_r^2 + \sigma_e^2)^2} \left\{ (1 - \rho_C)^2 \mathrm{var}(\hat{\sigma}_s^2) + \rho_C^2 [\mathrm{var}(\hat{\sigma}_r^2) + \mathrm{var}(\hat{\sigma}_e^2) + 2\mathrm{cov}(\hat{\sigma}_r^2, \hat{\sigma}_e^2)] \right.$$
$$\left. -2\rho_C(1 - \rho_C)[\mathrm{cov}(\hat{\sigma}_s^2, \hat{\sigma}_r^2) + \mathrm{cov}(\hat{\sigma}_s^2, \hat{\sigma}_e^2)] \right\}. \qquad (12.36)$$

In the above approximation, the estimates of the variance components as well as their variances and covariances are obtained from the fitted model.

For finding a confidence bound for ρ_C, we can use the methodology already available for the usual two-way ANOVA model with random effects. See Exercise 12.16.

12.6 CASE STUDIES

12.6.1 Two Raters with Two Categories

Consider the dichotomous classification of physicians and nurses of 1025 Medicare beneficiaries introduced in Section 12.3.2.2. Two types of complications were considered for determining the degree of agreement.

For decisions on surgical issues, 71.69% of the physicians and 81.56% of the nurses found complications and McNemar's χ^2 test that tests for symmetry of disagreement or equivalently $H_0 : p_{1\cdot} = p_{\cdot 1}$ strongly rejects it with a p-value of under 0.0001. The sample kappa, $\hat{\kappa}$, given by (12.12), is 0.3588 and the 95% lower confidence limit based on the variance estimate in (12.13) and asymptotic normality is 0.2847. This is a situation where there is a rater bias and the sample kappa value is low even though the physicians and nurses agree on 76.72% of the cases examined.

For decisions on medical complications, 37.14% of the physicians and 40.57% of the nurses responded "Yes." McNemar's χ^2 test that tests $H_0 : p_{1\cdot} = p_{\cdot 1}$ fails to reject it with a p-value of 0.3035. The sample kappa, $\hat{\kappa}$, given by (12.12), is 0.5916. Had we assumed no rater bias and used the maximum likelihood estimate of the intraclass version of kappa using (12.18), $\hat{\kappa}_I$ would have been 0.5911. The 95% lower confidence limit based on the variance estimate in (12.13) and the assumption of asymptotic normality is 0.4889. This is a situation where there is hardly any rater bias and the sample kappa value is higher; further, the physicians and nurses agree on 80.57% of the cases examined.

12.6.2 Weighted Kappa: Multiple Categories

In Section 12.3.2.3, we introduced an example on agreement between two neurologists where the ratings were measured on an ordinal scale. Earlier, we provided a graphical representation using Bangdiwala's agreement graph for these data in Section 12.3.3.

The sample kappa coefficient for the multi-category ($c = 4$) rating scale is 0.2570 with an estimate of the standard error of 0.0429. This does not indicate a good level of agreement between the two neurologists in their classification of the 218 cases presented. Neurologist 1 (from Winnipeg) has classified 23.9%, 29.8%, 26.1%, and 20.2% of the patients into categories 1, 2, 3, and 4, respectively. In contrast, the corresponding proportions for the second neurologist (from New Orleans) are 43.6%, 30.3%, 10.1%, and 16.1%. These marginal sample proportions may tempt one to naively infer that Winnipeg and New Orleans neurologists disagree a lot while classifying a patient into either category 1 or 3; but perhaps agree to a substantial extent with category 2 or 4. A look at Table 12.3 in Section 12.3.2.3 indicates that, in the case of category 2, there is substantial disagreement; 36 of the subjects identified as category 2 by the first neurologist have been rated as 1 by the second. When we compute the kappa coefficients by dichotomizing the categories as t versus non-t, $t = 1, 2, 3$, and 4, the corresponding sample kappa coefficients are $0.4001, 0.0507, 0.0666$, and 0.5221, respectively. These values indicate that the two neurologists agree the most when there is extreme evidence while showing hardly any agreement beyond chance in the intermediate cases.

Since we have ordinal ratings, it is very appropriate that weighted kappa coefficient be used to assess the degree of agreement between the two neurologists. With absolute distance weight function (given in (12.33)), $\hat{\kappa}^w = 0.4406$ and its estimated standard error is 0.0413. With quadratic weight function in (12.33), the estimate of κ^w and its estimated standard error are 0.5887 and 0.0459, respectively. When compared to the simple (unweighted) κ estimate of 0.2570, we see substantial increase in these estimates, but the standard error estimates remain quite stable. A random effect ANOVA model with ratings as the response variable provides an estimate of 0.5891 for the intraclass correlation coefficient; as anticipated it is very close to the $\hat{\kappa}^w$ obtained from the use of the quadratic weight function.

12.7 MODELS FOR EXPLORING AGREEMENT

12.7.1 Conditional Logistic Regression Models

Suppose there are two raters where each one classifies a subject into one of two categories. We considered this situation in Section 12.4 where the kappa coefficient was introduced. There we assumed that the subjects form a random sample or that the joint probabilities p_{ij} remain the same across the subjects. But the classification probabilities may depend on known covariates. Now we present a simple model that assumes the following: (i) κ remains constant across the subjects, (ii) the marginal probabilities $p_{1.}$ and $p_{.1}$ are the same for each subject but these probabilities vary across subjects; and (iii) the logit function $\log\{p_{1.}/(1 - p_{1.})\}$ is related to the covariates through a linear relationship. With $p_{1.} = p_{.1} = \theta_1$, we use the reparameterization defined in (12.9) to obtain

$$p_{11} = \theta_1^2 + \kappa\theta_1(1 - \theta_1); p_{12} = p_{21} = (1 - \kappa)\theta_1(1 - \theta_1); p_{22} = (1 - \theta_1)^2 + \kappa\theta_1(1 - \theta_1).$$
$$(12.37)$$

Since the discordant probabilities are the same, the 2×2 cells in our multinomial trial can be reduced to three categories by combining the two discordant cells. To elaborate, we assign subjects with both ratings of 1 to cell 1, with discordant ratings to cell 2, and with both ratings of 2 to cell 3 with respective probabilities $\theta_1^2 + \kappa\theta_1(1-\theta_1)$, $2(1-\kappa)\theta_1(1-\theta_1)$, and $(1-\theta_1)^2 + \kappa\theta_1(1-\theta_1)$.

For a subject i, let $V_{il} = 1$ if the subject is placed in cell l, and 0 otherwise, for $l = 1, 2, 3$, and $i = 1, \ldots, n$. Further, let $\mathbf{x}_i = (1, x_{i1}, \ldots, x_{ip})^T$ be the covariate vector associated with the ith subject and it is related to the probability θ_1 above such that

$$\log\left(\theta_{1i}/(1-\theta_{1i})\right) = \mathbf{x}_i^T\boldsymbol{\beta} \text{ or } \theta_{1i} = \frac{\exp\{\mathbf{x}_i^T\boldsymbol{\beta}\}}{1 + \exp\{\mathbf{x}_i^T\boldsymbol{\beta}\}}.$$

Here κ is the parameter of our interest while $\boldsymbol{\beta} = (\beta_0, \ldots, \beta_p)^T$ is the nuisance parameter vector in the problem. The multinomial likelihood is given by

$$\prod_{i=1}^{n} \frac{\exp(\mathbf{x}_i^T\boldsymbol{\beta})}{\{1 + \exp(\mathbf{x}_i^T\boldsymbol{\beta})\}^2} \{\exp(\mathbf{x}^T{}_i\boldsymbol{\beta}) + \kappa\}^{v_{i1}} \{2(1-\kappa)\}^{v_{i2}}\}\{\exp(-\mathbf{x}_i^T\boldsymbol{\beta}) + \kappa\}^{v_{i3}}$$

$$= \prod_{i=1}^{n} \frac{\{\exp(\mathbf{x}_i^T\boldsymbol{\beta}) + \kappa\}^{v_{i1}} \{2(1-\kappa)\}^{v_{i2}}\}\{\exp(-\mathbf{x}_i^T\boldsymbol{\beta}) + \kappa\}^{v_{i3}}}{\exp(\mathbf{x}_i^T\boldsymbol{\beta}) + \kappa + 2(1-\kappa) + \exp(-\mathbf{x}_i^T\boldsymbol{\beta}) + \kappa}.$$

This multinomial likelihood is equivalent to that of a conditional logistic regression model arising in a *matched case-control* study. For that representation, three observations are created for each subject i, and the outcome variable indicates which of the three cells l ($l = 1, 2, 3$) actually was realized; that is, the one for which $V_{il} = 1$. The observation l that corresponds to $V_{il} = 1$ is taken as the *case*, and the other two are labeled as *control*. To describe the relative risk function for the underlying conditional logistic model, define covariate $\mathbf{z}_i = \mathbf{x}_i, 0, -\mathbf{x}_i$, and $w_i = 1, -2, 1$, respectively, for $l = 1, 2, 3$ for the ith subject. The relative risk function for that subject is then given by

$$r_i = \exp(\mathbf{z}_i^T\boldsymbol{\beta}) + w_i\kappa - \frac{(w_i - 1)}{3} = \begin{cases} \exp(\mathbf{x}_i^T\boldsymbol{\beta}) + \kappa, & \text{if } l = 1, \\ 2(1-\kappa), & \text{if } l = 2, \\ \exp(-\mathbf{x}_i^T\boldsymbol{\beta}) + \kappa, & \text{if } l = 3. \end{cases} \tag{12.38}$$

Software available for the conditional logistic models can then be used to obtain estimates of κ and its standard error.

12.7.2 Log-Linear Models

When the number of categories c exceeds 2, log-linear models have been used to explore the nature of agreement and association. We now introduce two simple models that are useful for the exploration of agreement for the nominal and ordinal categories.

As before, let p_{ij} denote the joint probability of a subject being rated as category i and j, respectively, by the first rater (A) and second rater (B) for $i, j = 1, \ldots, c$. In the $c \times c$ contingency table, resulting from n subjects, let $\mu_{ij} = np_{ij}$ denote the expected frequency in the (i, j)th cell. Consider the log-linear model

$$\log(\mu_{ij}) = \mu + \lambda_i^A + \lambda_j^B + \delta_{ij}, \tag{12.39}$$

where

$$\delta_{ij} = \begin{cases} \delta_i, & \text{if } j = i, i = 1, \ldots, c, \\ 0, & \text{otherwise.} \end{cases}$$

The parameter δ_i included for the (i, i)th diagonal cell represents agreement beyond expected by chance for category i if raters A and B were to independently choose that category. Now if $\delta_i = \delta$ for all i, the parameter δ can be viewed as a single measure of agreement beyond chance and can be used as a measure in place of κ. The measure δ has an interesting connection to $\log(\tau_{ij})$ where

$$\tau_{ij} = \frac{p_{ii}p_{jj}}{p_{ij}p_{ji}} = \left\{ \frac{p_{ii}/(p_{ii}+p_{ji})}{1 - p_{ii}/(p_{ii}+p_{ji})} \right\} \Big/ \left\{ \frac{p_{ij}/(p_{jj}+p_{ij})}{1 - p_{ij}/(p_{jj}+p_{ij})} \right\}. \tag{12.40}$$

For $i \neq j$ the numerator in the second form for τ_{ij} in (12.40) represents the odds that the rating by A is i rather than j when the rating by B is i and the denominator is nothing but the odds that the rating by A is i rather than j when the rating by B is j. Under the model given by (12.39) with $\delta_i = \delta$, $\log(\tau_{ij}) = 2\delta$. Thus, δ has another meaningful interpretation as an agreement measure. Its estimation and associated inference based on ML method can be carried out using commonly available log-linear model procedures in the statistical packages.

When categories are ordinal in nature, a parsimonious model that would account for a measure of agreement and a *linear-by-linear association* is given by

$$\log(\mu_{ij}) = \mu + \lambda_i^A + \lambda_j^B + \beta u_i u_j + \delta_{ij}, \; i, j = 1, \ldots, c, \tag{12.41}$$

where $0 < u_1 < \ldots < u_c$ are fixed scores assigned to the c categories and $\delta_{ij} = \delta$ for $i = j$ and is 0, otherwise. The scores $u_i = i$ are commonly used. This model is unsaturated for $c > 2$ and when fit, the residual degrees of freedom is $(c - 1)^2 - 2$. Further, the τ_{ij} defined in (12.40) has the form $\log(\tau_{ij}) = \beta(u_j - u_i)^2 + 2\delta$. In particular, when $u_i = i$, $\log(\tau_{i(i+1)}) = \beta + 2\delta$ expresses the distinguishability of adjacent categories i and $i+1$. The null hypothesis of independence corresponds to $\beta = \delta = 0$ in the model given in (12.41). The null hypothesis that $\delta = 0$ corresponds to the assumption that there is no additional agreement beyond the baseline association caused by the linear-by-linear association term involving β in (12.41). These hypotheses can be tested by using the likelihood ratio tests available in software that handles log-linear models. Of course, our interest is in the point and interval estimation of δ and β.

12.7.3 A Generalized Linear Mixed-Effects Model

Suppose there are n randomly chosen subjects from a large population of subjects being rated on a binary scale (category 1 or 2) by a group of J randomly chosen raters from a large rater population. Let Y_{ij} be the rating of rater j of subject i, $j = 1, \ldots, J; i = 1, \ldots, n$, and $P(Y_{ij} = 1) = \theta_{ij}$. Since the subjects and raters are randomly chosen, the probability θ_{ij} can be modeled using a link function $g(\cdot)$ of the form $g(\theta_{ij}) = \eta + U_i + V_j$ where η is the intercept and U_i and V_j are independent normal random variables with mean 0 and respective variances σ_U^2 and σ_V^2. A popular link function is the probit link function; that is, $g(\cdot) = \Phi^{-1}(\cdot)$, where Φ is the standard normal cdf. This specifies a generalized linear mixed-effects model for our rating experiment.

Under the above model, the prevalence of rating 1 in the population is given by

$$
\begin{aligned}
P_1 \equiv P(Y_{ij} = 1) &= E(\Phi(\eta + U_i + V_j)) = P(Z \leq \eta + U_i + V_j) \\
&= P(Z - U_i - V_j \leq \eta) = \Phi(\eta_0).
\end{aligned}
\tag{12.42}
$$

In (12.42), Z is an independent standard normal variable,

$$
\eta_0 = \eta / \sqrt{(1 + \sigma_U^2 + \sigma_V^2)},
\tag{12.43}
$$

and the last assertion follows from the fact that $Z - U_i - V_j$ is normally distributed with mean 0 and variance $(1 + \sigma_U^2 + \sigma_V^2)$.

The probability of agreement between raters j_1 and j_2 while rating subject i can also be represented in terms of the parameters of the generalized linear mixed-effects model. Note that

$$
\begin{aligned}
P_o &\equiv P(Y_{ij_1} = Y_{ij_2}) = 1 - P(Y_{ij_1} \neq Y_{ij_2}) = 1 - 2P(Y_{ij_1} = 1, Y_{ij_2} = 2) \\
&= 1 - 2E\left\{ \Phi(\eta + U_i + V_{j_1})(1 - \Phi(\eta + U_i + V_{j_2})) \right\}.
\end{aligned}
\tag{12.44}
$$

Now, upon conditioning with respect to $U_i = u$, first we see that,

$$
\begin{aligned}
\Phi(\eta + u + V_{j_1})(1 - \Phi(\eta + u + V_{j_2})) &= P(Z - V_{j_1} \leq \eta + u)P(Z - V_{j_2} > \eta + u) \\
&= \Phi\left(\frac{\eta + u}{\sqrt{1 + \sigma_V^2}} \right) \left(1 - \Phi\left(\frac{\eta + u}{\sqrt{1 + \sigma_V^2}} \right) \right).
\end{aligned}
$$

Upon averaging this quantity with respect to the pdf of U_i, the expectation on the right side of (12.44) can be simplified further as

$$
\int_{-\infty}^{\infty} \Phi\left(\frac{z\sqrt{\rho} + \eta_0}{\sqrt{1 - \rho}} \right) \left\{ 1 - \Phi\left(\frac{z\sqrt{\rho} + \eta_0}{\sqrt{1 - \rho}} \right) \right\} \phi(z)dz,
\tag{12.45}
$$

where $\rho = \sigma_U^2/(1 + \sigma_U^2 + \sigma_V^2)$ and η_0 is given above in (12.43). A measure of chance agreement can be represented by $P_c = 1 - 2P_1(1 - P_1)$ where P_1, the expected prevalence, is given by (12.42). Finally, a model-based expression for Cohen's kappa coefficient that provides a chance adjusted measure of agreement between two randomly chosen raters can be given as

$$
\kappa_M = \frac{P_o - P_c}{1 - P_c} = 1 - \frac{\int_{-\infty}^{\infty} \Phi\left(\frac{z\sqrt{\rho} + \eta_0}{\sqrt{1 - \rho}} \right) \left\{ 1 - \Phi\left(\frac{z\sqrt{\rho} + \eta_0}{\sqrt{1 - \rho}} \right) \right\} \phi(z)dz}{\Phi(\eta_0)(1 - \Phi(\eta_0))}.
\tag{12.46}
$$

Statistical packages that handle generalized linear mixed-effects models can be used to obtain estimates of κ_M for this probit model and bootstrapping technique can be used for the lower confidence limit.

12.8 DISCUSSION

In this chapter we considered categorical rating scale and discussed some basic measures of agreement with an emphasis on agreement between two raters. The kappa coefficient was considered in detail and its properties were discussed. We also computed sample kappa in our case studies but never actually said whether the kappa on hand represents excellent agreement or weak agreement. We will take up that question now. As we do, it is worth recalling that the value of $\hat{\kappa}$ is affected by the estimated prevalence and rater bias.

There is substantial discussion in the literature about attaching a qualitative statement to the kappa coefficient obtained from an agreement study. Let us consider the dichotomous case with two raters. Landis and Koch (1977a) provide some guidance when they suggest that $\hat{\kappa} > 0.80$ can be taken to represent "almost perfect" agreement, and $\hat{\kappa}$ in the range of 0.61 to 0.80 corresponds to "substantial" agreement. Further, ranges 0.41–0.60 and 0.21–0.40 represent, respectively, "moderate" and "fair" agreement. This guidance is simplistic as the range of values for $\hat{\kappa}$ depend on other features of the collected data.

Instead, we can use the proportion of agreement $\hat{\theta}$ and the associated upper bound on the value of $\hat{\kappa}$ based on the bound on κ for a given θ, displayed in Figure 12.2 of Section 12.4. So, it is instructive to provide the maximum possible value for $\hat{\kappa}$ given the observed $\hat{\theta}$ in the sample data. For example, for the case study presented in Section 12.6.1, $\hat{\theta}$ values are 81% and 77%, respectively, for medical and surgical complications. Using the bounds given in (12.8), we conclude that the maximum possible value for $\hat{\kappa}$ is 0.63 for medical and 0.56 for surgical complications. While an observed $\hat{\kappa}$ of 0.59 compares favorably with 0.63, 0.36 appears to be too low in comparison with 0.56. Further, as noted earlier for continuous ratings, an agreement problem is multidimensional and consequently knowledge of sample prevalence rates $\hat{p}_{1\cdot}$ and $\hat{p}_{\cdot 1}$ along with $\hat{\kappa}$ would be more helpful in assessing agreement. Also, more informative would be the upper bounds for $\hat{\kappa}$ that use the sample prevalence rates and (12.10). This exercise yields the upper limit to be 0.73 for medical complications and 0.93 for surgical complications, again showing good agreement for the former and poor one for the latter. In any case, when $\hat{\kappa}$ is close to 0 or negative, we know the agreement is no better than that occurs by just chance alone, and when it is very close to 1, almost perfect agreement is established. These conclusions hold even when we have multiple categories.

Interpreting the value of $\hat{\kappa}$ in multi-category case is more complex and the situation is further involved when there are multiple raters. In these circumstances, many models assume unbiased raters and then $\hat{\kappa}$ is close to the intraclass correlation estimate in a suitably chosen continuous ANOVA model, and hence $\hat{\kappa}$ can be interpreted as an intraclass correlation. In such cases, properties of κ or κ^w are linked to the comparison of within subject variation across raters and between subject variation.

One can consider modeling the entire bivariate or multivariate categorical data using the various modeling approaches available and by incorporating an appropriate parameter that can be interpreted as a measure of agreement. We have briefly discussed three such models, the conditional logistic regression model, log-linear models, and a probit model that can be directly linked to κ. Latent class models and Rasch models have also been used.

12.9 CHAPTER SUMMARY

1. Measuring agreement within and between raters while subjects are rated on a nominal or ordinal scale is an important problem.

2. Cohen's κ, a chance-corrected measure of agreement, provides an important measure for this purpose for nominal categories.

3. Since the range of possible values for κ is constrained by other parameter values, one should be cautious in interpreting it.

4. With multiple categories and multiple raters interpretation of κ as a measure of agreement becomes tenuous.

5. With unbiased raters, intraclass version of the κ coefficient, κ_I, is used.

6. The κ coefficient is closely linked to the CCC used for continuous data.

7. For ordinal categories, weighted κ provides a measure of agreement but is sensitive to the weights chosen.

8. For the two-rater two-category setup, conditional logistic regression models, and for more general setups, general log-linear models that incorporate parameters that measure the degree of agreement exist.

9. Probit and logit generalized mixed-effects models can be used to develop κ coefficients for measuring agreement between two randomly chosen raters using a binary scale.

12.10 BIBLIOGRAPHIC NOTE

Bangdiwala (1985) introduced a chart that illuminates the inter-rater bias as well as the strength of agreement between them. Cohen (1960) introduced the sample κ coefficient as a chance-corrected measure of agreement for a sample consisting of two raters and two categories. A large-sample estimate of $\mathrm{var}(\hat{\kappa})$ was obtained by Fleiss, Cohen, and Everitt (1969) for c categories for weighted and unweighted κ coefficients. We have used their estimates in (12.13) and (12.32). When there are two raters and two categories, Lee and Tu (1994) considered four methods for finding a confidence interval for κ. Their recommended method, while maintaining the nominal level even for small samples, is rather complex to implement; hence it perhaps is not commonly used. Bloch and Kraemer (1989) introduced the concept of intraclass kappa (κ_I) and derived the approximation to its variance that is given in (12.19). The agreement index π suggested by Scott (1955) for the multi-category case is this κ_I for two categories, and is the κ coefficient computed under the assumption of homogeneity of the marginal distribution of the raters. Kraemer et al. (2002) propose a simplification that groups the subjects based on the number of positive classifications and uses the jackknifing procedure to reduce bias in the estimate of κ. Cochran (1950) proposed the statistic Q given in (12.21) that can be used to test for possible bias across multiple raters. ANOVA approach resulting in the estimate given by $\hat{\kappa}_I$ in (12.25) is due to Landis and Koch (1977b); in the definition of BMS, we have followed the recommendation of Fleiss et al. (2003) and have used the divisor n in place of $n-1$ suggested by them. Barlow et al. (1991) showed through simulation that the estimate of κ^* given in (12.26) with weights $C_j = n_j$ has smaller bias and mean square error under a variety of settings than the estimate that uses the reciprocal of the variances as these weights. The discussion of the comparison of m independent intraclass κ measures using a χ^2 test statistic with better power properties for smaller sample sizes is taken from Donner et al. (1996). Donner et al. (2000) handle the problem of testing two dependent κ measures with two raters and two categories of ratings under the intraclass kappa model. Andrés and Marzo (2005) introduce a conditional probability model for the two rater agreement problem with multiple categories and use it to propose five chance-corrected indices that are not sensitive to marginal totals and also depend on whether one of the raters is the gold standard. The closeness between $\hat{\kappa}^w$ and the moment estimate of the intraclass correlation coefficient in a two-way random effects model when $1 - w_{ij} \propto (i - j)^2$, noted in Section 12.5.2, was pointed out by Fleiss and Cohen (1973). The material on multiple raters and multiple categories in Section 12.5.3 is inspired by Landis et al. (2011), Kraemer et al. (2002), and Fleiss (1971). Chapter 1 of Fleiss (1986) provides an excellent introduction to doing inference on intraclass correlation in the context of reliability studies with normally distributed data.

The conditional logistic model introduced in Section 12.7.1 is due to Barlow (1996), which contains further details. Use of log-linear models for agreement studies began with the work of Tanner and Young (1985). Agresti (1992) provides an excellent overview of these models in his survey of modeling agreement and disagreement between raters using categorical rating scales. Section 12.7.3 on the generalized linear mixed-effects model approach to the kappa coefficient is adapted from Nelson and Edwards (2008). The recent review by Landis et al. (2011) provides a nice overview of the connection between the kappa measure, the intraclass correlation, and CCC. It presents a methodological framework for studying multilevel reliability and agreement measures.

A number of packages in the statistical software system R provide functionality for inference on κ and related measures. They include irr (Gamer et al., 2012), psych (Revelle, 2016), and vcd (Meyer et al., 2015) packages. The stats and lme4 (Bates et al., 2015) packages in R can, respectively, be used to fit log-linear and generalized linear mixed-effects models.

Data Sources

The data on agreement between meta analyses and subsequent randomized clinical trials is taken from LeLorier et al. (1997). Weingart et al. (2002) contains the data on the agreement between physicians and nurses. Westlund and Kurland (1953) is the source of the data on agreement in multiple sclerosis assessment. Their data, given for two groups of patients separately, have been studied extensively; see, for example, Landis et al. (2011) and references therein.

EXERCISES

12.1 Bangdiwala (1985) proposed an agreement measure that is closely related to the agreement plot introduced in Section 12.3.3. In terms of the notation developed in the creation of the plot, it is given by

$$\hat{B} = \frac{\sum_{i=1}^{c} n_{ii}^2}{\sum_{i=1}^{c} n_{i\cdot} n_{\cdot i}}. \tag{12.47}$$

(a) Show that $\hat{B}$ is always between 0 and 1. When does it take on the boundary values? Explain.

(b) Compute $\hat{B}$ for the data in Table 12.3.

(c) The $c \times c$ categorization of a subject by the two raters can be seen as a multinomial experiment with p_{ij} being the probability that the subject is classified by rater 1 into category i and by rater 2 into j. Suppose the data from the n subjects can be assumed to be a random sample from this multinomial population. Show that under this model $\hat{B}$ defined in (12.47) is the ML estimator of

$$\beta = \frac{\sum_{i=1}^{c} p_{ii}^2}{\sum_{i=1}^{c} p_{i.} p_{.i}},$$

where $p_{i.} = \sum_{i=1}^{c} p_{ij}$ and $p_{.i} = \sum_{j=1}^{c} p_{ji}$ provided $0 < p_{ii} < 1$ for all i. Does the ML estimator of β exist when a $p_{ii} = 1$ or when some or all of the p_{ii} are 0?

(d) Draw the agreement plot given in Figure 12.1.

12.2 (a) Determine conditions on the p_{ij} that yield (i) $\theta = 0$ and (ii) $\theta = 1$, where θ is defined by (12.2).

(b) Determine conditions on the p_{ij} that yield (i) $\theta_0 = 0$ and (ii) $\theta_0 = 1$, where θ_0 is defined by (12.3).

(c) What is θ when $\theta_0 = 0$, and when $\theta_0 = 1$? What happens to $(\theta - \theta_0)/(1 - \theta_0)$ in these two cases?

12.3 Let

$$g(x) = \frac{2\theta - 1 + x}{1 + x}, 0 \le \theta \le 1; -\theta^2 \le x \le (1 - \theta)^2.$$

(a) Show that $g(x)$ is monotonically increasing on its support.

(b) Determine the minimum and maximum values of $g(x)$ in terms of θ.

12.4 Let $\theta_1 = p_{11} + p_{12}$ and $\theta_2 = p_{11} + p_{21}$, where the p_{ij} are defined in (12.1).

(a) Show that κ can be expressed as

$$\kappa = \frac{2(p_{11} - \theta_1 \theta_2)}{\theta_1 + \theta_2 - 2\theta_1 \theta_2}.$$

(b) Using the constraints that $p_{ij} \ge 0$ and the expressions in (12.9), establish the upper and lower bounds for κ in terms of θ_1 and θ_2 that are given in (12.10).

(c) Determine the range of possible values for κ when (i) $\theta_1 = \theta_2 = 0.5$; (ii) $\theta_1 = 0.25, \theta_2 = 0.75$; (iii) $\theta_1 = \theta_2 = 0.75$. Comment on your findings.

(d) Construct contour and surface plots of the upper and lower bounds for κ in terms of given θ_1 and θ_2 as these parameters vary in the interval $(0, 1)$.

(This exercise is based on Lee and Tu, 1994.)

12.5 Show that, with the notation introduced in Section 12.4.1, the denominator $1 - \theta_0$ in the definition of κ in (12.4) can also be expressed as $1 - \theta_0 = p_{1.} p_{.2} + p_{.1} p_{2.}$. This easily interpretable expression represents $P(Y_1 \ne Y_2)$ under the assumption of independence of raters and results in another expression for κ.

12.6 (a) Show that when rater 1 is the gold standard and prevalence (θ_1), sensitivity (η_1), and specificity (η_2) are known, κ can be expressed as given in (12.15).

(b) Show that the probability of agreement θ always lies between η_1 and η_2.

(c) Show that when η_1 and η_2 are given, the maximum value of κ is given by (12.16), and that it is achieved when the prevalence is

$$\theta_1 = \frac{\sqrt{1 - \eta_2}}{\sqrt{1 - \eta_1} + \sqrt{1 - \eta_2}}.$$

(This exercise is based on Thompson and Walter (1988) and Feuerman and Miller (2008).)

12.7 The κ coefficient can be used as a measure of reliability of a test that produces one of two categories, 1 and 2. Let γ be the prevalence of category 1 in a dichotomous population. Consider a test with sensitivity (η_1) and specificity (η_2). Also assume that the two applications of the test produce independent results.

(a) Show that $p_{11} = \gamma\eta_1^2 + (1 - \gamma)(1 - \eta_2)^2$ and $p_{1.} = \gamma\eta_1 + (1 - \gamma)(1 - \eta_2)$.

(b) Determine an expression for κ in terms of γ, η_1, and η_2. [Hint: Recall intraclass kappa.]

12.8 In Exercise 12.7, suppose we have two tests with possibly different sensitivities and specificities. Find an expression for κ in terms of these sensitivities, specificities, and prevalence γ for category 1. (This exercise generalizes the setup in Section 12.4.3.)

12.9 Verify the equivalence of the two expressions for the statistic Q in (12.21).

12.10 (a) Show that (12.24) holds for the random effect one-way ANOVA model given by (12.22) where BMS and WMS are given in (12.23).

(b) Thus, show that the method of moments approach for estimating the variance components results in the estimator $\hat{\kappa}_I$ of κ_I, given by (12.25).

(c) Is $\hat{\kappa}_I$ unbiased?

12.11 (a) Let κ_t be the kappa coefficient when there are two raters and their ratings are dichotomized as t and non-t for $t = 1, \ldots, c$. Let $p_{tt}, p_{t.}$, and $p_{.t}$, respectively, be the probabilities that both raters, rater 1, and rater 2 will rate a subject as category t. Using Exercise 12.4 or otherwise show that

$$\kappa_t = \frac{2(p_{tt} - p_{t.}p_{.t})}{1 - (1 - p_{t.})(1 - p_{.t})}.$$

(b) Using the above relationship express $(p_{tt} - p_{t.}p_{.t})$ as a weighted function of κ_t.

(c) Show that when there are $c \ (\geq 3)$ categories, the overall κ defined in (12.29) can be expressed as $\kappa = \sum_{t=1}^{c} w_t \kappa_t$, where the weight w_t is given by (12.30).

(d) Show that $\sum_{t=1}^{c} w_t = 1$.

(e) Verify that $\hat{\kappa} = \sum_{t=1}^{c} \hat{w}_t \hat{\kappa}_t$ holds for the example considered in Section 12.3.2.3 when we use ML estimators for their respective parameters.

12.12 Show that if $1 - w_{ij} \propto (j - i)^2$, and $p_{i.} = p_{.i}$ for all i, then the expression for κ^w in (12.31) reduces to the Pearson correlation between two identically distributed random variables with support $\{1, \ldots, c\}$ and joint pmf given by p_{ij}. (Cohen, 1968)

12.13 As noted in Section 12.3.2.3, multiple sclerosis (MS) has debilitating effects on the activities of patients' daily life. In order to investigate the agreement of fitness-to-drive decisions made by referring physicians and by the on-road assessors in MS subjects, Ranchet et al. (2015) collected data from 218 MS patients. The choice of physician was at the discretion of the subject and the on-road assessors were either an occupational or physical therapist who followed a standardized protocol. Table 12.5 provides the distribution of "Pass" or "Fail" decisions by these two types of raters.

Physician	On-road Assessor Response	
Response	Pass	Fail
Pass	189	10
Fail	15	4

Table 12.5 Fitness-to-drive evaluation data for Exercise 12.13.

(a) Is there a bias between physicians and on-road assessors in terms of fitness-to-drive decisions?

(b) Determine the sample κ statistic and interpret it.

(c) Determine 95% lower confidence bounds for the population kappa coefficient using (i) the basic formula based on normal approximation (ii) bootstrapping methodology.

12.14 This exercise introduces other parameters discussed in the agreement literature for categorical ratings (e.g., Byrt et al., 1993). In a 2×2 agreement problem, (i) $|p_{12} - p_{21}|$ is called the *bias index* (BI), (ii) $|p_{11} - p_{22}|$ is called the *prevalence index* (PI) (iii) $2(p_{11} + p_{22}) - 1 \equiv 2\theta - 1$ is called the *prevalence adjusted, bias adjusted kappa index* (PABAK).

(a) Find the range for each of the above indices.

(b) Establish the following relationship between κ and them:

$$\kappa = \frac{PABAK - PI^2 + BI^2}{1 - PI^2 + BI^2}.$$

12.15 International Classification of Diseases, Tenth Revision (ICD-10), developed by the World Health Organization, contains codes and classifications for patient medical conditions and are followed all over the world. Chen et al. (2009) have measured agreement on 32 conditions between data from an ICD-10 administrative database and from chart reviews of 4008 discharges from four hospitals in Alberta, Canada. The data presented in Table 12.6 on three conditions is extracted from their Table 2.

(a) Compute the sample estimates of κ, BI, PI, and PABAK for each of the three medical conditions.

(b) In each case, compare the estimates of κ and PABAK and comment on the degree of agreement between the discharge charts and the corresponding ICD-10 database.

Condition	Chart(+) ICD-10(+)	Chart(−) ICD-10(+)	Chart(+) ICD-10(−)	Chart(−) ICD-10(−)
Hypertension	826	61	384	2737
Cardiac Arrhythmias	341	24	533	3110
Solid Tumor (Without Metastasis)	175	123	206	3504

Table 12.6   Frequencies of observed classifications for disease classification data for Exercise 12.15.

12.16 Consider the two-way random effects model given in (12.34) and assume normality. Define the following random variables:

$$\overline{Y}_{i\cdot} = \sum_{j=1}^{J} Y_{ij}/J, \quad \overline{Y}_{\cdot j} = \sum_{i=1}^{n} Y_{ij}/n, \quad \text{and} \quad \overline{Y}_{\cdot\cdot} = \sum_{i=1}^{n}\sum_{j=1}^{J} Y_{ij}/nJ.$$

(a) Write down the ANOVA table that includes the sources of variation (Between Subjects, Between Raters, Error, and Total), associated degrees of freedom, and sum of squares in terms of the above averages. Denote the mean sum of squares by SMS for subjects, RMS for raters, and EMS for the error.

(b) Determine the expected values for SMS, RMS, and EMS.

(c) Using method of moments, determine the estimates of the variance components σ_s^2, σ_r^2, and σ_e^2.

(d) Let $\hat{\rho}_C$ be the estimate of ρ_C defined in (12.35). Show that

$$\hat{\rho}_C = \frac{n(SMS - EMS)}{nSMS + J \cdot RMS + \{n(J-1) - J\}EMS}.$$

(e) Define $F = RMS/EMS$ and

$$\nu = \frac{(n-1)(J-1)\left(J\hat{\rho}_C F + n\{1 + (J-1)\hat{\rho}_C\} - J\hat{\rho}_C\right)^2}{(n-1)J^2\hat{\rho}_C^2 F^2 + \left(n\{1 + (J-1)\hat{\rho}_C\} - J\hat{\rho}_C\right)^2}.$$

Note that ν is random, data dependent, and may be a non-integer.

(f) Let F_0 denote 95th percentile of an F distribution with degrees of freedom $n - 1$ and ν. Show that an approximate 95% lower confidence bound for ρ_C is given by

$$\frac{n(SMS - F_0 EMS)}{nSMS + F_0\{J \cdot RMS + \{n(J-1) - J\}EMS\}}.$$

[Hint: See the discussion in Fleiss and Shrout, 1978.]

12.17 Fleiss (1971) presents an example where each of 30 patients were evaluated by six psychiatrists, and different psychiatrists participated in the evaluation of distinct subjects. Each rater classified a patient into one of five mutually exclusive categories:

Patient	Depression (1)	Personality Disorder (2)	Schizophrenia (3)	Neurosis (4)	Other (5)
1	0	0	0	6	0
2	0	3	0	0	3
3	0	1	4	0	1
4	0	0	0	0	6
5	0	3	0	3	0
6	2	0	4	0	0
7	0	0	4	0	2
8	2	0	3	1	0
9	2	0	0	4	0
10	0	0	0	0	6
11	1	0	0	5	0
12	1	1	0	4	0
13	0	3	3	0	0
14	1	0	0	5	0
15	0	2	0	3	1
16	0	0	5	0	1
17	3	0	0	1	2
18	5	1	0	0	0
19	0	2	0	4	0
20	1	0	2	0	3
21	0	0	0	0	6
22	0	1	0	5	0
23	0	2	0	1	3
24	2	0	0	4	0
25	1	0	0	4	1
26	0	5	0	1	0
27	4	0	0	0	2
28	0	2	0	4	0
29	1	0	5	0	0
30	0	0	0	0	6

Reprinted from Fleiss (1971) with permission from American Psychological Assocation.

Table 12.7   Frequencies of observed evaluations of six psychiatrists for 30 patients for Exercise 12.17.

depression, personality disorder, schizophrenia, neurosis, and other. The data are summarized in Table 12.7.

(a) Write down the two-way random effects model given in (12.34) for these data.

(b) Assuming the model given above in (a), find the intraclass correlation ($\hat{\rho}_C$) representing the association between two ratings of the same subject using standard ANOVA methods.

(c) For the multi-rater, multi-category rating setup, Fleiss (1971) introduced sample overall κ coefficient with the following formula:

$$\hat{\kappa}_O = \frac{\sum_{i=1}^{n} \sum_{j=1}^{c} m_{ij}^2 - nJ[1 + (J-1)\sum_{j=1}^{c} \hat{p}_j^2]}{nJ(J-1)(1 - \sum_{j=1}^{c} \hat{p}_j^2)}.$$

Here n is the number of subjects; J is the number of raters, each rating every subject into one of c categories; and m_{ij} is the number of raters out of J that are classifying ith subject into jth category. Further, $\hat{p}_j = \sum_{i=1}^{n} m_{ij}/nJ$. Determine $\hat{\kappa}_O$ for the data given in Table 12.17 representing the m_{ij} for the 30 patients.

(d) Compare the intraclass correlation $\hat{\rho}_C$ obtained using the ANOVA model, and $\hat{\kappa}_O$.

(e) Obtain a 95% lower confidence bound for ρ_C using the methodology described in Exercise 12.16.

12.18 (a) Establish that var$(\hat{\rho}_C)$ for the model given in (12.34) can be approximated by the expression in (12.36). [Hint: Use bivariate Taylor series approximation for the variance of a ratio of random variables.]

(b) Give an estimate of the standard error of $\hat{\rho}_C$ for the data given in Exercise 12.17 using this formula.

12.19 (a) Establish the expression given in (12.45) for the probit generalized linear mixed-effects model.

(b) Show that the expression for κ_M simplifies to the one given in (12.46).

(c) Develop an expression for the Cohen's kappa coefficient for a logit generalized linear mixed-effects model for binary data. (See Nelson and Edwards, 2008.)

12.20 The sample size formula (12.28) can also be used in conjunction with testing agreement hypotheses (1.13) based on common agreement measures for continuous data. Further simplification of the formula is possible if $\widehat{\text{var}}(\hat{\kappa})$, which equals $\hat{\sigma}^2/n$ in the formula, can be replaced by its upper bound. For z-transformed CCC (see, page 80, Section 3.3.3), an approximate upper bound for the variance estimate is $1/(n-2)$ (Lin et al., 2011, Section 4.2).

(a) Show that using this bound in (12.28) yields the following sample size formula for inference on CCC:

$$n = \frac{(z_{1-\alpha} + z_{1-\beta})^2}{\{\tanh^{-1}(\text{CCC}_0) - \tanh^{-1}(\text{CCC}_1)\}^2} + 2,$$

where $\tanh^{-1}(\text{CCC}_0)$ and $\tanh^{-1}(\text{CCC}_1)$, respectively, represent the null and alternative values of Fisher's z-transformation of CCC.

(b) Use the above formula to compute the sample size necessary for a 5% level test of hypotheses (1.13) based on CCC to have 80% power when $\text{CCC}_0 = 0.90$ represents the boundary for insufficient agreement and $\text{CCC}_1 = 0.98$ is the anticipated high level of agreement.

REFERENCES

Agresti, A. (1992). Modeling patterns of agreement and disagreement. *Statistical Methods in Medical Research* **1**, 201–218.

Alanen, E. (2010). Everything all right in method comparison studies? *Statistical Methods in Medical Research* **21**, 297–309.

Altman, D. G. and Bland, J. M. (1983). Measurement in medicine: The analysis of method comparison studies. *The Statistician* **32**, 307–317.

Altman, D. G. and Bland, J. M. (1987). Comparing methods of measurement [Letter]. *Applied Statistics* **36**, 224–225.

Altman, D. G. and Bland, J. M. (2002). Commentary on quantifying agreement between two methods of measurement [Letter]. *Clinical Chemistry* **48**, 801–802.

Andrés, A. M. and Marzo, P. F. (2005). Chance-corrected measures of reliability and validity in $K \times K$ tables. *Statistical Methods in Medical Research* **14**, 473–492.

Arellano-Valle, R. B., Bolfarine, H. and Lachos, V. H. (2005). Skew-normal linear mixed models. *Journal of Data Science* **3**, 415–438.

Atkinson, G. and Nevill, A. (1997). Comment on the use of concordance correlation to assess the agreement between two variables. *Biometrics* **53**, 775–777.

Bablok, W., Passing, H., Bender, R. and Schneider, B. (1988). A general regression procedure for method transformation. Application of linear regression procedures for method comparison studies in clinical chemistry, Part III. *Journal of Clinical Chemistry and Clinical Biochemistry* **26**, 783–790.

Bangdiwala, S. I. (1985). A graphical test for observer agreement. In *International Statistical Institute Centenary Session 1985*, pp. 307-308, International Statistical Institute, Amsterdam.

Barlow, W. (1996). Measurement of interrater agreement with adjustment for covariates. *Biometrics* **52**, 695–702.

Barlow, W., Lai, M.-Y. and Azen, S. P. (1991). A comparison of methods for calculating a stratified kappa. *Statistics in Medicine* **10**, 1465–1472.

Barnett, R. N. (1965). A scheme for the comparison of quantitative methods. *American Journal of Clinical Pathology* **43**, 562–569.

Barnett, R. N. and Youden, W. J. (1970). A revised scheme for the comparison of quantitative methods. *American Journal of Clinical Pathology* **54**, 454–462.

Barnhart, H. X. and Williamson, J. M. (2001). Modeling concordance correlation via GEE to evaluate reproducibility. *Biometrics* **57**, 931–940.

Barnhart, H. X., Haber, M. J. and Lin, L. I. (2007a). An overview on assessing agreement with continuous measurement. *Journal of Biopharmaceutical Statistics* **17**, 529–569.

Barnhart, H. X., Haber, M. J. and Song, J. (2002). Overall concordance correlation coefficient for evaluating agreement among multiple observers. *Biometrics* **58**, 1020–1027.

Barnhart, H. X., Kosinski, A. S. and Haber, M. J. (2007b). Assessing individual agreement. *Journal of Biopharmaceutical Statistics* **17**, 697–719.

Barnhart, H. X., Lokhnygina, Y., Kosinski, A. S. and Haber, M. J. (2007c). Comparison of concordance correlation coefficient and coefficient of individual agreement in assessing agreement. *Journal of Biopharmaceutical Statistics* **17**, 721–738.

Barnhart, H. X., Song, J. and Haber, M. J. (2005). Assessing intra, inter and total agreement with replicated readings. *Statistics in Medicine* **24**, 1371–1384.

Bartko, J. J. (1994). Measures of agreement: A single procedure. *Statistics in Medicine* **13**, 737–745.

Bartlett, J. W. and Frost, C. (2008). Reliability, repeatability and reproducibility: Analysis of measurement errors in continuous variables. *Ultrasound in Obstetrics and Gynecology* **31**, 466–475.

Bates, D. and Maechler, M. (2015). *Matrix: Sparse and Dense Matrix Classes and Methods*. R package version 1.2-3.

Bates, D., Mächler, M., Bolker, B. and Walker, S. (2015). Fitting linear mixed-effects models using lme4. *Journal of Statistical Software* **67**, 1–48.

Blackwood, L. G. and Bradley, E. L. (1991). An omnibus test for comparing 2 measuring devices. *Journal of Quality Technology* **23**, 12–16.

Bland, J. M. and Altman, D. G. (1986). Statistical methods for assessing agreement between two methods of clinical measurement. *Lancet* **i**, 307–310.

Bland, J. M. and Altman, D. G. (1990). A note on the use of the intraclass correlation coefficient in the evaluation of agreement between two methods of measurement. *Computers in Biology and Medicine* **20**, 337–340.

Bland, J. M. and Altman, D. G. (1995a). Comparing two methods of clinical measurement: A personal history. *International Journal of Epidemiology* **24**, S7–S14.

Bland, J. M. and Altman, D. G. (1995b). Comparing methods of measurement: Why plotting difference against standard method is misleading. *Lancet* **346**, 1085–1087.

Bland, J. M. and Altman, D. G. (1999). Measuring agreement in method comparison studies. *Statistical Methods in Medical Research* **8**, 135–160.

Bland, J. M. and Altman, D. G. (2003). Applying the right statistics: Analyses of measurement studies. *Ultrasound in Obstetrics and Gynecology* **22**, 85–93.

Bland, J. M. and Altman, D. G. (2007). Agreement between methods of measurement with multiple observations per individual. *Journal of Biopharmaceutical Statistics* **17**, 571–582.

Bloch, D. A. and Kraemer, H. C. (1989). 2 × 2 kappa coefficients: Measures of agreement or association. *Biometrics* **45**, 269–287.

Bowling, L. S., Sageman, W. S., O'Connor, S. M., Cole, R. and Amundson, D. E. (1993). Lack of agreement between measurement of ejection fraction by impedance cardiography versus radionuclide ventriculography. *Critical Care Medicine* **21**, 1523–1527.

Bradley, E. L. and Blackwood, L. G. (1989). Comparing paired data: A simultaneous test for means and variances. *The American Statistician* **43**, 234–235.

Brockwell, P. J. and Davis, R. A. (2002). *Introduction to Time Series and Forecasting*, 2nd edn. Springer, New York.

Broemeling, L. D. (2009). *Bayesian Methods for Measures of Agreement*. Chapman & Hall/CRC, Boca Raton, FL.

Brulez, K., Choudhary, P. K., Maurer, G., Portugal, S. J., Boulton, R. L., Webber, S. L. and Cassey, P. (2014). Visual scoring of eggshell patterns has poor repeatability. *Journal of Ornithology* **155**, 701–706.

Byrt, T., Bishop, J. and Carlin, J. B. (1993). Bias, prevalence and kappa. *Journal of Clinical Epidemiology* **46**, 423–429.

Carrasco, J. L. and Jover, L. (2003). Estimating the generalized concordance correlation coefficient through variance components. *Biometrics* **59**, 849–858.

Carrasco, J. L., Caceres, A., Escaramis, G. and Jover, L. (2014). Distinguishability and agreement with continuous data. *Statistics in Medicine* **33**, 117–128.

Carrasco, J. L., Jover, L., King, T. S. and Chinchilli, V. M. (2007). Comparison of concordance correlation coefficient estimating approaches with skewed data. *Journal of Biopharmaceutical Statistics* **17**, 673–684.

Carrasco, J. L., King, T. S. and Chinchilli, V. M. (2009). The concordance correlation coefficient for repeated measures estimated by variance components. *Journal of Biopharmaceutical Statistics* **19**, 90–105.

Carroll, R. J. and Ruppert, D. (1988). *Transformation and Weighting in Regression*. Chapman & Hall, New York.

Carroll, R. J. and Ruppert, D. (1996). The use and misuse of orthogonal regression in linear errors-in-variables models. *The American Statistician* **50**, 1–6.

Carstensen, B. (2010). *Comparing Clinical Measurement Methods: A Practical Guide*. John Wiley, Chichester, UK.

Carstensen, B., Gurrin, L., Ekstrom, C. and Figurski, M. (2015). *MethComp: Functions for analysis of agreement in method comparison studies.* R package version 1.22.2.

Carstensen, B., Simpson, J. and Gurrin, L. C. (2008). Statistical models for assessing agreement in method comparison studies with replicate measurements. *The International Journal of Biostatistics* **4**, article 16.

Casella, G. and Berger, R. (2001). *Statistical Inference*, 2nd edn. Duxbury Press, Pacific Grove, CA.

Chen, C.-C. and Barnhart, H. X. (2008). Comparison of ICC and CCC for assessing agreement for data without and with replications. *Computational Statistics and Data Analysis* **53**, 554–564.

Chen, G., Faris, P., Hemmelgarn, B., Walker, R. L. and Quan, H. (2009). Measuring agreement of administrative data with chart data using prevalence unadjusted and adjusted kappa. *BMC Medical Research Methodology* **9**, article 5.

Cheng, C.-L. and Van Ness, J. W. (1999). *Statistical Regression with Measurement Error*. John Wiley, Chichester, UK.

Chinchilli, V. M., Martel, J. K., Kumanyika, S. and Lloyd, T. (1996). A weighted concordance correlation coefficient for repeated measurement designs. *Biometrics* **52**, 341–353.

Choudhary, P. K. (2007). Semiparametric regression for assessing agreement using tolerance bands. *Computational Statistics and Data Analysis* **51**, 6229–6241.

Choudhary, P. K. (2008). A tolerance interval approach for assessment of agreement in method comparison studies with repeated measurements. *Journal of Statistical Planning and Inference* **138**, 1102–1115.

Choudhary, P. K. (2009). Interrater agreement. In *Methods and Applications of Statistics in the Life and Health Sciences*, pp. 461-480, Balakrishnan, N. (Editor), John Wiley, Hoboken, NJ.

Choudhary, P. K. (2010). A unified approach for nonparametric evaluation of agreement in method comparison studies. *The International Journal of Biostatistics* **6**, article 19.

Choudhary, P. K. and Nagaraja, H. N. (2005a). Assessment of agreement using intersection-union principle. *Biometrical Journal* **47**, 674–681.

Choudhary, P. K. and Nagaraja, H. N. (2005b). Selecting the instrument closest to a gold standard. *Journal of Statistical Planning and Inference* **129**, 229–237.

Choudhary, P. K. and Nagaraja, H. N. (2005c). A two-stage procedure for selection and assessment of agreement of the best instrument with a gold standard. *Sequential Analysis* **24**, 237–257.

Choudhary, P. K. and Nagaraja, H. N. (2007). Tests for assessment of agreement using probability criteria. *Journal of Statistical Planning and Inference* **137**, 279–290.

Choudhary, P. K. and Ng, H. K. T. (2006). A tolerance interval approach for assessment of agreement using regression models for mean and variance. *Biometrics* **62**, 288–296.

Choudhary, P. K. and Yin, K. (2010). Bayesian and frequentist methodologies for analyzing method comparison studies with multiple methods. *Statistics in Biopharmaceutical Research* **2**, 122–132.

Choudhary, P. K., Sengupta, D. and Cassey, P. (2014). A general skew-t mixed model that allows different degrees of freedom for random effects and error distributions. *Journal of Statistical Planning and Inference* **147**, 235–247.

Chow, S.-C. and Liu, J.-P. (2008). *Design and Analysis of Bioavailability and Bioequivalence Studies*, 3rd edn. Chapman & Hall/CRC, Boca Raton, FL.

Cochran, W. G. (1950). The comparison of percentages in matched samples. *Biometrika* **37**, 256–266.

Cohen, J. (1960). A coefficient of agreement for nominal scales. *Educational and Psychological Measurement* **20**, 37–46.

Cohen, J. (1968). Weighted kappa: Nominal scale agreement with provision for scales disagreement of partial credit. *Psychological Bulletin* **70**, 213–220.

Cornbleet, P. J. and Gochman, N. (1979). Incorrect least-squares regression coefficients in method-comparison analysis. *Clinical Chemistry* **25**, 432–438.

Cotes, P. M., Doré, C. J., Yin, J. A., Lewis, S. M., Messinezy, M., Pearson, T. C. and Reid, C. (1986). Determination of serum immunoreactive erythropoietin in the investigation of erythrocytosis. *New England Journal of Medicine* **315**, 283–287.

Cressie, N. A. C. (1993). *Statistics for Spatial Data*. John Wiley, New York.

Dahl, D. B. (2015). *xtable: Export Tables to LaTeX or HTML*. R package version 1.8-0.

Davidian, M. and Giltinan, D. M. (1995). *Nonlinear Models for Repeated Measurement Data*. Chapman & Hall/CRC, Boca Raton, FL.

Davison, A. C. and Hinkley, D. V. (1997). *Bootstrap Methods and Their Application*. Cambridge University Press, New York.

Deming, W. E. (1943). *Statistical Adjustment of Data*. John Wiley, New York.

Dewitte, K., Fierens, C., Stöckl, D. and Thienpont, L. M. (2002). Application of the Bland-Altman plot for interpretation of method-comparison Studies: A critical investigation of its practice [Letter]. *Clinical Chemistry* **48**, 799–801.

Diggle, P. J., Heagerty, P., Liang, K.-Y. and Zeger, S. L. (2002). *Analysis of Longitudinal Data*, 2nd edn. Oxford University Press, Oxford, UK.

Donner, A., Eliasziw, M. and Klar, N. (1996). Testing the homogeneity of kappa statistics. *Biometrics* **52**, 176–183.

Donner, A., Shoukri, M. M., Klar, N. and Bartfay, E. (2000). Testing the equality of two dependent kappa statistics. *Statistics in Medicine* **19**, 373–387.

Dunn, G. (2004). *Statistical Evaluation of Measurement Errors*, 2nd edn. John Wiley, Chichester, UK.

Dunn, G. (2007). Regression models for method comparison data. *Journal of Biopharmaceutical Statistics* **17**, 739–756.

Dunn, G. and Roberts, C. (1999). Modelling method comparison data. *Statistical Methods in Medical Research* **8**, 161–179.

Edland, S. D. (1996). Bias in slope estimates for the linear errors in variables model by the variance ratio method. *Biometrics* **52**, 243–248.

Efron, B. and Tibshirani, R. J. (1993). *An Introduction to the Bootstrap*. Chapman & Hall, New York.

Eksborg, S. (1981). Evaluation of method-comparison data [Letter]. *Clinical Chemistry* **27**, 1311–1312.

Eliasziw, M., Young, S. L., Woodbury, M. G. and Fryday-Field, K. (1994). Statistical methodology for the concurrent assessment of interrater and intrarater reliability: Using goniometric measurements as an example. *Physical Therapy* **74**, 777–788.

Escaramis, G., Ascaso, C. and Carrasco, J. L. (2010). The total deviation index estimated by tolerance intervals to evaluate the concordance of measurement devices. *BMC Medical Research Methodology* **10**, article 31.

Fay, M. P. (2005). Random marginal agreement coefficients: Rethinking the adjustment for chance when measuring agreement. *Biostatistics* **6**, 171–180.

Fernholz, L. T. (1983). *von Mises Calculus for Statistical Functionals*. Springer, New York.

Feuerman, M. and Miller, A. R. (2008). Relationships between statistical measures of agreement: Sensitivity, specificity and kappa. *Journal of Evaluation in Clinical Practice* **14**, 930–933.

Finney, D. J. (1996). A note on the history of regression. *Journal of Applied Statistics* **23**, 555–557.

Fitzmaurice, G. M., Laird, N. M. and Ware, J. H. (2011). *Applied Longitudinal Analysis*, 2nd edn. John Wiley, Hoboken, NJ.

Fleiss, J. L. (1971). Measuring nominal scale agreement among many raters. *Pychological Bulletin* **76**, 378–382.

Fleiss, J. L. (1986). *The Design and Analysis of Clinical Experiments*. John Wiley, New York.

Fleiss, J. L. and Cohen, J. (1973). The equivalence of weighted kappa and the intraclass correlation as measures of reliability. *Educational and Psychological Measurement* **33**, 613–619.

Fleiss, J. L. and Shrout, P. E. (1978). Approximate interval estimation for a certain intraclass correlation coefficient. *Psychometrika* **43**, 259–262.

Fleiss, J. L., Cohen, J. and Everitt, B. S. (1969). Large sample standard errors of kappa and weighted kappa. *Psychological Bulletin* **72**, 323–327.

Fleiss, J. L., Levin, B. and Paik, M. C. (2003). *Statistical Methods for Rates and Proportions*, 3rd edn. John Wiley, Hoboken, NJ.

Gamer, M., Lemon, J., Fellows, I. and Singh, P. (2012). *irr: Various Coefficients of Interrater Reliability and Agreement*. R package version 0.84.

Geistanger, A., Berding, C., Vorberg, E. and Herlan, M. (2008). Local regression: A new approach for measurement system comparison analysis. *Clinical Chemistry and Laboratory Medicine* **46**, 1211–1219.

Gelman, A. and Hill, J. (2007). *Data Analysis Using Regression and Multilevel/Hierarchical Models*. Cambridge University Press, New York.

Genz, A. (1992). Numerical computation of multivariate normal probabilities. *Journal of Computational and Graphical Statistics* **1**, 141–149.

Genz, A., Bretz, F., Miwa, T., Mi, X., Leisch, F., Scheipl, F. and Hothorn, T. (2015). *mvtnorm: Multivariate Normal and t Distributions*. R package version 1.0-3.

Gilbert, P. and Varadhan, R. (2015). *numDeriv: Accurate Numerical Derivatives*. R package version 2014.2-1.

Giraudeau, B. and Mary, J. Y. (2001). Planning a reproducibility study: How many subjects and how many replicates per subject for an expected width of the 95 per cent confidence interval of the intraclass correlation coefficient. *Statistics in Medicine* **20**, 3205–3214.

Graybill, F. A. (2001). *Matrices with Applications in Statistics*, 2nd edn. Cengage Learning, Belmont, CA.

Grubbs, F. E. (1948). On estimating precision of measuring instruments and product variability. *Journal of the American Statistical Association* **43**, 243–264.

Guo, Y. and Manatunga, A. K. (2007). Nonparametric estimation of the concordance correlation coefficient under univariate censoring. *Biometrics* **83**, 164–172.

Guttman, I. (1988). Statistical tolerance regions. In *Encyclopedia of Statistical Sciences*, **9**, pp. 272-287, Kotz, S., Johnson, N. L. and Read, C. B. (Editors), John Wiley, New York.

Haber, M. J. and Barnhart, H. X. (2006). Coefficients of agreement for fixed observers. *Statistical Methods in Medical Research* **15**, 255–271.

Haber, M. J. and Barnhart, H. X. (2008). A general approach to evaluating agreement between two observers or methods of measurement from quantitative data with replicated measurements. *Statistical Methods in Medical Research* **17**, 151–169.

Haber, M. J., Barnhart, H. X., Song, J. and Gruden, J. (2005). Observer variability: A new approach in evaluating interobserver agreement. *Journal of Data Science* **3**, 69–83.

Hardin, J. W. and Hilbe, J. M. (2012). *Generalized Estimating Equations*, 2nd edn. Chapman & Hall/CRC, Boca Raton, FL.

Harris, I. R., Burch, B. D. and St. Laurent, R. T. (2001). A blended estimator for measure of agreement with a gold standard. *Journal of Agricultural, Biological, and Environmental Statistics* **6**, 326–339.

Hawkins, D. M. (2002). Diagnostics for conformity of paired quantitative measurements. *Statistics in Medicine* **21**, 1913–1935.

Hedayat, A. S., Lou, C. and Sinha, B. K. (2009). A statistical approach to assessment of agreement involving multiple raters. *Communications in Statistics - Theory and Methods* **38**, 2899–2922.

Hiriote, S. and Chinchilli, V. M. (2011). Matrix-based concordance correlation coefficient for repeated measures. *Biometrics* **67**, 1007–1016.

Ho, H. J. and Lin, T. I. (2010). Robust linear mixed models using the skew t distribution with application to schizophrenia data. *Biometrical Journal* **52**, 449–469.

Hollis, S. (1996a). Analysis of method comparison studies [Guest editorial]. *Annals of Clinical Biochemistry* **33**, 1–4.

Hollis, S. (1996b). Author's reply to Stöckl, D. (1996). *Annals of Clinical Biochemistry* **33**, 577.

Hothorn, T., Bretz, F. and Westfall, P. (2008). Simultaneous inference in general parametric models. *Biometrical Journal* **50**, 346–363.

Hsu, J. C. (1996). *Multiple Comparisons: Theory and Methods*. Chapman & Hall/CRC, Boca Raton, FL.

Hutson, A. D. (2010). A multi-rater nonparametric test of agreement and corresponding agreement plot. *Computational Statistics and Data Analysis* **54**, 109–119.

Hutson, A. D., Wilson, D. C. and Geiser, E. A. (1998). Measuring relative agreement: Echocardiographer versus computer. *Journal of Agricultural, Biological, and Environmental Statistics* **3**, 163–174.

Igic, B., Hauber, M. E., Galbraith, J. A., Grim, T., Dearborn, D. C., Brennan, P. L. R., Moskat, C., Choudhary, P. K. and Cassey, P. (2010). Comparison of micrometer- and scanning electron microscope-based measurements of avian eggshell thickness. *Journal of Field Ornithology* **81**, 402–410.

Jaech, J. L. (1971). Further tests of significance for Grubbs's estimators. *Biometrics* **27**, 1097–1101.

Johnson, R. A. and Wichern, D. W. (2002). *Applied Multivariate Statistical Analysis*, 5th edn. Prentice Hall, Upper Saddle River, NJ.

Kelly, G. E. (1985). Use of structural equations model in assessing the reliability of a new measurement technique. *Applied Statistics* **34**, 258–263.

Kelly, G. E. (1987). Author's reply to Altman and Bland (1987). *Applied Statistics* **36**, 225–227.

King, T. S. and Chinchilli, V. M. (2001a). A generalized concordance correlation coefficient for continuous and categorical data. *Statistics in Medicine* **20**, 2131–2147.

King, T. S. and Chinchilli, V. M. (2001b). Robust estimators of the concordance correlation coefficient. *Journal of Biopharmaceutical Statistics* **11**, 83–105.

King, T. S., Chinchilli, V. M. and Carrasco, J. L. (2007a). A repeated measures concordance correlation coefficient. *Statistics in Medicine* **26**, 3095–3113.

King, T. S., Chinchilli, V. M., Wang, K.-L. and Carrasco, J. L. (2007b). A class of repeated measures concordance correlation coefficients. *Journal of Biopharmaceutical Statistics* **17**, 653–672.

Kraemer, H. C., Periyakoil, V. S. and Noda, A. (2002). Kappa coefficients in medical research. *Statistics in Medicine* **21**, 2109–2129.

Krippendorff, K. (1970). Bivariate agreement coefficients for reliability of data. *Sociological Methodology* **2**, 139–50.

Krishnamoorthy, K. and Mathew, T. (2009). *Statistical Tolerance Regions: Theory, Applications, and Computation*. John Wiley, Hoboken, NJ.

Krouwer, J. S. (2008). Why Bland-Altman plots should use X, not (Y+X)/2 when X is a reference method [Letter]. *Statistics in Medicine* **27**, 778–780.

Krummenauer, F. (1999). Intraindividual scale comparison in clinical diagnostic methods: A review of elementary methods. *Biometrical Journal* **41**, 917–929.

Krummenauer, F., Genevriere, I. and Nixdorff, U. (2000). The biometrical comparison of cardiac imaging methods. *Computer Methods and Programs in Biomedicine* **62**, 21–34.

Kummell, C. H. (1879). Reduction of observation equations which contain more than one observed quantity. *The Analyst* **6**, 97–105.

Kutner, M., Nachtsheim, C., Neter, J. and Li, W. (2004). *Applied Linear Statistical Models*, 5th edn. McGraw-Hill/Irwin, Chicago.

Lai, D. and Shiao, S.-Y. (2005). Comparing two clinical measurements: A linear mixed model approach. *Journal of Applied Statistics* **32**, 855–860.

Lakshminarayanan, M. Y. and Gunst, R. F. (1984). Estimation of parameters in linear structural relationships: Sensitivity to the choice of the ratio of error variances. *Biometrika* **71**, 569–573.

Landis, J. R. and Koch, G. (1977a). The measurement of observer agreement for categorical data. *Biometrics* **33**, 159–174.

Landis, J. R. and Koch, G. (1977b). A one-way components of variance model for categorical data. *Biometrics* **33**, 671–679.

Landis, J. R., King, T. S., Choi, J. W., Chinchilli, V. M. and Koch, G. G. (2011). Measures of agreement and concordance with clinical research applications. *Statistics in Biopharmaceutical Research* **3**, 185–209.

Lange, K. (2010). *Numerical Analysis for Statisticians*, 2nd edn. Springer, New York.

Lee, J. J. and Tu, Z. N. (1994). A better confidence interval for kappa (κ) on measuring agreement between two raters with binary outcomes. *Journal of Computational and Graphical Statistics* **3**, 301–321.

Lehmann, E. L. (1998). *Elements of Large-Sample Theory*. Springer, New York.

LeLorier, J., Grégoire, G., Benhaddad, A., Lapierre, J. and Derderian, F. (1997). Discrepancies between meta-analyses and subsequent large randomized, controlled trials. *New England Journal of Medicine* **337**, 536–542.

Lewis, P. A., Jones, P. W., Polak, J. W. and Tillotson, H. T. (1991). The problem of conversion in method comparison studies. *Applied Statistics* **40**, 105–112.

Liao, J. (2009). Sample size calculation for an agreement study. *Pharmaceutical Statistics* **9**, 125–132.

Lin, L. I. (1989). A concordance correlation coefficient to evaluate reproducibility. *Biometrics* **45**, 255–268. Corrections: 2000, **56**, 324-325.

Lin, L. I. (1992). Assay validation using the concordance correlation coefficient. *Biometrics* **48**, 599–604.

Lin, L. I. (2000). Total deviation index for measuring individual agreement with applications in laboratory performance and bioequivalence. *Statistics in Medicine* **19**, 255–270.

Lin, L. I. (2008). Overview of agreement statistics for medical devices. *Journal of Biopharmaceutical Statistics* **18**, 126–144.

Lin, L. I. and Chinchilli, V. M. (1997). Rejoinder to the letter to the editor from Atkinson and Nevill. *Biometrics* **53**, 777–778.

Lin, L. I., Hedayat, A. S. and Wu, W. (2007). A unified approach for assessing agreement for continuous and categorical data. *Journal of Biopharmaceutical Statistics* **17**, 629–652.

Lin, L. I., Hedayat, A. S. and Wu, W. (2011). *Statistical Tools for Measuring Agreement*. Springer, New York.

Lin, L. I., Hedayat, A. S., Sinha, B. and Yang, M. (2002). Statistical methods in assessing agreement: Models, issues, and tools. *Journal of the American Statistical Association* **97**, 257–270.

Lin, S. C., Whipple, D. M. and Ho, C. S. (1998). Evaluation of statistical equivalence using limits of agreement and associated sample size calculation. *Communications in Statistics - Theory and Methods* **27**, 1419–1432.

Linnet, K. (1990). Estimation of the linear relationship between the measurements of two methods with proportional errors. *Statistics in Medicine* **9**, 1463–1473.

Linnet, K. (1993). Evaluation of regression procedures for method comparison studies. *Clinical Chemistry* **39**, 424–432.

Linnet, K. (1998). Performance of Deming regression analysis in case of misspecified analytical error ratio in method comparison studies. *Clinical Chemistry* **44**, 1024–1031.

Linnet, K. (1999). Limitations of the paired t-test for evaluation of method comparison data [Letter]. *Clinical Chemistry* **45**, 314–315.

Liu, J.-P. and Chow, S.-C. (1997). A two one-sided tests procedure for assessment of individual bioequivalence. *Journal of Biopharmaceutical Statistics* **7**, 49–61.

Liu, Q. and Pierce, D. A. (1994). A note on Gauss-Hermite quadrature. *Biometrika* **81**, 624–629.

Ludbrook, J. (2010). Confidence in Altman-Bland plots: A critical review of the method of differences. *Clinical and Experimental Pharmacology and Physiology* **37**, 143–149.

Luiz, R. R., Costa, A. J. L., Kale, P. L. and Werneck, G. L. (2003). Assessment of agreement of a quantitative variable: A new graphical approach. *Journal of Clinical Epidemiology* **56**, 963–967.

Maloney, C. J. and Rastogi, S. C. (1970). Significance test for Grubbs's estimators. *Biometrics* **26**, 671–676.

Mandel, J. (1978). Accuracy and precision: Evaluation and interpretation of analytical results. In *Treatise on Analytical Chemistry, Part I, Theory and Practice*, 2nd edition, volume 1, pp. 243-298, Kolthoff, I. M. and Elving, P. J. (Editors), John Wiley, New York.

Mandel, J. and Stiehler, R. D. (1954). Sensitivity – a criterion for the comparison of methods of test. *Journal of Research of the National Bureau of Standards* **53**, 155–159.

Marshall, G. N., Hays, R. D. and Nicholas, R. (1994). Evaluating agreement between clinical assessment methods. *International Journal of Methods in Psychiatric Research* **4**, 249–257.

Martin, R. F. (2000). General Deming regression for estimating systematic bias and its confidence interval in method-comparison studies. *Clinical Chemistry* **46**, 100–104.

McCulloch, C. E., Searle, S. R. and Neuhaus, J. M. (2008). *Generalized, Linear, and Mixed Models*, 2nd edn. John Wiley, Hoboken, NJ.

McGraw, K. O. and Wong, S. P. (1996). Forming inferences about some intraclass correlation coefficients. *Psychological Methods* **1**, 30–46.

Meeker, W. Q., Hahn, G. J. and Escobar, L. A. (2017). *Statistical Intervals: A Guide for Practitioners and Researchers*, 2nd edn. John Wiley, Hoboken, NJ.

Meyer, D., Zeileis, A. and Hornik, K. (2015). *vcd: Visualizing Categorical Data*. R package version 1.4-1.

Morgan, W. A. (1939). A test for the significance of the difference between the two variances in a sample from a normal bivariate population. *Biometrika* **31**, 13–19.

Müller, R. and Büttner, P. (1994). A critical discussion of intraclass correlation coefficients. *Statistics in Medicine* **13**, 2465–2476.

Nawarathna, L. S. and Choudhary, P. K. (2013). Measuring agreement in method comparison studies with heteroscedastic measurements. *Statistics in Medicine* **32**, 5156–5171.

Nelson, K. P. and Edwards, D. (2008). On population-based measures of agreement for binary classifications. *Canadian Journal of Statistics* **36**, 411–426.

Nickerson, C. A. (1997). Comment on "A concordance correlation coefficient to evaluate reproducibility". *Biometrics* **53**, 1503–1507.

Nix, A. B. J. and Dunston, F. D. J. (1991). Maximum likelihood techniques applied to method comparison studies. *Statistics in Medicine* **10**, 981–988.

Olsson, J. and Rootzén, H. (1996). Quantile estimation from repeated measurements. *Journal of the American Statistical Association* **91**, 1560–1565.

Osborne, C. (1991). Statistical calibration: A review. *International Statistical Review* **59**, 309–336.

Pan, Y., Haber, M., Gao, J. and Barnhart, H. X. (2012). A new permutation-based method for assessing agreement between two observers making replicated quantitative readings. *Statistics in Medicine* **31**, 2249–2261.

Passing, H. and Bablok, W. (1983). A new biometrical procedure for testing the equality of measurements from two different analytical methods. Application of linear regression procedures for method comparison studies in clinical chemistry, Part I. *Journal of Clinical Chemistry and Clinical Biochemistry* **21**, 709–720.

Passing, H. and Bablok, W. (1984). Comparison of several regression procedures for method comparison studies and determination of sample sizes. Application of linear regression procedures for method comparison studies in clinical chemistry, Part II. *Journal of Clinical Chemistry and Clinical Biochemistry* **22**, 431–445.

Perez-Jaume, S. and Carrasco, J. L. (2015). A non-parametric approach to estimate the total deviation index for non-normal data. *Statistics in Medicine* **34**, 3318–3335.

Pinheiro, J. C. and Bates, D. M. (2000). *Mixed-Effects Models in S and S-PLUS*. Springer, New York.

Pinheiro, J. C., Bates, D., DebRoy, S., Sarkar, D. and R Core Team (2015). *nlme: Linear and Nonlinear Mixed Effects Models*. R package version 3.1-122.

Pinheiro, J. C., Liu, C. and Wu, Y. N. (2001). Efficient algorithms for robust estimation in linear mixed-effects models using the multivariate t distribution. *Journal of Computational and Graphical Statistics* **10**, 249–276.

Pitman, E. J. G. (1939). A note on normal correlation. *Biometrika* **31**, 9–12.

Pollock, M. A., Jefferson, S. G., Kane, J. W., Lomax, K., MacKinnon, G. and Winnard, C. B. (1992). Method comparison—A different approach. *Annals of Clinical Biochemistry* **29**, 556–560.

Quiroz, J. (2005). Assessment of equivalence using a concordance correlation coefficient in a repeated measurements design. *Journal of Biopharmaceutical Statistics* **15**, 913–928.

Quiroz, J. and Burdick, R. K. (2009). Assessment of individual agreements with repeated measurements based on generalized confidence intervals. *Journal of Biopharmaceutical Statistics* **19**, 345–359.

R Core Team (2015). *R: A Language and Environment for Statistical Computing*. R Foundation for Statistical Computing. Vienna, Austria.

Ranchet, M., Akinwuntan, A. E., Tant, M., Neal, E. and Devos, H. (2015). Agreement between physician's recommendation and fitness-to-drive decision in multiple sclerosis. *Archives of Physical Medicine and Rehabilitation* **96**, 1840–1844.

Revelle, W. (2016). *psych: Procedures for Psychological, Psychometric, and Personality Research*. R package version 1.6.4.

Rifkin, R. D. (1995). Effects of correlated and uncorrelated measurement error on linear regression and correlation in medical method comparison studies. *Statistics in Medicine* **14**, 789–798.

Rocke, D. M. and Lorenzato, S. (1995). A two-component model for measurement error in analytical chemistry. *Technometrics* **37**, 176–184.

Roy, A. (2009). An application of linear mixed effects model to assess the agreement between two methods with replicated observations. *Journal of Biopharmaceutical Statistics* **19**, 150–173.

Rubin, D. B. (1983). Iteratively reweighted least squares. In *Encyclopedia of Statistical Sciences*, **4**, pp. 272-275, Kotz, S., Johnson, N. L. and Read, C. B. (Editors), John Wiley, New York.

Ryan, T. P. and Woodall, W. H. (2005). The most-cited statistical papers. *Journal of Applied Statistics* **32**, 461–474.

Sarkar, D. (2008). *Lattice: Multivariate Data Visualization with R*. Springer, New York.

Sarkar, D. and Andrews, F. (2013). *latticeExtra: Extra Graphical Utilities Based on Lattice*. R package version 0.6-26.

Schluter, P. J. (2009). A multivariate hierarchical Bayesian approach to measuring agreement in repeated measurement method comparison studies. *BMC Medical Research Methodology* **9**, article 6.

Scott, W. (1955). Reliability of content analysis: The case of nominal scale coding. *Public Opinion Quarterly* **19**, 321–325.

Searle, S. R., Casella, G. and McCulloch, C. E. (1992). *Variance Components*. John Wiley, New York.

Sengupta, D., Choudhary, P. K. and Cassey, P. (2015). Modeling and analysis of method comparison data with skewness and heavy tails. In *Ordered Data Analysis, Modeling and Health Research Methods*, pp. 169-187, Choudhary, P. K., Nagaraja, C. H. and Ng, H. K. T. (Editors), Springer, New York.

Sharpsteen, C. and Bracken, C. (2015). *tikzDevice: R Graphics Output in LaTeX Format*. R package version 0.9.

Shoukri, M. M. (2010). *Measures of Interobserver Agreement and Reliability*, 2nd edn. Chapman & Hall/CRC, Boca Raton, FL.

Shyr, J. Y. and Gleser, L. J. (1986). Inference about comparative precision in linear structural relationships. *Journal of Statistical Planning and Inference* **14**, 339–358.

St. Laurent, R. T. (1998). Evaluating agreement with a gold standard in method comparison studies. *Biometrics* **54**, 537–545.

Stöckl, D. (1996). Beyond the myths of difference plots [Letter]. *Annals of Clinical Biochemistry* **33**, 575–576.

Stöckl, D., Cabaleiro, D. R., Uytfanghe, K. V. and Thienpont, L. M. (2004). Interpreting method comparison studies by use of the Bland-Altman plot: Reflecting the importance of sample size by incorporating confidence limits and predefined error limits in the graphic [Letter]. *Clinical Chemistry* **50**, 2216–2218.

Stöckl, D., Dewitte, K. and Thienpont, L. M. (1998). Validity of linear regression in method comparison studies: Is it limited by the statistical model or the quality of the analytical input data? *Clinical Chemistry* **44**, 2340–2346.

Stroup, W. W. (2012). *Generalized Linear Mixed Models: Modern Concepts, Methods and Applications*. Chapman & Hall/CRC, Boca Raton, FL.

Tan, C. Y. and Iglewicz, B. (1999). Measurement-methods comparisons and linear statistical relationship. *Technometrics* **41**, 192–201.

Tanner, M. A. and Young, M. A. (1985). Modeling agreement among raters. *Journal of the American Statistical Association* **80**, 175–180.

Thompson, W. D. and Walter, S. D. (1988). Kappa and the concept of independent errors. *Journal of Clinical Epidemiology* **41**, 969–970.

Tsai, M.-Y. (2015). Comparison of concordance correlation coefficient via variance components, generalized estimating equations and weighted approaches with model selection. *Computational Statistics and Data Analysis* **82**, 47–58.

Twomey, P. J. (2006). How to use difference plots in quantitative method comparison studies. *Annals of Clinical Biochemistry* **43**, 124–129.

van der Vaart, A. W. (1998). *Asymptotic Statistics*. Cambridge University Press, New York.

Vardeman, S. B. (1992). What about the other intervals? *The American Statistician* **46**, 193–197.

Verbeke, G. and Lesaffre, E. (1996). A linear mixed-effects model with heterogeneity in the random-effects population. *Journal of the American Statistical Association* **91**, 217–221.

von Eye, A. and Mun, E. Y. (2004). *Analyzing Rater Agreement: Manifest Variable Methods*. Lawrence Earlbaum Associates, Mahwah, NJ.

Vonesh, E. F. and Chinchilli, V. M. (1997). *Linear and Nonlinear Models for the Analysis of Repeated Measures*. Marcel Dekker, New York.

Wang, W. (1999). On equivalence of two variances of a bivariate normal vector. *Journal of Statistical Planning and Inference* **81**, 279–292.

Wang, W. and Hwang, J. T. G. (2001). A nearly unbiased test for individual bioequivalence problems using probability criteria. *Journal of Statistical Planning and Inference* **99**, 41–58.

Weingart, S. N., Davis, R. B., Palmer, R. H., Cahalane, M., Hamel, M. B., Mukamal, K., Phillips, R. S., Davies, D. T. J. and Lezzoni, L. I. (2002). Discrepancies between explicit and implicit review: Physician and nurse assessments of complications and quality. *Health Services Research* **37**, 483–498.

Wellek, S. (2010). *Testing Statistical Hypotheses of Equivalence and Noninferiority*, 2nd edn. Chapman & Hall/CRC, Boca Raton, FL.

Westgard, J. O. and Hunt, M. R. (1973). Use and interpretation of common statistical tests in method-comparison studies. *Clinical Chemistry* **19**, 49–57.

Westlund, K. B. and Kurland, L. T. (1953). Studies on multiple sclerosis in Winnipeg, Manitoba, and New Orleans, Louisiana I. Prevalence; comparison between the patient groups in Winnipeg and New Orleans. *American Journal of Hygiene* **57**, 380–396.

Woodman, R. J. (2010). Bland-Altman beyond the basics: Creating confidence with badly behaved data [Editorial]. *Clinical and Experimental Pharmacology and Physiology* **37**, 141–142.

Yin, K., Choudhary, P. K., Varghese, D. and Goodman, S. R. (2008). A Bayesian approach for sample size determination in method comparison studies. *Statistics in Medicine* **27**, 2273–2289.

Young, D. S. (2010). An R package for estimating tolerance intervals. *Journal of Statistical Software* **36**, 1–39.

Zhang, D. and Davidian, M. (2001). Linear mixed models with flexible distributions of random effects for longitudinal data. *Biometrics* **57**, 795–802.

DATASET LIST

The following compilation consists of 34 of the datasets discussed in the book, and it provides the page number of their first appearance and reference source. First, datasets given in the book are listed; those marked with an asterisk (*) are also available on the companion website. Next, datasets given on the website are noted. Datasets available from other sources are given at the end.

In the book

1. Plasma volume data* (Bland and Altman, 1999), page 26

2. Potato weights data (Dunn, 2004), page 48

3. IPI angle data (Luiz et al., 2003), page 48

4. Fat content data* (Bland and Altman, 1999), page 49

5. Oxygen consumption data (Atkinson and Nevill, 1997), page 66

6. Cardiac output data (Müller and Büttner, 1994), page 110

7. Kiwi eggshell data* (Igic et al., 2010), page 113

8. Knee joint angle data* (Eliasziw et al., 1994), page 138

9. Cardiac ejection fraction data* (Bland and Altman, 1999), page 138

10. Peak expiratory flow rate data* (Bland and Altman, 1986), page 140

Measuring Agreement: Models, Methods, and Applications. By P. K. Choudhary and H. N. Nagaraja
Copyright © 2017 John Wiley & Sons, Inc.

11. Coronary artery calcium score data* (Haber et al., 2005), page 140

12. Fractional area change data (Hutson, 2010), page 201

13. Gull eggshell thickness data* (provided by P. Cassey), page 228

14. Crab claws data* (Choudhary et al., 2014), page 276

15. Meta analyses versus randomized clinical trials data (LeLorier et al., 1997), page 290

16. Medicare chart review data (Weingart et al., 2002), page 291

17. Multiple sclerosis (MS) assessment data (Westlund and Kurland, 1953), page 291

18. Fitness-to-drive evaluation data (Ranchet et al., 2015), page 315

19. Disease classification data (Chen et al., 2009), page 315

20. Psychiatric evaluation data (Fleiss, 1971), page 316

On the companion website

In addition to the datasets marked with an asterisk (*), the following datasets are also available on the website.

21. Oxygen saturation data (Bland and Altman, 1986), page 24

22. Vitamin D data (Hawkins, 2002), page 26

23. VCF data (Bland and Altman, 1986), page 49

24. Cyclosporin data (Hawkins, 2002), page 143

25. Cholesterol data (Chinchilli et al., 1996), page 143

26. Replicated blood pressure data (Bland and Altman, 1999), page 203

27. Blood pressure data (Carrasco and Jover, 2003), page 214

28. Percentage body fat data (Chinchilli et al., 1996), page 231

29. Unreplicated blood pressure data (Bland and Altman, 1995b), page 259

From other resources

30. Oximetry data, page 113, available in MethComp package of Carstensen et al. (2015)

31. Visceral fat data, page 140, available in MethComp package of Carstensen et al. (2015)

32. Subcutaneous fat data, page 175, available in MethComp package of Carstensen et al. (2015)

33. Tumor size data, page 180, available in Broemeling (2009, Chapter 6)

34. Standardized uptake value data, page 202, available in Broemeling (2009, page 202)

INDEX

accuracy, 4
agreement
    chart, 292
    evaluation, 5, 12, 17, 59, 64, 88, 98, 123,
        151, 164, 190, 211, 241, 258, 293,
        303
        controversies, 14, 44
        inappropriate use of tests, 34
        nonparametric, 253
    hypotheses, 16, 60
    limits of, *see* limits of agreement
    meaning, 6
    measures, 12, 54, 60, 62, 64, 88, 293, 303
    perfect, 6
AIC, 84
autocorrelation, 76, 238, 240

BIC, 84
bivariate normal model, 21, 97, 107
    data with covariates, 211
    diagnostics, 97
    heteroscedastic data, 162, 211
Bland-Altman
    approach, 60
    criterion, 59, 61
    limits of agreement, *see* limits of agreement
    method, 23
    plot, 23, 25–27, 45
Bonferroni inequality, 200
bootstrap, 81, 110, 129, 298, 315

case study
    categorical data, 305, 306
    data from multiple methods, 192, 195
    data with covariates, 214
    heteroscedastic data, 152, 165
    longitudinal data, 242
    nonparametric approach, 259, 263
    paired measurements data, 99, 101, 103,
        165
    repeated measurements data, 126, 129, 152,
        214
    sample size determination, 282
CCC, 44, 54, 65, 89, 108, 135, 200, 226, 249,
    272, 286
    as statistical functional, 274
    confidence band, 160, 169, 223, 246
    connection with kappa, 297
    data from multiple methods, 190, 213
    data with covariates, 212, 213
    definition, 55
    Fisher's z-transformation, 80
    generalization, 56
    heteroscedastic data, 152, 165, 212, 213
    hypotheses testing, 56
    influence function, 270
    limitations, 56
    longitudinal data, 241
    lower confidence bound, 56, 259
    nonparametric estimator, 258
    paired measurements data, 98, 212

properties, 55
repeatability, 125, 126, 152, 191, 192, 213
repeated measurements data, 124, 190, 212, 213
sample size determination, 283, 286
unreplicated data, 190, 213
concordance correlation, *see* CCC
confidence band, 83, 151
   CCC, 160, 169, 223, 246
   mean difference, 245
   precision ratio, 158, 222
   TDI, 160, 169, 223, 246
   variance ratio, 168
confidence bound, 17, 78
   bootstrap, 82
   CCC, 56
   CP, 63
   kappa, 298
   MSD, 54
   nonparametric, 258, 270
   simultaneous, 80, 178, 191
   TDI, 63, 259
confidence interval, 18, 78
   bootstrap, 81
   nonparametric, 258
   simultaneous, 79, 178, 191
correlation, 6, 10, 14, 20, 55, 235
   concordance, *see* CCC
   Fisher's z-transformation, 35
   intraclass, *see* intraclass correlation
   model, 235, 237
      autoregressive, 238
      compound symmetry, 237
      exponential, 239
      semivariogram, 239
      spatial, 238
      time series, 238
   test for zero value, 34, 240
coverage probability, *see* CP
CP, 62, 66, 286
   comparison with TDI, 63
   definition, 62
   hypotheses testing, 63
   lower confidence bound, 63
   normal distribution, 63
   sample size determination, 286

data
   categorical, 289
   from multiple methods, 177, 208
   heteroscedastic, 141, 146, 207, 208
   longitudinal, 112, 229
   method comparison, 84, 85
      steps in analysis, 39
   paired measurements, 95, 141, 173, 208
   repeated measurements, 111, 141, 146, 171, 186, 208
      linked, 111, 112
      unlinked, 111, 112

unreplicated, 184, 208
   with covariates, 205
datasets, 331

empirical distribution, 255
equivalence, 15
estimation
   best linear unbiased, 74
   least squares, 30, 33
   ML, 74
      large-sample properties, 76
   nonparametric, 255, 271
   orthogonal least squares, 32, 33

fixed bias, 3, 11

gold standard, 5, 298

influence function, 258, 268, 271
intraclass correlation, 4, 65, 125, 126, 192, 299, 304, 305

kappa, 290, 311
   bounds, 295
   connection with CCC, 297
   definition, 295
   hypotheses testing, 298
   interpretation, 309
   intraclass, 299, 301
   lower confidence bound, 298
   multiple categories, 303
   multiple experiments, 301
   multiple raters, 300
   properties, 295
   random raters, 304
   sample, 297
   sample size determination, 302
   test of homogeneity, 302
   weighted, 303

limits of agreement, 23, 44, 60, 65, 135
   comparison with prediction and tolerance intervals, 62
   data from multiple methods, 191, 214
   data with covariates, 214
   definition, 60
   heteroscedastic data, 152, 165, 214
   longitudinal data, 241, 242
   paired measurements data, 98
   repeatability, 125, 126, 192
   repeated measurements data, 124, 191
   unreplicated data, 191
Lin's probability criterion, 59, 62

mean model, 206, 234, 237
mean squared deviation, *see* MSD
mixed-effects model, 71, 89
   BLUP, 73, 92
   data from multiple methods, 184, 186, 209, 210

data with covariates, 209, 210
diagnostics, 75
estimated BLUP, 74
estimation, 74
fitting, 74
general form, 72
heteroscedastic data, 148, 209, 210
longitudinal data, 236
method comparison data, 86
paired measurements data, 20, 95, 106
repeated measurements data, 118, 121, 186, 187, 209, 210
unreplicated data, 184, 210
model
bivariate normal, *see* bivariate normal model
classical linear, 3
comparison, 84
AIC, 84
BIC, 84
likelihood ratio test, 84
conditional logistic regression, 306
correlation, *see* correlation model
evaluation, 123, 150, 164, 189, 211, 240
generalized linear mixed-effects, 308
Grubbs, 20, 41
linear mixed-effects, *see* mixed-effects model
log-linear, 307
mean, *see* mean model
measurement error, 9, 19
nonparametric, 253
one-way random effect, 300
test theory, *see* test theory model
two-way random effects, 305
variance, *see* variance model
MSD, 54
definition, 54
generalization, 54
hypotheses testing, 54
upper confidence bound, 54

notation, 1

plot
Bland-Altman, *see* Bland-Altman plot
box, 179
interaction, 116
Q-Q, 76
residual, 75
scatter, 6
trellis, 39
precision, 4
precision ratio, 98, 123, 190
confidence band, 158, 222
definition, 12
heteroscedastic data, 152, 212
modified, 124, 190
prediction, 73

best, 73
best linear, 73
best linear unbiased, 73
BLUP, 73
error, 73
interval, *see* prediction interval
mean absolute error, 90
mean squared error, 73
mixed-effects model, 73, 92
unbiased, 73
prediction interval, 57, 66
definition, 57
normal distribution, 58
prevalence, 299
proportional bias, 3, 11

regression, 29
Deming, 31, 41, 42
ordinary linear, 29, 33
orthogonal, 32, 33
Passing-Bablok, 43
reliability, 4, 15, 125
repeatability, 15, 124
evaluation, 124, 152, 191, 213
measure, 124
standard deviation, 3
reproducibility, 15
residuals
normalized, 75, 240
standardized, 75
studentized, 75

sample size determination, 279, 286, 302
CCC, 283, 286, 318
CP, 286
kappa, 302
limits of agreement, 286
paired measurements design, 281
repeated measurements design, 281
TDI, 283, 286
semivariogram, 238
sensitivity
categorical data, 298
continuous data, 4, 12, 43
ratio, 12
similarity
evaluation, 5, 11, 12, 18, 88, 98, 123, 151, 164, 190, 211, 241, 258
measures, 11, 12, 88
specificity, 298
statistical functional, 255, 271

TDI, 62, 66, 89, 108, 135, 200, 226, 249, 272, 286
as statistical functional, 274
comparison with CP, 63
confidence band, 160, 169, 223, 246
connection with tolerance interval, 63
data from multiple methods, 190, 213

data with covariates, 212, 213
definition, 62
heteroscedastic data, 152, 165, 212, 213
hypotheses testing, 63
influence function, 270
log transformation, 80
longitudinal data, 241, 242
nonparametric confidence bound, 259, 270
nonparametric estimator, 258
normal distribution, 63
paired measurements data, 98, 212
repeatability, 125, 126, 152, 191, 192, 213
repeated measurements data, 124, 190, 212, 213
sample size determination, 283
unreplicated data, 190, 213
upper confidence bound, 63, 259, 270
test
Bradley-Blackwood, 36, 43
Cochran's Q, 300
for homoscedasticity, 151, 164
for zero correlation, 34, 240
for zero intercept and unit slope, 38
intersection-union, 68
likelihood ratio, 84
McNemar's, 300
of equivalence, 15
of homogeneity, 83, 302
paired t, 36
Pitman-Morgan, 36, 43
significance, 15
test theory model, 11
congeneric, 11
essential tau-equivalence, 11
parallel, 11
tau equivalence, 11
tolerance interval, 57, 60, 63, 66
definition, 57
normal distribution, 58
total deviation index, *see* TDI
transformation
CCC, 80
Fisher's z, 35, 80
log, 80
logit, 80
parameter, 80
TDI, 80
variance, 80

variance
between-subject, 3
error, 3
log transformation, 80
model, 144, 149, 163, 207
exponential, 146, 154, 166
power, 146, 154, 166, 218
ratio, 98
confidence band, 168
heteroscedastic data, 165, 212
test for homoscedasticity, 151, 164
within-subject, 3